Frederike Offizier
The Biosecurity Individual

T0402300

Frederike Offizier works as a lecturer and researcher in the American Studies Department at Universität Potsdam, where she also completed her PhD with the project "Help Yourself, So Help You Science". Part of her research was conducted as a Fulbright Scholar at the University of Washington, Seattle. Her MA thesis "DeComposing the Self" was awarded the Hans-Jürgen-Bachorski-Preis. Her research focuses on biocultural studies, affect theory, performance studies, ecocriticism, and disaster narratives.

Frederike Offizier

The Biosecurity Individual

A Cultural Critique of the Intersection between Health, Security, and Identity

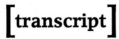

This work was accepted as a PhD thesis by the Faculty of Arts at the University of Potsdam in November 2021 with the title "Help Yourself, So Help You Science: Security, Biology, and Identity Construction." The PhD thesis was supervised by Prof. Dr. Rüdiger Kunow and Prof. Dr. Marc Priewe.

This publication was supported by funds from the Publication Fund Open Access Monographs of the Federal State of Brandenburg, Germany.

Bibliographic information published by the Deutsche Nationalbibliothek
The Deutsche Nationalbibliothek lists this publication in the Deutsche Nationalbibliografie; detailed bibliographic data are available in the Internet at https://dnb.dnb.de/

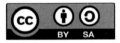
First published in 2024 by transcript Verlag, Bielefeld
© Frederike Offizier

Cover design: Antonia Offizier – lol studio berlin
Printed by: Majuskel Medienproduktion GmbH, Wetzlar
https://doi.org/10.14361/9783839471456
Print-ISBN: 978-3-8376-7145-2
PDF-ISBN: 978-3-8394-7145-6
ISSN of series: 2747-4372
eISSN of series: 2747-4380

Printed on permanent acid-free text paper.

What happens to a dream deferred?

Does it dry up
Like a raisin in the sun?
Or fester like a sore–
And then run?
Does it stink like rotten meat?
Or crust and sugar over-
Like a syrupy sweet?

Maybe it just sags
Like a heavy load.

Or does it explode?

Langston Hughes

Contents

Part II: Fictions of Biosecurity

Acknowledgements

This book would never have been possible without the help and support of many people. I would like to use this space to acknowledge those who have helped me along this journey with their interesting ideas and thoughts, their time, their trust, their friendship, and love.

I would like to thank Professor Rüdiger Kunow for his intellectual support and trust in my work, but first and foremost for the intellectual and academic home he created. Marked by an open door, hours of conversation, and academic debate this intellectual upbringing shaped my thinking beyond the scope of this project. I would also like to thank Professor Marc Priewe for supervising this project and for his attentive and detailed commentary in the editing process, as well as Professor Nicole Waller for providing a stable place for me to finish this project.

Furthermore, I would like to thank Dr. Ariane Schröder for her helpful critique, intellectual and emotional support, and for being the most patient editor, colleague, and friend, without whom this project would never have been completed. I am also thankful to Justine Hancock for her swift and thorough editing support and the time she made for this in her tight schedule.

Last but not least, I would like to thank my family for their love, support, and understanding. I am especially grateful to Ned, Nell and Esther, for their sacrifices and for bearing with me, most of all though, for their love.

Introduction: Health, Security, and Identity

> Everyone who is born holds dual citizenship, in the kingdom of the well and in the kingdom of the sick. Although we all prefer to use only the good passport, sooner or later each of us is obliged, at least for a spell, to identify ourselves as citizens of that other place.
> *Susan Sontag*

Susan Sontag suggests in *Illness as Metaphor* that health and disease constitute two different countries, two nations in which everybody holds citizenship, though only begrudgingly to the "kingdom of the sick." She uses this image of two different nations to open her seminal study on the metaphorical understanding of disease. It was written in the late 1970s just before the emergence of AIDS at a time when disease and the body were still largely neglected in the study of culture. Sontag criticizes the dominant view that sickness can be understood purely in biological terms emphasizing its dependence on cultural frameworks and narratives. She asserts that illness is not a purely physiological experience and cautions that "it is hardly possible to take up one's residence in the kingdom of the ill unprejudiced by the lurid metaphors with which it has been landscaped" (Sontag, *Illness and Metaphor* 3). She thus articulates one of the central premises of the field of biocultures, namely that biological and cultural understandings are intimately intertwined.[1]

More importantly, the national metaphor, which Sontag uses to introduce her study of cancer and tuberculosis, expresses two further components which are in essence what I will attempt to explore more thoroughly with my study of the confluence of health, security, and identity. Sontag reiterates the understanding of health and biology as inflected in terms of national security – in her study most crucially through the metaphor of warfare and battle. With the image of kingdoms and citizenship, she represents health as

---

1   In 2007 Lennard Davis and David B. Morris wrote the "Biocultures Manifesto" defining the perspective of the nascent field. Their declaration is based on assumptions already formulated by critics such as Philipp Sarasin and Michel Foucault, namely that science is not factually objective but that the findings are always inflected by culture and cultural narratives.

a closed "space" that can be secured and protected by the appropriate authority over security. It is imagined as a space that can be separated from other territories. Furthermore, her introduction echoes the commonly held misconception that being healthy is the norm and the normal which everybody should experience with few and temporarily limited exceptions. This assumption reflects a pervasive "cultural imaginary" (Fluck) of biological security, as I will argue, that was produced by the rise of medical and scientific normative power since the 19th century. At the same time, her image of a dual citizenship antagonizes this expectation of security produced by what I will analyze as the messianic narrative of scientific and medical salvation and the promise of radical self-empowerment, which still dominate cultural beliefs today.

Today the border between the two countries of healthy and sick, to stick to Sontag's metaphor, is more arbitrary and untenable than it seemed in the 1970s and 1980s. At the same time, it represents a highly securitized zone with border guards and high-tech security equipment enforcing the borderlands. The all-encompassing reach of medicalization and biomedicalization[2] has significantly changed the understanding and experience of health and disease. Both "states" cannot be distinguished in a clearly delineated binary opposition discerned by a person feeling healthy or the presence of disease. Biotechnological developments have allowed for the diagnosis of presymptomatic illness, so for the detection of a disease before the body expresses symptoms. They have altered the "medical gaze" (Foucault, *Birth* xii) and understanding of the body. Contemporary surveillance medicine[3] "has redrawn the boundaries between health, illness, and disease to promote a regime of total health" (Earle et al. 96). This imaginary of total health promises security through the controllability of the body, while at the same time rendering health a "precarious state" (Armstrong 397) that one can never be quite sure of. This "problematization of the normal" (Armstrong 395) produces an "always precarious normality" (Luhmann vii) which dominates the experience of biological security. The "kingdom of the well," thus, describes rather a transitional zone that everybody holds only a visa for. And this visa needs to be certified and renewed regularly and can be revoked at any point.

Biology and health have not only metaphorically been increasingly understood in terms of security and risk. In addition to detecting diseases earlier and in their molecular stages, biotechnological developments have progressively focused on uncovering disease potentials in the form of increased susceptibility, such as the risk for breast cancer, diabetes, or depression. It has therefore become crucial to know one's risks and to identify one's security status. Such a diagnosed risk does not describe a change in terms of health but in terms of security, or rather a future state of security. Nonetheless, increased risks, as well as presymptomatic illness, initiate an "anticipatory mode of patienthood" (Nye

---

2   Medicalization is commonly understood as "the processes through which aspects of life previously outside the jurisdiction of medicine come to be construed as medical problems" (Clarke et al., "Biomedicalization" 161). Biomedicalization, which started in the mid 1980s is conceptualized as the *"transformations* of such medical phenomena and of bodies, largely through sooner-rather-than-later technoscientific interventions not only for treatment but also increasingly for enhancement" (Clarke et al., "Introduction" 2).

3   Armstrong asserts that medical practice today needs to be understood as surveillance medicine, which relies on techniques different from other medical practices and forges a distinct relation between individual, the body, and illness (Armstrong 402).

105) that demands the individual to act. In fact, the risk of falling ill becomes in this context a "diseaselike state in itself" (Fosket 331).

Most Americans, thus, live in a space between the two kingdoms, in the borderland that "is a constant state of transition" (3) as Gloria Anzaldúa describes it in a different context. This is a fearful space, as every transgression seems to constitute a security threat – for the individual as much as for the community at large – representing punishable offences. "[S]elf-techniques" (Rose, *Politics* 24) to ensure one's security in terms of biology are therefore paramount. "Under this regime, the individual is not just subjected to the technologies of medical surveillance but is expected to engage in the practice of self-surveillance" (Earle et al. 96), making security practices and logics an inherent part of understanding the body and the self. It is therefore the understanding of biological security rather than merely health, as I will argue, that demands attention and critical thinking, especially in the United States of America.

Historically, security has been an important concept for the self-understanding of the United States of America. Framed in the terminology of freedom and liberty, which was inseparable from the understanding of security at the time (Reid 70), it was the ideal of the American Revolution and became enshrined as a "God given Right" in the Declaration of Independence. With shifting meanings, security has remained a central part of U.S. American self-perception and representation. Today, John T. Hamilton even asks in *Security: Politics, Humanity and the Philology of Care* if we are living in an "age of security" (2). But security is not just one of the leading topics of today's discussion in terms of national and international measures; it also pervades American society and culture in a more intimate manner. Security, or rather the contemporary understanding of security is increasingly central to the understanding of biology and health, as well as the conception of what "good life" is. In this book I will examine the biologically inflected understanding of security as an increasingly central paradigm in American culture and society.

The intersection of security and biology is commonly understood and studied in terms of biosecurity designating governmental practices that protect the nation from contagious disease outbreaks.[4] Biosecurity has become such an important cultural and political paradigm that its study has established the burgeoning field of Biosecurity Studies. Especially following the Covid-19 outbreak this association is more fixed and more tangible than it was just a couple of years ago. And President Trump's repetitive use of the term "China-Virus" and his blame campaign against China show how closely connected national security and disease are. The pandemic also exposed how biosecurity affects the most private and intimate spaces of life. Private bodies are not only public texts but are understood as public threats and are regulated and defined within the

---

4   There is a decisive definitional difference between biosafety and biosecurity in the US: biosafety refers to measures taken in laboratories; biosecurity refers to infectious disease outbreaks (as terrorist attacks or naturally occurring). In Europe biosecurity is focused on food security and in Oceania on imported agrarian practices and species that endanger indigenous flora and fauna. (Bingham and Hinchliffe 173)

responsibilities of "biological citizenship" (Rabinow and Rose 197).[5] Though in the U.S. American context, biosecurity as a term is used predominantly to refer to contagious diseases, epidemics, and bioterrorism, the logics of security have also been integrated in the understanding of biology and health outside of contagious diseases. I therefore wish to argue that the term can and should be extended to include the biomedicalization of U.S. American society. With this book I aim to show that security holds a central position in U.S. American culture that extends beyond questions of national security to the biological, applying the same logics to the individual body and life as to the nation at large. In applying the term biosecurity to non-contagious disease contexts I want to imply both that many of the measures and practices of "official" biosecurity find ample use and are rather routinely applied to individual bodies (such as surveillance) as well as that the logics, rhetoric and images used to represent biological security of the individual body are inflected by logics of national security: most importantly prevention and pre-emption.

The confluence of these logics with biotechnological and biomedical possibilities, I will argue, facilitates or produces new and renewed identity formations, collectively as well as individually. Pre-emptive and preventive security logics determine the way the body is understood and encountered, influencing the understanding of self and identity. They produce new relations between the individual and their body, engendering new biosecurity identities or "biosecurity individuals" as I will call them. When Pathway Genomics as a global genetic testing laboratory, for instance, advertises their genetic tests with the promise to decode not only the biological make-up of the body but the fate of the targeted consumer,[6] the relation of body and self becomes inherently interconnected and attached to a new logic of bodily security. Life is here not represented as a fateful and given fact, but rather as a controllable process that can be optimized and maximized – that can be secured. And it is the responsibility of the biologically self-empowered biosecurity individual to engage in the proper security practices and to take advantage of their right to choose. This responsibility for the self is a crucial expression of "biological citizenship" (Rabinow and Rose 197) which is framed as fundamentally American. It is represented as an essential part of the freedom and liberty which allows the self-reliant individual to take part in the American Dream. Knowing one's risks and therefore knowing one's security status has thus become an increasingly important part of understanding body and self, that goes far beyond medical practice and health, and which seems to have become a precondition for a successful and happy life. "To live well today is to live in the light of biomedicine" (Rose, "Human Sciences" 7). Biological security is therefore an insightful object of research representing a dominant paradigm of culture as well as a crucial vantage point on how "good life" is conceptualized and shaped in U.S. America today. With the analysis of literary and cultural representations I aim to explore how the bio-

---

5   Nikolas Rose and Carlos Novas define this term in the homonymous article as the new and old ways of understanding citizenship as well as who is excluded from such a designation ("Citizenship").

6   Pathway Genomics advertises their genetic test-kit on their homepage with the claim "This is about gaining more knowledge about yourself." Similar claims can be found in the self-representation and the promises of 23andMe.

logically inflected understanding of security determines life and identity constructions, structuring U.S. American society and producing new paradigms of difference.

It would be suggestive to assume that security in the context of biology is simply health. Both – security and health – are usually regarded as fixed properties or characteristics. Security is most frequently understood as a clearly defined goal and endpoint, which serves as motivation and legitimization (Brunner et al. 856). A closer look reveals, however, that security is rarely a fixed property or characteristic. It has to be produced by convincing narratives in order to be intelligible and to develop its cultural force. Similarly, health is often talked and written about as if it was a definitive condition or a natural state that can be protected. But as Georges Canguilhem already argued in *The Normal and the Pathological*, health is a relational concept defined in opposition to its antonym the "pathological." Rather than understanding health as a definable fixed state he described it as "life lived in the silence of the organs" (*Writings* 43), which depends on individual experience.[7] Despite Canguilhem's critique, the understanding of the body as machine, which either works or is broken and has to be fixed, prevails and has been further exacerbated by the rise of the "Biomedical TechnoService Complex, Inc." (Clarke et al., "Biomedicalization" 162). In the current state of biomedicalization the understanding of the "normal" depends on the expectations of security. And these expectations are commonly organized in narratives that serve to make security and risk intelligible and represent them as manageable.

The processes of biomedicalization and its securitizing trends are predominantly analyzed within a sociological framework in terms of biopolitics. In contrast to the leading focus on the practices of securing health in these studies I wish to examine the narratives that facilitate such practices in the first place. Instead of focusing on the increasing normative power of biomedicine only, I would like to question how the understanding of biological security is constructed and made pervasive. And here my primary contention is that it is made culturally present in narrative form. I therefore propose to analyze biological security within the framework of performativity stressing that the understanding of biological security relies on narratives. I will thus regard biological security not as a determined end point but as a condition which has to be defined to become meaningful and acquire its culturally constructed meaning. In that sense, notions of security deeply depend on narratives that make a particular understanding of security intelligible and pervasive in a way that compels people to recognize it and to act or react accordingly. I regard security thus not as a stable state or self-evident object, but as a moving target that has to be narratively fixed. This narrative construction is all the more pertinent in the context of biological security, which often relies on highly professionalized and specialized knowledge. Since biosecurity is located in a "high technological frontier" (Giddens 3) where diagnosis of susceptibilities and predispositions are not experientially present to the person concerned – besides the medical procedures that go along with it – these narratives become all the more crucial.

---

7   Canguilhem focused on genealogical studies – similar to Foucault – looking at the history of the production of knowledge to understand contemporary practices. His study aims to "destabilize . . . a system of knowledge that has proclaimed itself to be the only fount of truth" (*Writings on Medicine* 6).

The understanding and study of security as narrative is by now an established part of Security Studies, especially Feminist Security Studies (Wibben). Literary Studies have also started to engage in the field by forming an emerging "literary security studies," as Johannes Völz proclaims ("Aestheticizing" 616), attempting to find ways in which literature can illuminate something more about security in the United States. David Watson asserts in the special edition "Security Studies and American Literary History" that the field reveals how questions of security and the logics of pre-emption pervade contemporary literature. Völz cautions, however, that "literary security studies" should not limit itself to a form of "surface reading" which results in a form of "security realism" ("Aestheticizing" 619). Publications such as "In/Security" edited by Martina Deny and Elaine Morley are more centered on raising the question of an aesthetics of security responding to an "[a]tmosphere of fear" (1). Völz, in specific, asserts that literature contains the possibility to represent and understand security differently, facilitating an enabling and empowering understanding of security. Literature, he claims, turns to insecurity performing a form of "transvaluation" (Völz, "Aestheticizing" 619). But also, the focus on the aesthetic quality of security is discussed controversially, as negating the material realities and suffering produced by security practices (Watson, "Beautiful Walls").[8] Most of these studies predominantly include biological security only in a cursory statement which subsumes it under the wider analysis of governmental power controlling the public. With this book I wish to raise biological security from its position in a subordinate clause, as I am convinced that its impact on life and the understanding of the self is far greater than such a position indicates and allows for. I will argue that the security narrative established by the rise of science and medicine as the arbiter of biological security has established a forceful fiction of biosecurity, a pervasive "cultural imaginary," which relies on narrative and performative acts.

I will therefore study biosecurity as both, performance and performativity to fully understand the growing phenomenon of "cultures of biosecurity." This Performance Studies lens allows me to include and further understand the performances that surround and constitute the biosecurity identities I am studying. Judith Butler developed her theory of performativity in *Gender Troubles*, and extended as well as defended it in *Bodies that Matter* and *Precarious Life*. Performance and performativity have long become dominant theoretical paradigms in Literary and Cultural Studies. At the same time, her theoretical approach has been harshly criticized for negating materiality and foreclosing subjectivity. It therefore might seem paradoxical to turn to this particular theory. However, I consider Butler's approach to materiality and the body a promising vantage point to understanding biosecurity and the identities forged by its narratives. Her writing seems to search for something hidden to be recovered from behind a "social mask" (*Precarious* 37). Similarly, the studies of biomedicalization seem to struggle to secure the human threatened by nature and/or medical practice and biomedical definitions. Both approaches have considerable shortcoming, especially in regard to bodies that defy the biosecurity narrative of

---

8   David Watson responds to the critique by Völz, which was targeted at his edited journal edition, by emphasizing the dangers of reducing "security" to aesthetics by quoting Trump's description of the wall he attempts to build.

an intact able body remaining caught in the role as the threatening other.[9] Nonetheless, I consider performativity the most productive approach when turning to a field of scientifically defined security with a forceful truth claim to the objective description of biological states and processes.

This does not mean, however, that scientific results are not to be taken seriously nor do I mean to engage in a discourse of the post-factual or "fake news," which is diametrically opposed to my academic and ethical conviction. Rather, the theoretical approach aims to contribute to a productive reassessment of narratives represented as unquestionable truth by a field that seems to effectively "lose sight" of the conceptual cultural frameworks, which gave rise to the research, and which reiterate the biased assumptions and violence of the cultural narratives they are based on. Science does not establish natural categories of security, as I will show, but represents an ableist and healthist security discourse that is deeply influenced by social and cultural bias. Rather than diminishing the suffering of individuals as non-referential, this perspective facilitates the critique of security narratives and practices which influence the production of disparate securities and biosecurity individuals under the guise of the natural. As a Cultural Studies project the central concern is therefore not to define the elusive and intangible object of biological security but rather to analyze how security narratives are constructed and what the material effects they produce are.

Since biosecurity practices are not enforced but rely on the complicity of biosecurity individuals as self-reliant subjects, affects are crucial to studying these material effects. Security narratives rely on fear as well as desire and hope to legitimize the practices as a necessary means to maintain and protect a "good life." "[W]e can see that bioscience is not only about the production of truth: it can become invested with hope and optimism by citizens who have an active stake in their health and that of others" (Rose and Novas 28).[10] I therefore wish to explore biosecurity as a "desired object" in terms of affect theory predominantly based on Sara Ahmed and Lauren Berlant. Rather than relying on an a priori meaning and feeling, biological security relies on the attachment to fears and hopes to become pervasive constructs and performative scripts. Similarly to Völz, I therefore wish to emphasize how security narratives "appeal" (Foucault, *Security* 21) to the individual and how they compel people to act. While Völz seeks to investigate the "appeal" of the concept of security by analyzing the narratives provided in literary fiction, my own approach both widens and narrows the investigative scope. It widens it by looking at diverse discursive formations emphasizing the antagonisms, commonalities, and reciprocities of the different forms of biosecurity narratives, and it narrows the perspective by focusing on security in the context of biomedicine and biotechnology.

---

9   Tobin Siebers explains in "Disability in Theory" that the disabled body is a blind spot in theory – including the theory of performativity – where it is pushed to the margin as much as in society built for able bodied.

10   In a similar way Deborah Lupton points out that "[i]t is not the ways in which such discourses and practices seek overtly to constrain individuals' freedom of action that are the most interesting and important to examine, but the ways in which they invite individuals voluntarily to conform to their objectives, to discipline themselves, to turn the gaze upon themselves in the interest of their health" (*Imperative* 11).

In part I – "Framed by Theory: Security, Biomedical Science, and the Biosecurity Individual"– I will establish my theoretical approach to biological security narratives and identity formation and provide the historical context of biology and security in the United States. In chapter 1 I will first elaborate on security narrative as performative following theoretical approaches of John Langshaw Austin and Jacques Derrida. With the theoretical terminology at hand, I will then trace how the body and life became securitized by focusing on the historical processes of medicalization and biomedicalization to establish the "historical ideas" (Butler, "Performative" 521) that shape the understanding of biosecurity today. I will trace and highlight the security logics which form a development from prevention to pre-emption and total control, and show how the messianic narrative of scientific and medical salvation has become more and more forceful. In chapter 3 I will then show how the growing complex of biomedicalization and its adherence to logics of prevention and pre-emption define the relation of the individual to their body, producing new biosecurity identities. After establishing the historical genealogy of biosecurity culture and the individual in the present, in chapter 4 I will return to performativity to facilitate a more thorough understanding of the "new" biosecurity individuals in terms of identity theory.

In part II – Fictions of Biosecurity – I will turn to the analysis of biosecurity narratives as cultural form which pervade society and culture at every turn, creating an essential part of "biosecurity culture" and its necessary stories to understand the self. Analyzing biosecurity narratives in different discursive formations I will use the renderings in classical memoir, testimonies, documentary, and fiction to draw attention to the performativity of security and the material effects produced by the security narratives. I chose a wide variety of texts to argue that fictions of biosecurity and its intertextual dependence on the messianic narrative of scientific salvation are not restricted to fictional renderings but constitute an essential part of how we understand bodies and identities.

In chapter 5 I will examine Alice Wexler's memoir *Mapping Fate* focusing on an early expression of the biosecurity identity forged by the nascent possibilities of genetically testing for Huntington's disease and the security promised by this practice. I will show how the understanding of biological security as well as of her identity relies on narrative construction accomplished by the act of life writing. In chapter 6 I will read previvor testimonies of pre-emptive mastectomies, which are performed because of the diagnosis of hereditary breast and ovarian cancer risk, as paradigmatic examples of biosecurity individuals today. The identification of risk instigates and demands narratives that performatively produce both risk and security as present realities leading to changed understandings of the self and to invasive material effects. While the pre-emptive surgical interventions in the context of breast cancer produce the fiction of control and total security, in chapter 7 I will turn to the failure of such security promises and the possibility of escaping the seemingly all-encompassing regimen of biosecurity. In the analysis of Physician Assisted Dying represented in the documentary *How to Die in Oregon* by Peter Richardson I will focus most explicitly on the re-negotiation of the dominant narrative of scientific and medical salvation, as well as on what biological security in terms of good life really means. In the last analysis chapter I will turn to fictional accounts of biosecurity and its failure by examining Nathaniel Hawthorne's "The Birth-Mark" and Gary Shteyngart's *Super Sad True Love Story*. Analyzing these two texts of failed utopian attempts to establish perfection or total biological security together aims to highlight the continuities and changes in the imagination of biosecurity and the narratives that produce it.

Health and biology have become dominant paradigms in the study and understanding of U.S. American culture and identity. Sociologists have even pointed out that biology represents one of the "key sites for the fabrication of the contemporary self" (Rose, *Politics* 111). Also in the humanities the significance of health and biology has been widely acknowledged. Already in 2005, Priscilla Wald wrote that it is important to consider "how 'biology' is articulated within social institutions through narratives that can shift to incorporate new formulations into familiar hierarchical structures" and that "[t]he nation is an important site at which those narratives are produced" ("What's in a Cell" 220–1). She reasserted this focus in her 2009 presidential address to the American Studies Association when she called for American Studies to recognize the importance of this "turn" to biology, or bio-cultures, as a crucial lens and object of study ("American Studies" 186). With this book I wish to emphasize the underlying processes shaping the understanding of allegedly "natural" corporealities and fixed meanings that constitute the dominant apprehension of what "good life" is, and what it means to be human. By making visible the structures that help to make an understanding of biological security pervasive, I wish to provide a basis on which prevalent structures and ostensibly fixed meanings can be questioned, critiqued, and potentially challenged. My cultural critique of the intersection between health and security is committed to the efforts of Biocultural Studies, and that is the "bringing together of science and culture" – not to pit them against each other but to bifurcate each other. The study is thus intended to be more productive than a formulation of hostile *resentiments* against a field of academia that is clearly striving while the humanities, my own home ground, is struggling for legitimacy, funding, and relevance. Instead, I hope to show that cultural critique based on performance and performativity can raise questions that might also be productive in the life sciences. In "disarming the disciplinary firewalls" (Davis, "Biocultures" 950), literary and cultural analysis should not just serve as a way to humanize science, but should be consulted in bioethics commissions as well as in policy questions as both Jay Clayton and Lennard Davis point out: "Although there is now required ethical, legal, and social research and information that must accompany major federal grants in areas like genomics and nanotechnology, it isn't clear that there is also a cultural dimension that needs to be included" (Davis, "Biocultures" 950). This book turns to these cultural dimensions.

Part I: Framed by Theory: Security, Biomedical Science and the Biosecurity Individual

> They who can give up essential liberty to obtain a little temporary safety deserve neither liberty nor safety.
> *Benjamin Franklin*

Today, "security" is an overdetermined signifier in public as much as in academic discourse. It is usually understood within national security terms, which imply the notion of protection and control to guarantee freedom and liberty. According to most scholars, this rise of security as a central paradigm of protection was "predicated upon the nation-state" (Chilton 139). In fact, throughout the centuries security has become the main object of the state. The origins of security in that sense are most commonly fixed to liberal political theory and the protection of property, especially when discussing the expansions of the security state centered on surveillance and control.[1] But – as Benjamin Franklin's quote demonstrates – the founding fathers did not value security in the way it is predominantly understood and practised today. Franklin's famous phrase, originating from the failed negotiations in Britain before the Declaration of Independence, indicates the tension between security and freedom, particularly in the U.S. American context.[2] It

---

1   In "The Aspiration for Impossible Security" Völz asserts that it is a simplification to assume that "security constitutes both liberalism's ultimate legitimation of power and a distinctly liberal technology of rule" (13). He points out that with the foundation of the nation the liberal roots of security are in fact not based on governmental control but the right to overturn the government. Security in its contemporary sense represents a break from the understanding of security in the tradition of liberal thought.

2   Benjamin Franklin also embodies the strong connections between politics and science in the United States. However, his emphasis on the primacy of liberty over control and security did not translate to the relation of the self to the individual. In *The Autobiography of Benjamin Franklin*, he showcases the "self-made" individual based on a vigorous practice of self-control according to 13 virtues. Furthermore, he was a supporter of variolation against smallpox.

represents a balancing act between collective, national and individual security defined by freedom and liberty. It exemplifies the intimate interconnections of the private and the public, which are both also central to the understanding of biological security. As the nation-state rose to become the guarantor of political security, medicine and science became the arbiter of biological security.

The study of security has established its own field, namely that of Security Studies, which comprises various different disciplinary perspectives, most dominantly Political and Policy Studies, as well as Anthropological and Sociological perspectives. More recently, also Literary Studies has started to engage in the growing field studying this central paradigm of contemporary culture. The disciplinary focus of Security Studies, which had been almost exclusively dedicated to national security concerns, was broadened and challenged decisively after the Cold War. The work of scholars such as David A. Baldwin and Emma Rothschild is paradigmatic for this discursive shift of rethinking the state as the "primary referent object" of security (Kaltofen 37). Rothschild seeks to find a new conceptualization of security in adding "human security"[3] to the purview and defining it as reliant on "the distinctive self-consciousness principles" (Rothschild 54–5). Today, the concept of security finds many fields of application, which range from individual security to human or environmental security, as well as to national and domestic security. Yet, more radical and more important for my argument is another theoretical shift of the field. In the 1990s the study of security underwent "a radical, linguistically based 'constructivist turn'" (Burgess 2) establishing so-called Critical Security Studies.[4] This theoretical approach to security "focuses on the means by which security issues are constructed through language" (ibid.).

Similar to this "constructivist turn" in Security Studies, I will regard biological security not as a determined end point but as a condition, which has to be defined to become meaningful and acquire its culturally constructed meaning. Understanding security as performative helps to recognize that any representation of security is at the same time expressing, as well as (re-)producing, an understanding of security. I am not interested in defining or redefining security. Rather, I wish to study security as an operational term that does things. I will further argue that security narratives not only produce the understanding of security, but arrange people, positioning them toward the defined state of security. Unlike in a political-philosophical context, where the components that make up the ideal configuration of security are discussed, my own Cultural Studies perspective focuses on the way security is (made) culturally present. Instead of focusing on security mechanisms and practices as a form of governmental control and infringement on liberty and freedom only,[5] I wish to focus on the narratives of security as a productive force that articulates an imaginary of security and facilitates such practices in the first place.

---

3   "Human Security refers to both 'freedom from want' and 'freedom from fear'. . . . The core of Human Security is the concern for the holistic well-being of the individual human being. In other words, Human Security asserts that in order for an individual to be safe and secure both positive and negative peaces [sic] are necessary." (Von Feigenblatt 2)

4   Critical Security Studies are not exclusively focused on speech-act theory but also on other theoretical schools of Critical Theory. For a critical discussion of the use of the Frankfurt School in Critical Security Studies see Carolin Kaltofen "Engaging Adorno."

5   This is extensively done in anthropological and sociological studies following Foucault.

The "narrative constructedness" of security is understood by Security Studies scholars as "needed specification" to define a concept of security so as not to leave it a "useless category" (Baldwin 17).[6] More radically, I would suggest that security narratives are a form of storytelling and are therefore best analyzed with a Cultural Studies approach. Security narratives stabilize a social fiction which produces a "cultural imaginary" (Fluck; Iser) that cannot be described as a mimetic representation but is also always performative, relying on its aestheticization and reception. Studying biological security as performative allows for a more thorough understanding of the material effects that are produced by security narratives. With the performativity of security I refer to the theatrical as well as deconstructive sense of performativity, basing the perspective principally on John Langshaw Austin, Jacques Derrida, and Judith Butler, tracing the concept from speech to language, and finally to the body.

To establish my understanding of security and its reliance on narrative I will first turn to the central position of security narratives in the U.S. American cultural archive. In chapter 1 I will use the Declaration of Independence as the most iconic security narrative in the United States to explain my theoretical approach of performativity, and what it means to understand security as performative following the theory of Austin and Derrida. The Declaration of Independence is useful to highlight the structural and temporal characteristics of security which are central in biological security narratives. In chapter 2 I will show how science and medicine assumed normative power over life and its security, becoming in the Austinean sense the authoritative voices producing new security narratives. I will trace how body and life were increasingly securitized by focusing on the processes of medicalization and biomedicalization, as well as the shifting logics of security from prevention to pre-emption. I will use this historic overview to emphasize that the rise of biological security is not predicated on scientific findings only but on narrative practice and faith. In focusing on narrative construction I will argue that (bio)medical sciences as the arbiter of biological security establish a messianic narrative of scientific and medical salvation that represents the hope to control the body and correct nature's "mistakes."

In chapter 3 I will elaborate on the cornerstones of the theory of biomedicalization and show how biosecurity logics of prevention and pre-emption have become central for the understanding of individual biological security. I will discuss how biosecurity narratives define the relation of individuals to their body producing new biomedicalized identities: self-reliant biosecurity individuals, responsible and able to determine their own biological fate. In chapter 4 I will then focus on how to understand such biosecurity individuals in terms of identity theory. I will argue that biosecurity represents a further intersectionality that greatly impacts lives, structuring U.S. American society. To broaden the largely sociological Foucauldian-based understanding of biosecurity identities produced by governmentality, I will introduce Butler and the performativity of the body to facilitate a more thorough understanding of these "new" biosecurity individuals. Since security narratives are not only present in textual form in the traditional sense,

---

6   Baldwin proposes that "one could specify security with respect to the actor whose values are to be secured, the values concerned, the degree of security, the kinds of threats, the means for coping with such threats, the costs of doing so, and the relevant time period" (17).

but are also "written" on the body, Butler's concept of the performativity of the body is crucial, both in its deconstructive as well as theatrical sense. It allows a more comprehensive study of biologically inflected security narratives that define the materiality of these bodies, which are not perceived as intimate space (only) but are also always public.

1. "We hold these truths to be self-evident": Performativity and Security in the U.S. American Cultural Archive

> Gatsby believed in the green light, the orgiastic future that year by year recedes before us. It eluded us then, but that's no matter tomorrow we will run faster, stretch out our arms farther... And one fine morning
> —
> So we beat on, boats against the current, borne back ceaselessly into the past.
> *F. Scott Fitzgerald*

The concluding words of F. Scott Fitzgerald's novel describe the American Dream Jay Gatsby is chasing in his quest for happiness using the symbol of the green light. It represents a source of optimism, a goal to aim for and to live and understand his life by; a dream which remains unreachable and deferred "reced[ing] before us" (ibid.). This American Dream is one of the most famous and persistent U.S. American narratives and an extraordinary generator of individual stories. Already the Declaration of Independence (US 1776) gave shape to and stands paradigmatically for this national narrative of the American Dream – so much so that Craig Calhoun has claimed that the nation "declared itself as a dream" (159). The Declaration defines the American creed of "life, liberty, and the pursuit of happiness," and its promise of freedom has, as Eric Foner shows, "provided the most popular 'master narrative' for accounts of our past" (xiv). Though freedom and liberty are often understood as opposed to security (in its liberal and predominant understanding of control), they rely on the most iconic security narrative in American history, which established their understanding in the first place: The Declaration of Independence.[1] The document narrates the security of the future political society of the United States as well

---

[1] As "the most absolute principle in eighteenth-century constitutional theory" (Reid 68) security and liberty were interdependent, especially in the context of constitutionally secured rights. John Phillip Reid even attests that "[l]iberty and security were so interconnected in eighteenth-century political thought that today it is almost impossible to untangle them" (70).

as the threats against which it establishes itself. The Declaration exemplifies not only the centrality of security in U.S. American culture as a way of self-understanding, but that this ur-security narrative of the United States represents a performative act of security that articulates a "cultural imaginary" (Fluck; Iser). Furthermore, the understanding of security established in the Declaration of Independence is pivotal for the meaning of biological security and the rise of medicine as its arbiter in the United States, and it has remained a main reference point for the articulation of individual biological security narratives. Using the Declaration I will emphasize the importance of narrative to impact and form a reality rather than describing it. I will then turn to the temporal characteristics of security as a distinct relation between past, present, and future, and how the changes of understanding security can be described as a form of "deferral" (Derrida) which is produced by shifting horizons of security.

Making it New: Security as Speech Act

In the initial conceptualization of Austin's speech act theory, performatives describe a category of utterances that are not descriptive or expressive of a certain meaning but rather produce a reality (Austin 32). This speech act is exemplified by the wedding ceremony and the sentence "I hereby pronounce you husband and wife." With this sentence Austin describes the "creative function of language" (Culler 506), meaning a language that does not describe an existing state, but produces the reality it is referring to. Though security is not a magical act conjured up by the proper words, the performative act of security is nonetheless of utmost importance. This seems especially obvious when one considers the long history of declaring war or peace, an emergency or state of exception, or an epidemic. In that sense, security narratives produce rather than describe an understanding of security. Though not a "speech act" as such, the Declaration of Independence as a text pronounces rather than declares the independence of the English colonies in North America, as Derrida puts it ("Declaration"). While the document was adopted and signed on July 4th 1776, it took many more years of war for independence to be legally settled in the Treaty of Paris on September 3rd 1783. Independence did therefore not exist prior to, or at the time of the act of signing. "[T]he Declaration had announced independence at a time when it had yet to be achieved and when it was still under vigorous assault by Britain" (Armitage 3). The performativity of this instituting act, which Derrida fixes on the signatures, thus, "performs, it accomplishes, it does what it says it does" ("Declaration" 8).

Understood as a speech act, the Declaration performatively shifted the rebellion into a struggle for independence. Though the Declaration of Independence is not "the event" of independence itself as a singular exceptional moment – as Carl Becker asserts in his seminal study – it represents the narrative "in which the event was proclaimed and justified to the world" (qtd. in Armitage 13). The Declaration thus allows for a new meaning that had to be anchored in reality through narratives. Studies show that Thomas Jefferson worked diligently to make this "new" security narrative understandable and pervasive. He wrote and revised the draft of the Declaration of Independence thoroughly, carefully crafting each word as Becker shows in his study of the writing process. Jefferson was "chosen to draft the Declaration because he was known to possess a 'masterly pen'" (Becker 78). With editorial oversight from the Continental Congress he wrote a document that was to represent the legitimacy of separating from the governing power of the Crown of England. The carefully phrased security narrative shifted the rule of the Crown from security to threat by enumerating the tyrannies with which the English Crown had, according to the text, forfeited its God given right to rule. The Declaration thus most importantly affected a re-evaluation of who holds which rights and obligations. "Although occupying a subordinate place in the logical structure, the list of grievances is of the highest importance in respect to the total effect which the Declaration aims to produce" (ibid.). It created the legitimacy of the security practice, "[t]hat these united Colonies are, and of Right ought to be Free and Independent States."

More generally, in Security Studies, speech acts are understood as crucial in constructing "security issues" (Burgess 2):

> According to the theory, a given object becomes securitized by virtue of the pronouncement of a securitizing actor, appropriately positioned, permitting it to be shifted from the order of ordinary politics to one kind or another of exceptional politics. (ibid.)

The Declaration accomplishes exactly such a performative act. It moves the rule of England from one order (of the ordinary) to another (the exceptional). To do so the narrative has to establish a new order that allows for this shift. The Declaration of Independence articulated a new understanding of security that was set against the former security narrative of the legitimacy of and loyalty to the Crown. In form of a declaration and a manifesto (Armitage 50) the document expressed and challenged the understanding of what security means. It legitimized overthrowing a government by force: "it is their [the people's] right, it is their duty, to throw off such Government, and to provide new Guards for their future security." The security narrative defines the unjust tyranny in "a history of repeated injuries and usurpations" and provides a way to confront it. "It is a high literary merit of the Declaration that by subtle contrasts Jefferson contrives to conjure up for us a vision of the virtuous and long-suffering colonists standing like martyrs to receive on their defenseless heads the ceaseless blows of the tyrant's hand" (Becker 82). The text thus represents an example of what Sara Ahmed terms "narratives of injury" (Ahmed, *Politics* 32f) in which struggles for the public recognition of suffering are articulated. The "fears" and "suffering" associated with the rule of England in the Declaration of Independence are contrasted with the hopes invested in a new form of governance, a civil government, whose main object is the security of the inalienable rights of "life, liberty and the pursuit of happiness." The narrative of security thus establishes a new order that removes the Crown as a source of security and defines it as the origin of threat, while revolution and independence replace it as the "new" source of security.

The security narrative, condensed in the iconic sentence of "We hold these truths to be self-evident, that all men are created equal, that they are endowed by their Creator with certain unalienable Rights, that among these are Life, Liberty and the pursuit of Happiness", articulated the principles on which this new security is founded. It allowed for a new political subject which is defined by equality and inalienable rights.² Though the principles of the Declaration might seem intrinsic to today's readers, the new security narrative was not clear and logical to everyone at its time. Jeremy Bentham, who had been commissioned by the English government to formulate a response to the Declaration, described the claims as follows: "they attempt to establish a theory of Government; a theory, as absurd and visionary, as the system of conduct in defense of which it is established, is nefarious" (16).

The success of the security narrative set forth in the Declaration thus hinged on the question of authority. In *How We Do Things with Words* Austin defines rules that constitute a successful performative act, which he distinguishes as "happy" and "unhappy" (inter alia 21).³ He writes, that "the *circumstances* in which the words are uttered should be in some way, or ways *appropriate*" (Austin 8). "Appropriate" in this context refers to the speech act itself and its context, but it also refers to the relation of speaker and listener, or authors and reader in the case of the Declaration. According to Austin a performative act can only be accomplished if the utterance is meant truthfully and honestly.⁴ The truthfulness refers to both the veracity of the utterance as well as to its legitimacy. The performative act has to be imbued with the authority of the speaker to perform the given act. This authoritative voice is particularly crucial in security narratives, as they have to be pervasive and convince people of their truthfulness; they have to "appeal" as Foucault puts it (*Security* 21).

The ultimate legitimacy of the authoritative voice was of course contingent on the victorious outcome of the Revolutionary War. But the signatures on the Declaration of Independence represent the authority that Austin defines as a precondition for a successful performative act. In Derrida's elaborations the signatures take the place of the act of signing in the Austinean sense of a speech act. The signers – represented by their votes and later their signatures – provide the authority of the Declaration of Independence as "unanimous."⁵ They personified the elite of the colonies. But more than the political and social standing of this American elite assembled in the Continental Congress, the authority was derived from its representative function. The security narrative represented in the Declaration of Independence is produced by a new narrative authority – the signers as the representatives of the people.

Understanding the Declaration as a speech act necessarily directs the attention to the interlocutor highlighting the relational characteristic of security. The concept of the performative does not only rely on the utterance but also crucially on its reception. Emphasizing the position of the listener, Austin defines performatives as co-created. This

---

2   There were many groups excluded from the promises of the nation and the concept of the "political subject." Equality in this foundational document is thus more a promise than a reality.

3   While "happy" describes a successful performative act, "unhappy" refers to an unsuccessful performative act.

4   With this restriction Austin excludes lies and theatrically staged acts from the "appropriate circumstances" that lead to the production of the reality the utterance refers to (21–2).

5   Notwithstanding the fact that it is disputed if the Declaration was signed on the 4ᵗʰ of July, the signatures represent a crucial constituent of the performative act, as the debates among the signers of the document and later among scholars show (Becker, Warren).

means that the listener has to partake in the performative act, even if just by recognizing it, for the performative act to be accomplished. The Declaration of Independence, as most security narratives, has multiple addressees. Though the official addressee of the Declaration should have been the King of England, the Declaration of Independence was never sent to England by Congress. It was first published in London newspapers in August 1776. Rather, the world is the Declaration's intended audience as the text refers to "the opinions of mankind" and not to the King of England. The "opinions of Mankind" were, according to David Armitage, the more relevant interlocutor since "[a]s a document that announced the transformation of thirteen united colonies into the 'United States of America,' the Declaration marked the entry of those states into what would now be called international society" (16). The performative act of security relies like any performance on the relation between actor and audience to create the meaning of the performance (Fischer-Lichte),[6] making it an inevitably relational act.

Looking at the publication history of the Declaration of Independence, however, suggests that the primary and most immediate "interlocutor" and audience was the "American" public. After Congressional approval on the 4th of July, the document was printed the next day, to be distributed and performed all over the colonies, addressing the people which it represents and to a certain extent invents, as Derrida puts it ("Declaration" 11). The security narrative is thus not only productive in articulating a new and changed understanding of security; at the same time it produces a new "group identity." Though the Declaration is signed in the name of "the people," this "we" – as independence itself – "does not exist, before this declaration, not as such" (Derrida, "Declaration" 10). However, Armitage asserts that for the public this was the primary effect: "a contemporary report in August 1776 noted that when the Declaration was first read out to the Continental troops at Ticonderoga, in western Pennsylvania, 'the language of every man's countenance was, Now we are a people! We have a name among the states of this world!'" (Armitage 17–18). Derrida asserts that "[t]he obscurity, this undecidability between, let's say, a performative structure and a constative structure is *required* in order to produce the sought-after effect" (Derrida, "Declaration" 1). Clearly, the identity of "Americans" was not born over night with the publications and performances of the Declaration of Independence, nonetheless the security narrative of independence "named into being" (Butler, *Bodies* 13) the nation and its people. It represents a performative shift that changed the understanding of security, to be found in independence and revolution instead of loyalty to the crown, and this re-defined the "new" American.

The group identity "inaugurated" in the Declaration shows that security narratives serve to align people. The Declaration defines the security of the "new" self "counterpunctually" (Said 52) in opposition to the other. In that sense the Declaration of Independence does not just express an "imagined community" in terms of Benedict Anderson's the-

---

6   In Fischer-Lichte the co-presence of actor and audience is the most important constituent of a performance (47), which is not given here. Nonetheless, the performative act also in its temporally and spatially distant form relies on such a form of interaction to produce its effect.

ory of nationalism.[7] The produced group affiliation would be more fittingly described as "imagined communities of (in)security" (Völz, "A Nation" n.p.). The security narrative represents a group defined by their common position toward the object of security: the equality of men and their inalienable right of "life, liberty, and the pursuit of happiness."

Promising Futures – Haunting Pasts: Security and Reiteration

The equality of men and their innate right to "life, liberty, and the pursuit of happiness" is an understanding of security which was revolutionary in itself, in addition to legitimating the political and military revolution. The preamble created the vision of a new subject that would be celebrated as the true revolutionary act soon after independence. In his Fourth of July oration "American Principles" in 1821, John Quincy Adams argues that the "'principles' in the preamble to the Declaration—rather than the particular charges against the King—were the proper objects of celebration on the Fourth of July" (qtd. in Dyer 30). And although the new political subject defined in the Declaration was unquestionably revolutionary, it was by no means a radically "new" idea.

Both Austin and Derrida stress the necessity of already established meanings for performative acts to work. However, Derrida goes one step further. He divorces the concept of performativity of language from its strict adherence to a certain category of words and speech acts and applies it to language in general. He asserts that all communication is performative, not just in constructing a reality but in its relation to the referent object. The security that the Declaration of Independence represents is in that sense not referring to an a priori existing "reality," but rather to a cultural construction through which security is comprehended. Understanding language as non-referential and incapable of communicating "a thing itself" without relying on previously established meaning defines all language as a form of "citation" (Derrida "Signature" 17). And this citation is only understandable because it is based on the iterability of signs and on already established meanings. Language might try to approximate an extra-linguistic thing but will never be able to supersede or outstrip the cultural constructiveness that is inevitably expressed when using language.[8] Security narratives are in that sense always referring to established understandings. Though undoubtedly a revolutionary act and narrative that stands at the beginning of a "new global genre" as David Armitage asserts, the Declaration does not represent an isolated performance but refers to already circulating narratives. Jefferson himself wrote that he aimed to express "the American mind" (Jefferson 19). Independence as well as the principles on which it could be established had been debated, circulated and prepared for in the years leading up to the Declaration, and its history of meaning reaches back several centuries. The claims expressed in the preamble of the Declaration relied on well-known traditions of thinking: Enlightenment and Natural Law.

---

7   In his study of nationalism Benedict Anderson famously defines "imagined communities" and their sense of belonging as "a deep horizontal comradeship" (*Imagined* 7), which is made possible by print capitalism.

8   Derrida explains that language does not and cannot refer to an "a priori or exterior state of things" ("Signature" 14).

The histories of meaning in the Declaration of Independence are not difficult to discern and have been studied extensively.[9] The iconic phrase, "life, liberty, and the pursuit of happiness" represents, according to most scholars, a direct reference to, or citation of John Locke's *Two Treatises of Government* (1689). In fact, Jefferson was accused by Richard H. Lee of having produced merely a copy of said work. Lee had presented the preamble that led to the vote for the Declaration of Independence in Continental Congress on 2nd of July but was eclipsed by Jefferson's pre-eminence (Becker 15). Becker shows that the text was thus utterly dependent on English Philosophical tradition to articulate independence (34), and maybe even to conceive of it. First and foremost, the representation of a security narrative thus fixes a meaning or understanding by reiteration. And this meaning was, according to Becker, "commonly taken for granted" (15) by the contemporary American public.

The Declaration's assertion of the equality of men and their inalienable rights was an expression of natural law, which by the time of the Revolution had long surpassed ideas of eternal law (Becker 20). Most importantly, the Enlightenment thinking that is expressed in the Declaration gives the individual the power to rationally understand the truth that was expressed in nature. The world was understood as knowable, to be enlightened by rational discernment which "left men free to make their own laws with their reason" (Jayne 40). It reiterated the understanding that the values and rights of human existence were naturally given, which was seminal for demands of "human rights" formulated in the Revolutionary War and the Declaration of Independence (Brunner et al. 847).

The just government that is to be forged by independence is, according to the Declaration, responsible for the "Safety and Happiness" of its constituents. Safety of the governed as the main objective of the government had been a well-established part of political philosophy at the time of the revolution.[10] Also the inclusion of happiness as an objective of government is not surprising, considering the etymology of the term security. Already Cicero called security an "object of supreme desire," defining it as the "absence of anxiety upon which the happy life depends" (qtd. in Rothschild 61). Security was understood as a state of freedom from the natural drives, resulting in "happiness," or *beata vita* in Epicurean thought. Similarly, in Greek philosophy Aristotle defined the good life as eudaimonia, or happiness.[11] Happiness, according to the Enlightenment tradition, was not equitable with property as more modern inflections of the American Dream would have it. Rather happiness was understood in Epicurean or Aristotelian terms of eudaimonia,[12] reiterating the understanding of a good, virtuous and meaningful life that is

---

9   For a thorough study of the history of ideas see Carl Lotus Becker's paradigmatic study *Declaration of Independence: A Study on the History of Political Ideas.*

10   Already in Hobbes the *status civilis* established the legitimacy of the principalities (Fürstenstaat) in the relationality of (state) protection and (civil/subject's) security. This idea of protection, emblematically visualized on the title page of *Levianthan's* publication, increasingly became the key element of governmental objective (Brunner et al. 845).

11   The conceptual shift to the *sine cura* as indicating the freedom from sorrow wasn't introduced until Cicero and Lucretius. Cicero wrote "securitatem nunc appello vacuitatem aegritudinis, in qua vita beata posita est" (engl. "I call security the absence of sorrow, which makes the good life") (qtd. in Ritter and Gründer 745).

12   Concept of a state of "felicitude" and "beatitude."

above all balanced (Schlesinger 326). And, according to the Declaration of Independence, the security of this "good life" is the purpose of the new civil government that the Declaration promises. Happiness of men becomes the highest goal of the governments that are to be "instituted among Men," as it is understood as the highest form of being.

While the reiterated meanings used to describe security are important, equally important is the future-directedness of the security narrative. Rather than using past ideas to describe a present moment only, the Jeffersonian security narrative established a vision and a promise for the future. Neither independence, nor the Constitution and the Bill of Rights, which legally define the rules of the just government, existed. Jefferson himself called the Declaration "an instrument, pregnant with our own and the fate of the world" (qtd. in Armitage 1). The preamble that would be understood as an expression and testament of American exceptionalism, that "must forever stand alone, a beacon on the summit of the mountain, to which all the inhabitants of the earth may turn their eyes for a genial and saving light" (Adams 31) represented a promise, rather than describing a present reality.

As a promise the security narrative describes a future state that is made present performatively. The act of promising is itself a prime example Austin uses in the study of performative words/acts, which he returns to throughout his lectures. According to him, the act of promising is connected to an intentionality that "obliges me" (10) to truly follow up on what I promised. Promises and their obligating characteristics are widely conceptualized by many authors and philosophers (Gloyna n.p.). Rather than tracing the history of different conceptualizations I would like to focus briefly on the relation between promises and the promised object or event. The "futurity" of the promised event is a crucial constituent of the event itself. The promise creates the presence of a "reality" that is situated in the future. The promise of security establishes a future state of security *as if* it was present. It becomes an object of desire, which represents the aim and rationale behind processes, the motivation for action, such as the joint struggle for independence.

The particular promise of future security based on equality and freedom is a specific accomplishment of the Declaration. However, the promise is also a structural constituent when understanding security as performative. Derrida not only stresses the importance of past meanings in his theoretical considerations, he stresses that by creating the reality they describe, performatives appropriate a future. This temporal relation is compared by Derrida to the "future perfect" ("Declaration" 10), emphasizing the future-directedness of the performative act. Though the signing of the Declaration of Independence did not describe a de facto independence, the performative act creates a semblance of a present. Derrida describes this form of making present a state that is absent a *"simulacrum of the instant"* ("Declaration" 11; ital. orig.). The force of this "simulacrum of the instant" is part and parcel of how the performative act of security is understood.

Though the promises of the Declaration – independence, equality, pursuit of happiness – described a future, they also produced a semblance of the present in its different historic reiterations. For example, in his Gettysburg address, Abraham Lincoln declared: "Four score and seven years ago our fathers brought forth on this continent, a new nation, conceived in Liberty, and dedicated to the proposition that all men are created equal" (83). Thereby he "went so far as to identify the birth of the nation itself with the events of 1776" (Dyer xvii). This understanding is also reflected in the date chosen for the national holiday "Independence Day," which is celebrated on July 4th and represents a ritualized reiteration of the security narrative of the Declaration of Independence and its promises.

The Declaration expressed an optimistic sense of future and a form of utopianism. It aimed at affecting a future that reached beyond the security of independence, formulating a promise to serve the happiness of the people. Thomas Jefferson wrote in his letter for the semi-centennial of the Declaration: "May it be to the world, what I believe it will be, (to some parts sooner, to others later, but finally to all) the signal of arousing men to burst the chains, under which monkish ignorance and superstition had persuaded them to bind themselves, and to assume the blessings and security of self government" ("Fifty Years" 34–5). And indeed it was seen as a signal to other oppressed groups around the globe to fight for their independence.[13] However, the Declaration of Independence did not only incite men to break their shackles in the sense Jefferson primarily implied, which is the political struggle of the politically oppressed, but also expressed a general sentiment of optimism, a belief in progress toward an imaginary of security.

This general sentiment of optimism and the belief in the possibility to "burst the chains" as a God given right extended beyond political security to other fields and new horizons. The political revolutionary act was crucial for the American understanding and conception of the possibilities of a medical revolution that would strike against the other tyrannies wrongfully determining human existence: the chains of disease and nature. Benjamin Rush had risen to great eminence for his role in the 1793 yellow fever epidemic in Philadelphia (Shryock "Significance" 84). He also was one of five medical professionals who signed the Declaration of Independence, which at the outset indicates how closely related the revolutionary act and thought of the Declaration is with that of the coming medical revolution.[14] Rush describes the sentiment as follows:

> All the doors and windows of the temple of nature have been thrown open by the convulsions of the late American revolution [sic]. This is the time, therefore, to press upon her altars. We have already drawn from the discoveries in morals, philosophy, and government; all of which have human happiness for their object. Let us preserve the unity of truth and happiness, by drawing from the same source, in the present critical moment, a knowledge of antidotes to those diseases which are supposed to be incurable. (Rush 556)

The optimistic sense of future serving the cause of happiness was extended to health and the security of the body. Scientific research represented another beacon of Enlightenment illuminating a further corner of human existence, and was tightly connected to the security expounded in the Declaration of Independence. Rush, as well as Thomas Jefferson, and Thomas Paine believed that the health of the people "would flourish" and "was fostered by good social institutions" (Rosen 398), directly linking the political security promised in the Declaration with the biological security of the people and therefore the

---

13   Armitage elaborates on the many declarations of independence that followed the American one often citing the structure of the American Declaration of Independence.

14   "[T]wenty-six other doctors were members of the Continental Congress" (Starr 83).

nascent nation. And the medical revolution seemed to be following the political one. Benjamin Franklin marveled about the increasing possibilities of science: "The rapid progress true science now makes, occasions my regretting sometimes that I was born too soon. . . . all diseases may by sure means be prevented or cured, (not excepting even that of old age,) and our lives lengthened at pleasure, even beyond the antediluvian standard" ("Letter to Joseph Priestly"). But not only were both revolutions heir to the same school of thought and the hopes for a better future. The security narrative of the Declaration of Independence crucially influenced the development of medical knowledge, research, and practice in the U.S. and still does today, which I will explore further in the following chapters.

"What Happens to A Dream Deferred?":[15] Security and Deferral

In the time of the revolution the pursuit of happiness did not describe a dogmatic ideal imposed on individuals but represented the ability to practice one's individual definition of happiness. Security was framed in a private context and symbolized protection from interventions of the government, rather than a security that could be provided by governmental intervention. It hinged on "the conviction that good government is limited government" (K. Henry 16) and the ideal of the self-reliant individual. This personal freedom as "personal choice referred mainly to realms of democratic politics and religious affiliation" (Foner xviii). It guaranteed the right to live and represent one's individual ideas, as long as they did not infringe on others. The principle of small government has remained crucial throughout the centuries, significantly influencing also the history of medical practice and the way in which biological security has been understood and confronted in the United States.[16] However, rather than a fixed understanding, the imaginary of security established in the Declaration serves as a persistently shifting benchmark that the people and politics of the following centuries will try to catch up with. Understanding security as performative allows us to understand the changing meanings of security produced in the acts of reiteration, of actualizing and making present this historical concept in new and different specific historical moments.

These changes in the understanding of security mirror Derrida's concept of deferral. In his explanations of the non-referentiality of a word to an "outside" reality, Derrida elaborates on the temporality of deferral. In this temporality, the referent is always ahead of itself and similarly, security narratives such as the Declaration of Independence produce an imaginary of security that lies in the future. Derrida defines the failure of language to approximate the thing itself with his concept of *différance* (difference and deferral). In *Writing and Difference* as well as in the lecture "Différance" he defines this temporal relation as "the interposition of delay, the interval of a spacing and temporalizing that

---

15   The title is a quote from Langston Hughes's poem "Harlem," which reflects on the unfulfilled dream of equality and acceptance of African Americans throughout the centuries.

16   The most recent attempt to establish a general health care – the *Affordable Care Act* – and harsh critique as a fundamentally un-American program of an oppressive government, as well as its dismantling during the Trump Presidency, show the importance of this founding principle and its relation to biological security.

puts off until 'later' what is presently denied, the possible that is presently impossible" ("Différance" 278). Derrida establishes this temporality to describe the relation between word and referent object, which ends in an endless chain of constructions and approximations. I would suggest that security as a performative is fundamentally marked by this notion of constant deferral: on the one hand, it cannot approximate a presupposed real; on the other hand, the meaning of security is not static but ever-changing. Security as performative represents a moving target that is ahead of its realization, constantly retreating due to the shifting horizons of security. It is therefore marked by futurity and absence. While security narratives fix the meaning of security at least temporally, in the inevitable failure to approximate the referent it is deferred. Like Gatsby's green light, security "recedes before us" (Fitzgerald 115), remaining an elusive goal that motivates acts to meet the target which moves ever further away.

In a constant mode of "not yet," the promise that orients the people thus seems to violate the fundamental principal of promises and the act of promising ("Promises" n.p.). However, the futurity of the promised event is a crucial constituent of the event itself. The promised security as an object of desire represents the aim and rationale behind processes; the motivation for action despite (or precisely because of) its continual deferral. Laura Berlant describes a similar relationality of improbable accessibility in *Cruel Optimism*: "When we talk about an object of desire, we are really talking about a cluster of promises we want someone or something to make to us and make possible for us. This cluster of promises could be embedded in a person, a thing, an institution, a text, a norm, a bunch of cells, smells, a good idea – whatever" ("Cruel" 20). Her theory of "cruel optimism" seems in many instances fitting to describe the promise of security, and the hopes and fears invested in it. Security as "desired object" and a "cluster of promises" is marked by its perpetual absence. This perpetual absence is and has to be filled with promises that *make up* the object. Berlant makes clear that all "objects/scenes of desire are problematic" because they are projections rather than the thing themselves ("Cruel" 21). Understanding promised security as such a cluster of promises helps to understand the persistence of security narratives despite their continuous failure.

Over the centuries, minority and advocacy groups insisted on the founding principles of the nation in order to receive full citizen rights and gain equality. These groups often cited the Declaration of Independence, challenging and changing the understanding of security by rewriting the security narrative. "[A]ntislavery and women's rights activists in the nineteenth century routinely invoked the Declaration of Independence and the history of the nation's founding in their efforts to focus public attention on the plight of the disenfranchised" (K. Henry 25). The most famous and explicit examples for these narratives are probably the "Declaration of Sentiments" from the 1848 Seneca Falls Convention, or Frederick Douglass's "What to the Slave is the Fourth of July?". It is not particularly surprising that these claims to full citizen rights were invoking the Declaration of Independence. More importantly, as Katherine Henry points out, many of these demands were articulated as security-based arguments. She argues that the struggle for citizenship was based on a "rhetoric of protection" (1–24) "– not a challenge to the structure of thought that marked women and slaves as unfit for citizenship in the classical republican sense" (K. Henry 3). Similarly, Johannes Völz highlights in this context that "the invocation of '(in)security' was used to initiate a progressive political mobilization"

(Völz, "A Nation" n.p.). As the Declaration itself, also these revisions of the security narrative thus rely on a "narrative of injury" (Ahmed, *Politics* 32f) which represents a claim in the public for recognition. At the same time they create a "community of (in)security" (Völz, "A Nation" n.p.) crucial for the advance of the claims to protection.

The claims to protection articulate a changed understanding of security to that promised in the Declaration of Independence. Security as a private space from government coercion (the freedom from) was rhetorically turned into "being under the threat" and "in need of defense" (K. Henry 12).[17] This shift can also be found in the literature of the time, such as Stephen Crane's *Maggie: A Girl of the Streets*, or Upton Sinclair's *The Jungle*. And as the protection of civil rights became a core element of security, also health was more and more perceived as a right that had to be protected by government (Tomes, "Merchants" 530).[18] These changes in understanding security exemplify the importance of narratives to establish the meaning of security and show that security is not fixed but has to be retold and re-contextualized in the different historic movements.

The promise of security envisioned in the struggle for citizenship and voting rights, however, did not represent equality and equal access to "life, liberty, and the pursuit of happiness." The promised security represented by voting rights was deferred as for instance in the history of the African American "struggle for freedom." The promised security remained unattainable because of racist practices that undermined the established rights directly following the Fifteenth Amendment, such as literacy tests, grandfather-clauses, or poll-taxes.[19] Furthermore, voting rights, as the object of desire representing security, did not fully accomplish equality and equal access to the foundational promise. The rights to vote could not establish equality in a society and culture structured and saturated by racism and sexism, as the ongoing struggle for freedom and equality of the same groups today makes clear. In the iconic poem "Harlem" Langston Hughes expresses the frustrations of a people that sees their freedom and equality constantly deferred. But despite the continuous failure of the security narrative, the Declaration has remained a crucial reference in the African American civil rights movement. For instance in the iconic speech "I Have a Dream" Martin Luther King Jr. asserts that "we have come to cash a check" referring to the promise of the founding security narrative.[20] The American Dream and the Declaration of Independence have become an almost staple reference points of struggles for recognition and justice in the United States.

---

17   The example of the Abolition Movement and Women's Right Movement are paradigmatic for the change of understanding of security. A similar "rhetoric of protection" can be found in the representation of workers' rights as Eric Foner points out (125).

18   Protection did not refer to a form of universal health care but to government regulation of medical practice. Yet early biopolitical interventions such as the first vaccination laws (relating to smallpox) in 1855 were already abrogating the individual rights and freedoms of the Constitution. For a thorough study of the changes from positive to negative liberty in the U.S. see K. Henry or Eric Foner.

19   Only in the 1960s "did American constitutional doctrine begin to treat the right to vote as a fundamental constitutional right" (Pildes and Smith n.p.).

20   In fact, he calls the Declaration "a promissory note to which every American was to fall heir. This note was a promise that all men, yes, black men as well as white men, would be guaranteed the 'unalienable rights' of 'Life, Liberty, and the Pursuit of Happiness'" (King Jr.).

Many of these movements make the body and its health central to their cause. The Black Panthers set up a program for aging, and Martin Luther King Jr. asserted that, "[o]f all forms of inequality, injustice in health care is the most shocking and inhumane." Similarly, the Women's Movement with its famous claim of "Our Bodies, Our Selves!" was centrally concerned with medical practice, campaigning for birth control and abortion rights. The Declaration of Independence represents one of the foundational cultural (and political) objects of the security narrative that came to define the nation. Its promises of "life, liberty, and the pursuit of happiness" are foundational elements of the American national identity and the American Dream, which has come to include not only political sovereignty, equality and political participation, prosperity, and wealth, but also health. Though political and biological security seem to be vastly different fields of study at the first sight, I will argue in the next chapter that they are closely intertwined and structurally very similar. The political and biological security narratives are cut from the same cloth, both representing products of Enlightenment thinking and an adamant optimism in future progress. Furthermore, the principles and understandings of security formulated in the Declaration of Independence are central for the formation and understanding of the rise, expansion, and militarization of biological security.

2. Science as the Arbiter of Security: The Rise of Prevention and Pre-emption

How long, O Lord?
King James Bible, Ps. 13

While the Declaration of Independence defined the sovereign state as the guarantor of life liberty and pursuit of happiness, science became the arbiter of biological security. Medical science rose from a revolutionary movement and revolutionary ideas to an institutionalized normative power that has expanded to all aspects of life in its present and future form. The American pursuit of health was readily aligned with the God given rights promised in the Declaration of Independence as described previously. But the still nascent rise of science and medicine had not yet fully established its normative power over bodily security and life. Medical practices existed before and during the 19th century but in the United States they did not represent one professionalized field.[1] Though Cotton Mather is widely regarded as the "first significant figure in American medicine" (Shryock, "Medicine" 282) because of his study on smallpox and defense of variolation, diseases were nonetheless understood in a religious framework.[2]

---

1   When talking about medical practice and scientific knowledge I am referring to Western traditions. This does not mean that indigenous scientific and medical knowledge production did not exist at the time, nor should it dispute that in many areas the indigenous traditions were more advanced than the practices imported to the Americas, and had a great influence on Western medicine (Vogel). Much of these medical knowledges and practices were lost following the process of colonization. The indigenous medical traditions were largely eradicated all over the Americas, discursively reduced to the shamanistic rituals that were part of the healing practices (ibid. xi).

2   Cotton Mather performed clinical tests on smallpox inoculation in 1721 using "quantitative procedures" (Shryock "Medicine" 283) to prove that inoculation protected the individual from infection, but the findings were not further systematized. This example highlights also the cross-cultural exchange of knowledge that undermines the narrative of medicine as a purely "Western" achievement since Mather had the information of variolation from his slave Onesimus. For a discussion of the disputes over inoculation in 1721 see Shawn Buhr "To Inoculate or Not to Inoculate." For a thorough study of Mather as a Figure of Medicine see Otho T. Beall, Jr. and Richard H. Shryock *Cotton Mather: First Significant Figure in American Medicine*.

In this chapter I will illustrate the process by which medical science becomes in the Austinean sense the authoritative voice defining new narratives about biological security. Though this new authoritative voice was based on objective knowledge it also represents a movement of faith, belief, and ideology that is given shape in what I will call messianic narratives of medical salvation.[3] The security promised by medical and scientific developments becomes not a question of possibility but a question of time representing, as I will argue, a fervent belief in the "not yet" and the yet to come. I will trace the rise of science as the arbiter of security to establish the "historical ideas" (Butler, "Performative" 521) that define the understanding of biological security. With the historical overview of the rise, expansion, and militarization of (bio)medicalized security I will highlight the logics of security which form a development from prevention to pre-emption and total control.[4] Though representing a historical overview and following roughly traditional periods in U.S. American medical history (1880–1930; 1920–1980, 1980–now) these three processes do not neatly fit into closed time frames; they have at times coincided and overlapped. They represent three stages in the genealogy of the biosecurity narrative that greatly influences individual and collective identity formation today. I will argue that the revolution in medicine and science facilitated a biologically inflected "cultural imaginary" (Fluck; Iser) of security which expanded to further fields, shifting from fighting disease to securing health, life, and happiness itself. I will argue that this expansion of medical normative power incessantly relocates the horizon and thereby the understanding of biological security.

The Rise of Medicine as Normative Power: Biological Security and the Logic of Prevention

The rise of science as the normative power over biological security marks the transition from a moral to a scientific approach to disease, as George Canguilhem (*The Normal*) and others have pointed out.[5] It thereby marks a change in the narrative of security. This change describes the establishing of a new authoritative voice claiming the legitimacy

---

3   With Walter Benjamin I understand the originally religious term of the messianic as socially and historically fixed. The messianic in Benjamin, as well as in Derrida's use of it in *Specters of Marx*, does not describe a transcendental hope anymore, but a hope grounded in the experiential world of acting people in their specific historic and social context. "Once the classless society had become defined as an infinite task, the empty and homogeneous time was transformed into an anteroom, so to speak, in which one could wait for the emergence of the revolutionary situation with more or less equanimity" (Benjamin, "Concept" 402). In Benjamin this messianic act, thus, describes a relation of inaccessibility. The messianic "bears witness to a lack, an incompleteness" (Khatib 2) that motivates its specific time.

4   This is not an attempt at a complete historical analysis of U.S. medical history, public health, or its policies but rather a selection of events that exemplify the rise of science as arbiter over biological security in the United States. Though a narrative of supposed continual progress toward bodily security, the narrative is fractured, full of incongruences and misguided ideas and treatments, which I will attempt to do justice to.

5   This is not an absolute transition, since still today disease are reflected in moral categories as for example the representation of AIDS shows.

to write (or prescribe?) a "new" security narrative. The medical paradigm shift represents a revolution similar to the American political revolution and is based on the same philosophical ideas of Enlightenment, which defined nature and thus the body as legible truth. The new biological security narrative was based on the understanding of the body as a machine that can be studied and described, and therefore controlled, managed, and fixed. The concept of the body as machine, as Canguilhem criticizes it in the chapter "Diseases" (*Writing*) is not an invention of modern medicine. It is derived from Descartes's dualism of body and mind (Powell 209), which modern medicine is still predominantly based on. The systematic implementation of this understanding in medical practice is commonly exemplified with the foundation of the Paris School of Medicine at the end of the 18th century and the turn to observation-based medicine (Shryock, "Significance" 85). The threats to biological security were in this "new approach" classified and distinguished as specific diseases.[6] This new understanding of diseases was facilitated by the change from "bedside medicine" to "hospital medicine." The centralized treatment of patients in hospitals facilitated the systematic study of symptoms and pathologies (through surgery and autopsy).

Hospital medicine with its famous operating theatres opened up the body to the "clinical gaze," purportedly making "truth" (Foucault, *Birth* 155) accessible in performative acts.[7] Michel Foucault asserts that this "opening up of the concrete individual, for the first time in Western history, to the language of rationality, that major event in the relationship of man to himself and of language to things – was soon taken as a simple, unconceptualized confrontation of a gaze and a face, or a glance and a silent body" (Foucault, *Birth* xiv-xv).[8] The new structure of seeing has established the understanding of a direct access to "truth," or the natural. This claim to a truth instituted the authority of medicine over biological security replacing other traditions of practice and understanding. The rise of science and the normalization of medical practices challenged the "space in which the bodies and eyes meet" (Foucault, *Birth* xi). Foucault stresses that with this "medical gaze" a stable relation between sign and knowable fact was "forged" (xii), converting the body into a readable text, a truth hidden beneath the enigmatic signs of nature.

Through this medical gaze, the idea of the body as machine was reinforced as the defining element of the security narrative redirecting the focus from individual suffering to sickness. Ivan Illich claims that "[w]ithin this mechanized framework, pain turned into a red light and sickness into mechanical trouble" (*Nemesis* 58). And the understanding of sickness as "mechanical trouble" emphasized that these "troubles" could be controlled. It further defined biological security as a natural state that can be protected and returned to if the necessary knowledge is discerned. The creation of new disease categories thus

---

6   Before, speculative pathology was based on the assumption that illness was caused by "impure body fluids" (Shryock, "Medicine" 284) with no real distinction between diseases.

7   The operating theatre with its clear spatial analogy to a theatrical space stages performances of security on multiple levels: it stages an increasingly crucial security practice of surgery, and it stages a security practice to an audience with a didactic purpose and the goal of multiplying the practice and providing more security.

8   Foucault describes this structure already existing for earlier autopsies, however, in the nineteenth century the practice gained in legitimacy and normative power.

represents a first performative act of security that facilitates the protection of the natural and vulnerable body.

Science started to write its own declarations of independence: every description of pathology defined and identified a further tyranny of nature's mistakes that man had the right to rebel against. Every new category of normal and pathological represented a new security narrative, establishing first and foremost a new understanding and meaning of bodily states. These new normative understandings were facilitated by the generation and accumulation of knowledge and data, as both Canguilhem and Foucault point out. These knowledge categories which circumscribe the security and threats of the body were installed as "the natural," an incorruptible "truth" that could only be discerned by medical professionals. These new diagnostic categories significantly influence how bodies are understood. However, the pathological and the normal, that are represented as truth are not determined states but rather descriptions of what "ought to be" (*Normal* 125), which is influenced by historically changing value judgments as Canguilhem emphasizes and are therefore never purely objective.[9]

In the United States the shift to hospital and evidence-based medicine as well as the development of a certified professionalized field that facilitated this transition started significantly later than in Europe (Shryock, "Significance" 86, Starr). This delay has been put down to the resistance to regulations in general, legitimized on the basis of the Declaration of Independence. The rise of the medical security narrative emphasized the possibilities of control and protection through a professionalized elite, an ideal diametrically opposed to the ideals of the Declaration of Independence and the paradigm of self-reliance: "God helps those, who help themselves," as Franklin is supposed to have put it. From the colonial era onward a form of "medical self-reliance" had been the prevalent and often the only form of medical care available (Tomes, *Remaking* 20). Still, in the 19th and early 20th century the system Nancy Tomes terms "medical democracy" favored a "do-it-yourself approach" (ibid.). Richard Shryock stresses the importance of this particularity in U.S. American medical history. He quotes a senator in 1844 supporting licenses for irregular practitioners saying, "A people accustomed to governing themselves . . . want no protection but freedom of inquiry and freedom of action" (qtd. in Shryock, "Significance" 87).

The explicit involvement of governance with the health of the nation in the U.S. is most obviously rooted in the great epidemics, such as yellow fever and cholera in the 18th and mid 19th century, especially with regard to the growing population in urban areas.[10]

---

9   Canguilhem claims that the medical understanding of normal has incorporated moral metaphors in the experimental methods that produce their scientific findings and therefore influence the understanding of the disease. An example of this are the research biases that are contained in the experimental setup itself, such as the predominant study of mental illness in prisons leading to the correlation of criminality, violence, and certain conditions, or the gender and race bias that existed in clinical research up to 1993 when the Revitalization Act was passed. This Act requires 'that all federally funded clinical research prioritize the inclusion of women and minorities and that research participant characteristics be disclosed in research documentation" (Oh et al. 1).

10   In the 19th century, as for instance during the cholera epidemic of 1835, responding was the responsibility of the municipals and not federal agencies such as the Center for Disease Control and

Though medical practitioners held the explanatory authority over disease and were con-sulted in the events of epidemics even before the rise of bacteriology, they did not repre-sent a unified professionalized field yet. It was only in the last decades of the 19th century that medical science and its practitioners assumed the normative power over biological security in the United States as policy experts. "[T]he decades from 1880 to 1930 consti-tuted an economic and cultural watershed for the American medical profession" (Tomes, "Merchants" 524). The change coincided with the next big paradigm shift in medical his-tory: the turn to laboratory medicine and the rise of preventive medicine.

The shift of authoritative voice is on the grander scale of medical history assigned to the rise of bacteriology following Louis Pasteur's successful experiment immunizing an-imals in 1880 and Robert Koch's "discovery" of the mycobacterium tuberculosis in 1882. With the scientific evidence for the germ theory of disease the competing security narra-tive of miasma theory was abandoned (Shryock, "Significance" 85).[11] With the rise of bac-teriology, the jurisdiction over the biological security of the people in the United States was gradually taken over by medical science as the sole arbiter of security. The security narratives concerned with the health of the people in the United States had thus a new protagonist, and a new narrator and author.

This usurpation of normative power by medical science did not involve a radical change, however, but a gradual transition of passing over authority. During the Progres-sive Era (ca. 1890–1920) the nominal power over biological security and epidemics was still largely held by social reformers.[12] The Sanitary Movement and the Social Hygiene Movement are seen as pivotal in the history of early public health, and the practice of preventive medicine (Pivar 1, Duffy 167). In some areas, such as the prevention of syphilis, the social reformers held the normative power and authority in policy advice until the beginning of the 20th century. While the focus on preventive medicine had existed before, within a moralized discourse, with the evidence of the germ theory it was medicalized, consolidated, normalized, and most importantly professionalized.

The germ theory established microorganisms as the cause of disease and contagion – the transmission of microbes through contact – as the reason for its spread. The new understanding of what endangered the body produced a new security narrative based on the possibilities of visualizing that rendered the invisible threat of bacteria palpable (Wald, *Contagious* 136). The possibilities of visualizing bacteria through Gram stains (de-veloped in 1884) were yet another "opening up of the concrete individual" that Foucault has described for the study of anatomy. This turn from the organic to the microscopic further enforced the medical understanding of the body as machine and the need for experts who could "read" and interpret the (microscopic) data.

Though based on scientific discoveries, the security narrative that emerged from those findings also represented a question of faith. "Believing in the germ theory, as it was initially formulated from the experimental evidence available in the 1870s, required

---

Prevention (CDC) today (Fearnley 65). However, "public health is historically and legally a respon-sibility of state and local government" (ibid.).

11   The miasma theory proposed that diseases were caused by "foul and polluted air" (P. Mitchell 38).

12   The end of the 19th century saw the emergence of broad social movements in the U.S., which strove for policy interventions during the Progressive Era.

a considerable leap of faith that most physicians simply could not make" (*Gospel* 34). Nancy Tomes describes the rise of bacteriology as the rise of the "gospel of germs" – the title of her book – comparing the advent of the medical authority with a movement based on faith and conviction emphasizing the religious evangelical undertones in the "conversion" to the "gospel of germs" (*Gospel* 114). The rise of the "new" understanding of security thus relied on narratives that had to convince and appeal, which they had to far beyond the medical community.

What became unquestionably visible to scientists was not immediate to a general public. The findings had to be communicated in *understandable* security narratives in order to produce the desired effect of changing people's understandings and habits based on new security scripts. The authoritative voice of the performative needs its interlocutor and thus needs to be intelligible for this interlocutor. Nancy Tomes emphasizes the importance of communicating the new risks in narratives. She shows how the medical narrative used "preventive medicine" and the discourse of the Sanitary Movements to establish its findings in public practice (Tomes, *Gospel* 46). The initial security narrative of the germ theory was therefore represented as a logic extension to the discourse of the Sanitary Movement that had identified dirt as the source of disease. Germs were simply invisible dirt.

The preventive security narrative of bacteriology established a new order by defining the threat as invisible germs on everyday objects and individuals and explaining security practices to guard against them. Priscilla Wald stresses in this context the importance of the "outbreak narrative" (*Contagious* 2). It explains the origin of an epidemic marking its routes and possible containment, offering a way to narratively contain the rupture such an outbreak represents.[13] These narratives often reiterate already familiar literary forms, such as detective fiction to give shape to the new knowledges of biological security (Wald, *Contagious* 20). The epidemiologist became a "disease detective" chasing the culprit of infections – the microbial material and the individual spreader. Furthermore, the language used to describe this new order heavily relied on militarized language that emphasized the body under siege (Wald, *Contagious* 83). The narratives represent the threat of germs as a fearful specter of insecurity coming from the outside. The militarized language used already by Koch to describe processes in bacteriology established war metaphors "within the larger discourse and practice of medicine" (Nie 3) and therefore heavily influenced the understanding of biological security. In this narrative configuration medicine and scientific knowledge, or rather its practitioners are the saving protagonists that protect the security of the individual as well as the national body.

The security narrative focused on "lurking germs" circulated widely and occupied the public for the first decades of the 20ᵗʰ century. The "new risks" were often publicized in sensationalized, panic-inducing reports that evolved more and more centrally around the doctor and the individual spreader of disease (Wald, *Contagious*, Lepore). The fear of contagion was further increased by the discovery of "healthy carriers" such as the example

---

13   Wald asserts that "[t]he outbreak narrative . . . follows a formulaic plot that begins with the identification of an emerging infection, includes discussions of the global networks throughout which it travels, and chronicles the epidemiological work that ends with its containment" (*Contagious* 2).

of "'Typhoid Mary,'" who became the infamous exemplification for the myth of the immigrant stranger infecting the healthy American body (Wald, *Contagious* 9).[14] These fearful stories of looming infection made biological security more decisively the responsibility of the individual. However, at the same time the findings of medical science and the security narratives they were embedded in shifted the body as something private into a public matter, describing a "transformation of the most intimate into the most public" ("Community" 270) as Rüdiger Kunow points out. The individual was responsible for their own health as well as for the health of others they could potentially infect. Individual biological security was based on the health of the community, the "We, the people," which made it an increasingly important part of national security concerns.

The shift in the security narrative thus decisively influenced how national security, as well as identity were understood. While epidemics always functioned as a lens on defining the self and the other as Ariane Schröder shows in *Inf(l)ections of the American Dream*, the newly consolidated and professionalized security narrative of prevention made this biologically inflected distinction between self and other crucial also *outside* of epidemic crisis events. The biologized security narrative placed insecurity more firmly on the outside and located it within the other, as something foreign and hostile to the American body (Wald, *Contagious* 9). And this influenced legislative changes. The 1891 Immigration Act made medical inspections mandatory to the immigration process, most famously conducted on Ellis Island from 1892 onward. The Immigration Act of 1907 restricted the admission of physically or mentally disabled individuals and the sick to the U.S. These people were labeled as "defective persons" (Congress 1907), expressing the medicalized understanding of biological security. This conception forged new group identities, which legitimized the exclusion of individuals from the American "We."

As the example also shows, the rise of prevention did not exclusively focus on contagious disease. It represented a more wide-ranging mindset that was also regulating the people already in the country. As a repercussion of the new authoritative voice, the public space was sanitized from those who somehow did not fit the new mold of "biological Americanness." Ordinances that came to be called the "ugly laws" prohibited persons with visible disability or disease "to expose himself [or herself] to public view" (qtd. in Schweik 2). Susan Schweik describes how these ordinances emerged first in the 1860 and were then introduced in more and more places across the United States after 1880. In a general sentiment of progress and improvement, disease and disability had become an "unsightly" presence that disrupted the imaginary of security. The ordinances exemplify the broad influences that the security narrative of prevention had on the private and the public, restricting individual freedom.

---

14   Mary Malone first appeared as "Typhoid Mary" in 1909 in *New York American* (June, 20). Identified as the origin of typhoid outbreaks though she herself did not show any symptoms of being sick, led first to regulating Malone's possibilities of work, banning her from positions as a cook. Her transgression of these rules led to public intervention and her ultimate "incarceration" on an island where she was isolated (Walzer Laevitt, *Typhoid Mary* 18–19). Wald asserts that "[t]he idea of a healthy human carrier of disease was one of the most publicized and transformative discoveries of bacteriology" (Wald, *Contagious* 16).

Similarly, individual responsibility for performing security practices to prevent disease was not limited to contexts of deadly infections, but also extended to cases of normal flus and colds, as a pamphlet from New York City's Department of Health from 1929 shows (qtd. in American Center for History). Pamphlets such as this circulated the knowledges and practices of prevention, making preventive logics everyday performative acts. In that sense, every news story and every health campaign represents a narrative of security that explains the proper ways of being sick and staying healthy. "Cleanliness became not only a solution but a measure of citizenship" (Wald, *Contagious* 70).

The logic of prevention and its distribution of responsibility between government and individual is most poignant in the development of vaccines as the first "magic bullets" that promised the conquest of infectious disease (Tomes, *Gospel* 45). Variolation was performed long before the evidence of the germ theory was discovered, but with the professionalization of the knowledge followed the professionalization and proliferation of the practice.[15] The scientific evidence provided by Edward Jenner solidified vaccinations as "mechanisms of security" (Foucault *Security* 16) to control populations biologically. According to Foucault the techniques of systematized medical study added an "apparatus (dispositif) of security" (Foucault, *Security* 20) that emphasizes the logic of probabilities and costs which are based on statistical assessment. In changing the perspective from individual suffering to a numerical and collective understanding, the logic of the new security narrative dissolves the "binary division between permitted and prohibited" (Foucault, *Security* 19). Statistical assessment rather "establishes an average considered as optimal on the one hand, and, on the other, a bandwidth of the acceptable that must not be exceeded" (Foucault, *Security* 20). The assessments not only establish the status of security, they emphasize the "crucial notion of risk" that arises in calculating security (Foucault, *Security* 88). In the logic of preventive medicine, events and the future are therefore increasingly represented as predictable and therefore controllable. A lack of control signifies a lack of knowledge; the question of biological security is in the logic of prevention therefore a question of knowledge production.

At the same time security relies in this context more clearly on the production of narratives. In the context of preventive medicine, the biological security of the people becomes more decisively a national security concern and object of policy intervention outside of epidemic crisis events. Foucault emphasizes that "[i]n short it will no longer be the problem of exclusion, as with leprosy, or of quarantine, as with plague, but of epidemics and the medical campaigns that try to halt epidemic or endemic phenomena" (*Security* 23). Since the security practices such as vaccination aim at the prevention of an

---

15   Variolation was practiced widely in the U.S. in the fight against smallpox long before the scientific proof of the germ theory. The U.S. Vaccine Agency was established in 1813, and already in 1855 Massachusetts implemented mandatory smallpox vaccination for school children. Today, all states have adopted mandatory vaccination against most childhood diseases. However, most states allow exemptions for medical as well as religious and personal reasons, which has lead to increasing outbreaks of measles for instance. These exemptions can be overruled in some states during an outbreak (CDC, "Vaccination Law").

event, narratives are crucial to circulate the necessity of the security practices. The "medical campaigns" are indispensable to inform a wider public and to facilitate vaccination programs. The campaigns are further needed to reassert the urgency of a security practice such as vaccination in the absence of the experience of outbreaks. This necessity of narratives is as pertinent today as the recent measles outbreaks and emergency declarations from regions such as New York State at the beginning of 2019 make clear (Barbot), as well as the struggles to implement preventive measures against the spread of Covid-19 in 2020. Biological security is thus explicitly a question of information and its circulation, not merely of medical knowledge and practice. This circulation is needed to raise "biological awareness" and "scientific literacy" (Rose and Novas, "Citizenship" 443) to make the professionalized biological security narrative accessible and understandable, and to make it pervasive and appealing.

The preventive logic of biological security produced the need for new institutions in the United States that would facilitate the accumulation of data to provide the knowledge as the key to security. Toward the end of the 19th century the national institutions crucial for the overseeing and production of the required accumulation of data were founded, such as the predecessor of the National Institute of Health (NIH) in 1887,[16] the Food and Drug Administration (FDA) in 1906, and the Children's Bureau in 1912, to name but a few. All of these institutions mark the ascent of vital statistics and the belief in the calculability of biological security.[17] They institutionalize biological security education[18] and reiterate the messianic narrative of medical and scientific salvation, which aimed far beyond the infectious disease medicine was waging war on.

The rise of medicine as the arbiter of security at the turn of the century and the beginning 20th century was not only defined by scientific developments – as the revolution in microbiology could suggest. Its sweeping ascent was also marked by the hope and belief in continual progress facilitated by the new authoritative voice of science. It was a time when social problems were attempted to be fixed with the help of scientific solutions:

> As assorted elites in various countries sought to make sense of a world in flux, they increasingly turned not to religion but to science, which offered authority, rationality, and incisive explanatory power. Evolutionism, physical anthropology, and bacteriology could help diagnose, ameliorate, and perhaps even perfect society. (Stern 13)

Minna Stern indicates that the security narratives produced by medical sciences did not just promise to cure diseases. Rather, its promise was extended to most social problems turning science itself into a "magic bullet." An important aspect in the advances of the

---

16   Founded as the Hygienic Laboratory the institution was renamed Public Health Services in 1922 and was redesigned in 1930 as the NIH with the Randsdell Act.

17   For the rise of the use of statistics in psychiatric medicine see Allan V. Horwitz's and Gerald N. Grob's study of the history of American Psychiatric Epidemiology. For a brief history of medicine and statistics see Dan Meyer's "A Brief History of Medicine and Statistics."

18   Ruth Clifford Engs enumerates the rising number of educational platforms and publications that emerged in that time. The *Sanitarian* was an early public health publication which merged into the *Popular Science Monthly* (298). Its "masthead carried the statement 'Public Health is Public Wealth'" (297).

arbiter of biological security is, thus, based on belief and affective investment rather than factual knowledge or medicine's actual ability to protect the body.

This dynamic is most clearly reflected in the rise of eugenics in the United States. Instead of actual scientific findings, ideas and theories of inheritance and evolution and "faith" (Stern 6) marked the rising security narratives of eugenic population theory. With the consistent evocation of a better future (for "all") the eugenic "movement" represented a promise of national advancement, inextricably connecting individual biological security with national security. Eugenics was understood by its followers as "the prime duty – the inescapable duty – of the good citizen" as Theodore Roosevelt put it in a letter to Charles Davenport in 1913 (Roosevelt, "Letter"). Eugenics scientists, such as Davenport argued that eugenic measures such as forced sterilization were crucial to protect and improve the body of the nation. Eugenics based itself on a forceful security narrative that warned against maintaining the status quo, which would lead society to the doom of endlessly reproducing its weakness and suffering. They "demanded political action" (Hansen and King 49)[19] and delivered hope of averting an inhumane and threatening future by eugenic population control. The belief in scientific progress and the security narrative to improve society by "better breeding" reveals that eugenics was both an enforced oppressive practice as well as a practice that garnered a wide following. At its time, eugenics were "shining brightly" dominating many areas of biological, social and moral security narratives – not much unlike its succeeding heir genetics. Eugenics had its heyday in the U.S. in the 1920s during which it influenced federal policies such as the Supreme Court case *Buck v. Bell* and the introduction of the Johnson Reed Act in 1924.[20]

This faith-like belief in science at the beginning of the 20th century, and in biological science in particular, was famously articulated in J.B.S. Haldane's speech "Daedalus, or Science and the Future: A Paper Read to the Heretics" in 1923.[21] It epitomizes the glorification and unwavering faith that represented biological science as "humanity's best hope" (Bud, *Uses* 196). Haldane's speech represents the unwavering faith in a messianic narrative of scientific salvation and the coming of the "age of biology." Haldane

---

19   "Indiana was the first state to pass and adopt a sterilization law in 1907. Between 1907 and 1912 seven additional states (Washington, California, Connecticut, Nevada, Iowa, New Jersey, and New York) successfully passed laws. [...] Most states allowed for sterilization of institutionalized 'confirmed criminals, idiots, imbeciles, and rapists'" (Engs 111). Sterilization did not end with the condemnation of eugenics after WWII. In Oregon for instance, forced sterilization was still practices in 1983 (Stern 1). For a thorough and comprehensive discussion of the practice of sterilization in North America see Hansen and King *Sterilized by the State*.

20   The Supreme Court case *Buck v. Bell* ruled that compulsory sterilization of "unfit" individuals was not unconstitutional. The Johnson Reed Act in 1924 introduced a quota system regulating immigration to the United States based on national origin.

21   Haldane was a scientist who worked in various different fields, one of them evolutionary biology and genetics (Ronald Clark "*J.B.S.*"). Though an English scientist and a speech delivered in Cambridge, England, Haldane together with J.D. Bernal was central in publicizing and popularizing the belief in biological science in the scientific community in the U.S.. Harvard professor Bernard Davis asserts almost 60 years later in *Science Magazine* that "'Those of us who were entering biology in the 1930s were very much encouraged by the essays of J.D. Bernal and J.B.S. Haldane who predicted that the age of biology would soon emerge...'" (qtd. in Bud, *Uses* 196).

promises that science will save those who believe and prepare for its coming both technically, and ethically. His security narrative establishes biological science as the "magic bullet" against all evil and insists that "scientific knowledge is going to revolutionize human life" (20). The revolution that Haldane predicts is, however, not restricted to biological changes alone. It is ultimately linked to a social utopia as he ascribes to science the ability to eradicate inequalities (6). This messianic narrative of scientific salvation indicates that science did not just observe and describe biological matter and its security as a claim to truth but had started to describe the future with similar authority. The security narrative of prevention evolved more explicitly into a utopian tale of future securities.

And indeed, science seemed to deliver on its promises. The time between 1920 and 1960 is referred to as the "golden age" of American medicine and describes the moment when medicine rose to professional sovereignty and the United States to the leading place of medical research (Tomes, "Merchants" 524).[22] The security promise of the "mastery of disease" seemed to become more and more achievable as scientific progress proceeded with the discovery of the long anticipated "magic bullets,"[23] with the discovery of penicillin. Kaushik Sunder Rajan emphasizes the particular messianic rhetoric used to describe biomedical developments such as penicillin, which was celebrated as a "miracle drug." Similarly, when Merck released its new drug cortisone it was presented in a "structure of miracle" (*Biocapital* 187). But it is not just these "events" of discoveries that are given shape in a messianic narrative of scientific salvation. Sunder Rajan emphasizes the "structure of linear progress that is embedded and embodied in specific salvationary stories, heroic rescues of individual, extremely sick patients" (ibid.). He emphasizes the importance of individual stories that established and legitimized the provided security.

Furthermore, medical advances clearly started to affect people's lives as infant mortality decreased and life expectancy lengthened. Changes had started in 1900 but by the 1940s increased security was clearly notable. Life expectancy rose from 33 for Black Americans and 47.3 for White Americans in 1900, to 53.1 for Black Americans and 62.9 for Whites by 1940 (CDC, "Life Tables" 19). Census documents from the period also show how infectious and contagious diseases (such as measles, TB, and influenza) as the cause of death decreased because of antibiotics and more and more effective vaccines.[24] Ivan Illich asserts that in the 1930s it was "assumed that there was a strictly 'limited quantity of morbidity,' which if treated would result in a reduction of subsequent sickness rates" ("Medicalization" 73). And the rising longevity rates – the icon of medical *and* national progress – due to the mastery of infectious disease made the imaginary of biological security seem increasingly graspable. In the 1950s and 1960s it seemed that the continuous

---

22 The benchmark of independence from Europe as superseding it as a research power is emphasized in most accounts of American medical history, highlighting the importance of national(ist) narratives that are best studied as nationally distinct forms of security narratives despite their global points of conversion.

23 Sebastian G. B. Amyes discusses in *Magic Bullets, Lost Horizons* the rise and fall of antibiotics as magic bullets from a biochemical perspective highlighting the treacherous outcome of their widespread use in the rise of multi-resistant bacteria.

24 By the 1950s, vaccination against diphtheria, tetanus, pertussis, smallpox and polio was widely available. In the 1960s vaccines against measles, mums and rubella were developed (*History of Vaccines.org*).

progress of science had managed to control most major contagious disease problems in the nation. The advances led to the assumption that "life can be protected, if not absolutely then statistically, from the threat of both wars and disease" (Cooper 65). The coming of science and its promised security appeared imminent.

Changing Frames – Changing Expectations: the (Bio)Medicalization of Life and the Expansion of the Medical Security Narrative

The quest for biological security narrativized as the mastery of infectious disease did not lead to the control of mortality nor to the abolition of disease, much less to an end of ailments and suffering or a better and more just society. It did not lead to the "eradication of disease itself" as "Thurman B. Rice, a professor for sanitary science, predicted" in 1927 in "The Conquest of Disease" (Lepore 2). The advances in treating infectious diseases prolonged life and led to the rise of other diseases that are often correlated to lifestyle, consumption, and ageing, such as cardiovascular disease and cancer. As a consequence, the security of the body based on control and controllability receded, or was deferred as Derrida puts it. The sought-after security of control fails, not (necessarily) because older definitions are proven wrong, or because treatments were erroneous or even threatening, which they were.[25] It fails, because the proposed security articulated in the medical narratives does not describe an a priori existing thing, a natural state that can be protected and returned to, but rather a concept and a logic made pervasive by narratives. The messianic narrative of medical salvation temporarily fixes the moving target of security based on calculability and control. With the shifting horizon of security, however, medicine and science did not have any adequate knowledge or treatment for the rising number of patients with these "new" and often chronic diseases, which are the leading cause of death still today (CDC, "Death and Mortality"). The envisioned control of the body, which had seemed almost graspable "retreats" with every further approximation to the ideal. This shift from infectious to chronic and degenerative disease, as a deferral of biological security does not represent a disruption of the messianic narrative of medical salvation, but reinforces the temporality of "not yet," that propels the security narrative forward. It represents a changed frame of the security narrative, produced by medical and scientific progress as well as cultural changes. Increasingly, the security narrative of prevention extended its normative power from defining and treating disease to health and life.

The messianic narrative of medical salvation started to pervade the understanding of the body and life defining them increasingly in biological security terms. This process has been studied as "medicalization," which was initially defined by studies of Irv-

---

25   The medicalized understanding of race, gender, and sexuality for instance lead to misguided and violent forms of treatments such as isolation to treat "hysteria," electro shocks to treat "wrong" sexual orientation or the resistance to assigned social roles, or the systematic withholding of medical care and the abuse of individuals as guinea pigs for medical studies. But also other forms of treatment and medical knowledge have proved to be harmful over time, such as repeated x-ray treatment against acne, as one example among many.

ing Kenneth Zola and Ivan Illich, who both introduce "Medicine as an Institution of Social Control" (Zola). Peter Conrad defines it more broadly as "a process by which non-medical problems become defined and treated as medical problems, usually in terms of illness and disorders" (Conrad, *Medicalization* 4). This expansion of medicalized security narratives shifted the horizon of security changing frames and expectations. Already within the first three quarters of the 20th century increasingly more processes that were traditionally governed by social and cultural ritual became the object of medical security narratives. Science became the authority over life – not just disease – and the gatekeeper of its security. But it was also increasingly associated with individual possibilities to partake in the American Dream and the pursuit of happiness. This expansion from defining and curing disease to defining and securing health and life is particularly visible and profound in the changes of birthing practices in the United States. I will use the examples of pregnancy, birth, and childhood as returning thematic examples to highlight the expansion of the medical security narratives that took place in increasingly all processes of life.

Childbirth represents one of the earliest processes of life to be medicalized and marks the "passing power over the birth process from traditional female to professional male" (Mitford, *Birth* 51). Already by the turn of the 20th century birth was recognized as a pathological process, however, it was still predominantly experienced at home in the care of a midwife (Mitford, *Birth* 58). But "by 1939, 50 percent of all women and 75 percent of urban women chose hospitals for the purpose; by 1970, the figure had risen to close to 100 percent" (Mitford, *Birth* 47). In the U.S. the process of medicalization indicated in this statistic was so strong that midwifery nearly disappeared as a practice entirely.[26] This had nothing to do with the practices being more secure at that time. Instead, the wide circulation of science and medical practice as the arbiter of security had made the hospital and the obstetrician a seemingly natural authority over the birthing process. The doctor rose to "his role as a cultural hero" (Illich, "Medicalization" 73) and became the unquestionable authority in more and more life questions.

In birthing, the alleviation of pain became a central concern early on. The medical normative power over the security narratives had abolished the meaning in and of suffering as related to a higher meaning. Pain – a central part of labor – was perceived as meaningless and therefore useless and avoidable. Sedatives that had already revolutionized surgery had become more and more central in the treatment of birth. The new practices and security narrative defined women as incapable of leading the birthing process, as early practices of "twilight sleep" in the 1910s exemplify (Walzer Leavitt, "Birthing" 147). The birthing mother became a patient and was treated so she did "not remember" the labor and pains that were understood as a "birth trauma." In this preventive security practice the woman was rendered passive as the main protagonist of the new security narrative and performance is the doctor, not the laboring woman. The doctor delivered the

---

26   The practice recovered with the introduction of the "nurse midwife" and the midwife movement of Ina May Gaskin in the 1970s. But it is "again in jeopardy because of rising malpractice insurance costs, women's trust in technology, and, most recently, renewed efforts by physicians to once again prevent midwives from practicing" (Brodsky 48).

baby, as the saying goes.[27] Though this expansion of medical authority has often been described in a Foucauldian top-down power relation, most researchers also recognize that this transition of normative power and practice was desired. Hospital birth and routine medical interventions in the birthing process became the unquestionable and sought-after security. Mitford even describes the fast adoption as "a torrent" (*Birth*, 47). The medical practices were perceived as progress which happened in the assigned space of security: the hospital.[28]

Though medical care had become far more accessible and medical possibilities had undoubtedly improved life to a great extent as statistics stand to prove, it did not lead to people feeling more secure nor bound to one expert opinion. Medicalized security was available only to those able to pay the increasing prices of medical and hospitalized care. Treated as consumers, the patients acted early on as such, comparing treatment offers of different service providers as Tomes shows (*Remaking* 9). However, this also meant that the majority of people were "priced . . . right out" early on ("Merchants" 529) and the various health care strategies that have been implemented over the course of the century have not managed to close the medical care gap in the United States.[29] The chasm between medical possibility and accessibility of the services to the general public arose early on. Health seeking was a practice of the well-to-do center of society. But despite the exclusiveness of medical treatment, the possibilities of these practices had made a medicalized understanding of health and life a central topic in public discourse.

Over the course of the 20th century health and medical treatment had become something desirable in all contexts of life. Most researchers highlight in this context the commodification of health and medical care in the growing consumer culture of post-war America (Mitford, Shryock, Tomes, Illich, Clarke et al.). Tomes underlines the importance of advertising and pamphlets as early as the first half of the 20th century. She describes the rise of health as a consumer good, which was incremental for the wide circulation of preventive security narratives. This was possible because the "twentieth-century 'medical messiahs' could use mass media to promote themselves" (Tomes, "Merchants"

---

27   "In addition to forceps, physicians relied on opium, chloroform, chloral, cocaine, quinine, nitrous oxide, ergot, and ether to relieve pain, expedite labor, prevent injury" (Walzer Leavitt, "Birthing" 148). Today, pains of labor and their conscious experience are again recognized as necessary and important part of the birthing process for both child and woman. Nonetheless, "[t]echnology and obstetric interventions in normal childbirth continue, in spite of lack of evidence of their efficacy" (Brodsky 48).

28   The progress of medicine was not a utopian space of equality but structured by and perpetuating institutional racism in segregated hospitals. "[T]he new 'white palaces' of modern medicine remained white in a literal sense . . . . Segregated hospital care represented a form of medical Jim Crow common in both the South and the North well into the 1960s" (Tomes, "Merchants" 542).

29   Theodore Roosevelt's policies of the New Deal in 1934/5 instituted social security and defined its meaning in terms of *life insurance*, generalizing its principles of mutual risk exchange to the whole nation" (Cooper 7). But neither the New Deal, nor the Second New Deal or the Wagner Act included health care programs. Medicare for the elderly (65+) and Medicaid for the unemployed was only established with Johnson's "Great Society" in the 1960s. The proposals for these programs were initially resisted by the American Medical Association because of financial considerations and the assumption that it would inflate costs for treatment (Cohen 4).

534).[30] The accelerating adoption of medical security practices which started to pervade more and more aspects of life thus relied on the growth of mass media and capitalist consumer culture. The security narrative prescribed medical interventions, in the form of medical therapy but also in the form of consumption of medical goods as well as medical information: the "health in a bottle" and "health in a book" as Tomes puts it ("Merchants" 531–38). The normative power of experts reached deep into people's private lives though a majority did not frequent doctors nor were they able to pay for expensive hospital care.

The medical security narrative did not end with biological processes such as birth but expanded also to other areas of life and the understanding of the life course, such as the care of the infant and motherhood. Already in the first half of the 20th century advertisements targeted mothers urging them to adopt what Rima Apple has termed "Scientific Motherhood." The women were advised to follow medical suggestions in their childcare and child-rearing with slogans such as "[a]dd science to love and be a perfect mother" from 1938 (qtd. in Apple 173). The ad for information material promises "a hopeful future" (ibid.) that can be obtained by scientific help and by following scientific guidelines. Scientific knowledge is represented as necessary to facilitate the best possible future of the child and was therefore seemingly unquestionably desirable. Scientific motherhood implemented scientific understandings of child development as a security practice that would benefit mother and child. The focus, however, was more decisively the future of the child. The supposedly liberating and modern scientific motherhood did not re-evaluate the oppressed role of the women but cemented the cultural categories making mothers servants to changing ideals of child-rearing (Ehrenreich and English 126). Biological security was not established by the birth of a healthy baby anymore but started to encompass a widened horizon of security.

The medicalization of life represents the expansion of the security narrative of prevention to more and more fields of life, such as childhood, adolescence, sexuality, ageing, or dying. The establishing of more and more pathological categories that went hand in hand with this expansion was represented as a continuous progress toward biological security and a good life. All fields of life became object of the medical gaze, incessantly mapped out and estimated. In every field the medical definitions of pathologies also defined norms, as Canguilhem put it. In each diagnostic definition of a pathology a norm is performatively reiterated and re-established, and security is re-imagined. The continuous progress of medical science and practice thus renegotiates the normal and desirable state of being and thereby shifts the horizon of security. The promised security therefore retreats with every approximation of security. With their all-encompassing reach deeper into the individual lives, the security narratives describe increasingly what "good life" is, what it looks and feels like. The statistically determined norm of different life processes – the averages – become the normal healthy state in which a person "ought to" (Canguilhem, *Normal* 125) progress through life to become a productive member of society.

This medicalization of life is in more recent studies analyzed as a "pathologization of deviance," which also includes "alcoholism, mental disorders, opiate addictions, eat-

---

30   With this assertion Tomes confronts the myth of a "pure" science that became corrupted by market interests in the 1950s and 1960s while it occupied an exceptional role within the otherwise expanding consumer culture ("Merchants" 522–524).

ing disorders, sexual and gender difference, sexual dysfunction, learning disabilities, and child and sexual abuse" (Conrad, *Medicalization* 6). The list could be extended to book length and reflects how more and more human conditions became the object of the medical gaze, diagnosis, and treatment over the turn of the 20th century.[31] Conrad describes how giving unwanted behavior a "medical meaning" is "moving it from badness to sickness" (ibid.). He describes this transformation similar to a speech act that shifts a state of being into the field of medicalized security narrative. By moving it "from one order to the other," as Burgess puts it, the state of being is medicalized and therefore becomes the object of treatment and securitization.

This biologized understanding of security turns "human difference into pathologies" (Conrad, *Medicalization* 148), such as learning disabilities, delayed adolescence, premature puberty. The establishing of these diagnostic categories represents the first performative act of security that is aimed toward re-establishing the norm, including bodily matter as much as behavior and mental states. Once a state is pathologized, a medical model of disability is applied, which means that the diagnosed lack should be medically fixed if possible. For instance, Attention Deficit Hyperactivity Disorder (ADHD) was established as a diagnostic category in the 1950s, defined as a childhood disorder. By the 1960s Ritalin, the stimulant drug methylphenidate, was used to treat the disorder initiated by studies of American psychiatrist Charles Bradley. "By the mid-1970s it had become the most common childhood psychiatric problem (Gross and Wilson, 1974), and special clinics to identify and treat the disorder were established" (Conrad *Medicalization* 49f). The security narratives thus prescribe a norm that is increasingly achievable with professional help. Deviation is prevented by early detection and intervention.

But the medical salvation of the self can quickly turn into the damnation of the other. The narrative of medical salvation also applies to conditions and communities that themselves resist the ascription of lack, such as large parts of the Deaf Community that rejects cochlear implants.[32] The security narrative of preventive medicine and preventable disease prescribes that fitting the norm biologically and behaviorally – both inside and outside – is possible and therefore expected. The rising possibilities to intervene in normal bodily processes facilitated a medicalized normal that represents not only freedom from ailments but also a "considerable force of constraint" as Conrad puts it (*Medicalization* 25). It reinforces social pressures to "fit in," extending them to the biological.

According to Ivan Illich the "medicalization of life" was driven by "the belief in unlimited progress" (Illich, *Nemesis* 73). He defines the expansion of the medical normative power as a form of "medical imperialism" that colonizes life, imposing its system of meaning and thereby destroying the "natural" systems and processes. But Conrad and Carl Elliott, among others, show that doctors and science are not the only driving force

---

31   An example of such a book length list is the *Diagnostic and Statistical Manual of Mental Disorders* (DSM) which lists the categories of the different mental health afflictions and their treatment. It was first published in 1952, with the 5th edition published in 2013. The numbers of diagnostic categories grew from 106 in the first edition to 374 in its current form.

32   Harlan Lane shows in "Construction of Deafness" how Deaf Culture resist the ascription as disabled, instead representing a proud culture of sign language which is threatened by the biomedical practice of cochlear implants.

in the processes of medicalization. Corporate interests as well as "social groups and interest groups" (Conrad, "Shifting Engines" 4) also play a decisive role in the expansion of biological security. "Organized efforts were made to champion a medical definition for a problem or to promote the veracity of a medical diagnosis" (ibid.) as in the case of post-traumatic stress disorder (PTSD). Patient advocacy groups contributed to the "making of security" by promoting new medical definitions which allow for treatment as well as for the acknowledgment of suffering. In this sense biomedical security becomes also a question of "collective action" (Conrad, *Medicalization* 9),[33] which reiterate the belief in the messianic narrative of scientific salvation.

Additionally to expanding the medical security narratives to life, the "medical gaze" was directed deeper into the body with the rise of "new genetics"[34] in the 1950s and the growing molecularization and digitization of biomedical research and practice since then. Genetics further increased the stronghold of medical science as the arbiter of security over life in its entirety. Life and its security became largely reimagined as genetically determined. Findings in genetics reinforced the vision of control seemingly proving that in science "a problem clearly seen is already half solved" (7) as Lawrie Tatum, one of the first Nobel Prize Laureates for gene-related discoveries put it in 1958. The birth of new genetics is commonly associated with the discovery of the double helical structure in 1953 by James Watson and Francis Crick. The genetic revolution only really started with the discovery of the recombinant DNA technique by Cohen and Boyer in 1973. The circulation of the security narratives of new genetics began, nonetheless, immediately with the image of the model of the double helix, which has become a central symbol for science and the messianic promise it represents (de Chadarivan).

Tatum's Nobel Lecture on Dec. 11th 1958 marked as much as the prize itself the growing momentum of genetics and its vision for the future.[35] His speech embarks on a clear futurologist course, promising that "we will see the complete conquering of many of man's ills" and the goal is "not only to avoid structural or metabolic errors in the developing organism, but also to produce better organisms" (n.p.). Tatum expresses the belief that genetics would correct the mistakes of nature and make the human (biology) better, representing a promise of radical self-empowerment – a science utopia. Hence, long before genetics could really fix anything and provide security, it performatively established first and foremost the imaginary of security – the mastery of nature – as within reach. It

---

33   The same collective action is also central in the demedicalization of formerly medicalized categories, such as homosexuality. Homosexuality was only de-medicalized and removed as diagnosis from the second edition of the DSM by the American Psychiatric Association in 1973 under immense pressure from the gay movement. Homosexuality was excluded from the DSM III published in 1980 (Drescher 570).

34   The field of new genetics had to establish itself as distinct from its predecessor eugenics, divorcing itself from its haunting presence. The field rewrote its story of origin which "no longer starts with Mendel, but now begins with the 'discovery' of DNA by Watson and Crick" (van Dijck, *Imagenation* 35).

35   The Nobel Prize in 1958 was awarded for gene-related discoveries to George Wells Beadle, Edward Lawrie Tatum and Joshua Lederberg as joint laureates. It was the first genetics related prizes in Physiology or Medicine marking a new era of a genetically inflected security narrative (NobelPrize.org).

changed the understanding of the body and spurred the production of security narratives heralding the future security that the "molecular gaze" (Clarke et al., "Biomedicalization" 164) would facilitate. However, the shifting frontiers opened up by every new biomedical development further changed the horizon of security.

This temporality of "not yet" decisively allowed for the messianic promise of medical salvation to accelerate instead of falter. The dream deferred in biomedicine does not explode as Langston Hughes suggests, but it grows. Though by the 1970s the messianic narrative of scientific salvation had already obvious cracks,[36] the "wedding" of genetics and biotechnology (Bud, *Uses* 164–187) established both fields as the most promising sources of security.

The skepticism toward genetics received a new spin in the 1970s. The discovery of the process for reDNA by Cohen and Boyer in the early 1970s (patented in 1974) once again started the wider discussion about the amazing possibilities of genetics. But its promised possibilities also produced fear, this time leading geneticists such as Rollin Hotchkiss and Paul Berg warned against the dangers of unregulated research (Bud, *Uses* 170; van Dijck, *Imagenation* 68). In 1975 Berg, a later Nobel Laureate and reDNA researcher, hosted the famous Asilomar Conference, which led to a self-imposed research moratorium[37] "until NIH guidelines were available in mid-1976" (Bud, *Uses* 175). The growing field of bioethics thus started to play a major role in the fast emerging field of biotechnology (van Dijck, *Imagenation* 80) to safeguard the security practices of biomedical research. Though highly regulated, genetic research quickly turned into a dominant research paradigm promising the key to biological security.

At the same time as life was increasingly geneticized, the understanding of health broadened. It no longer described security by the absence of disease or non-normativity but by the absence also of discontent and unhappiness. Already in 1948 the World Health Organization adopted a definition of health that broadened the concept of health to an all-encompassing state of well-being.[38] The WHO's broadened approach includes well-being as a problem to be solved by science – it medicalizes well-being and subsumes it under a biological security narrative of protection and prevention. This broader understanding is also expressed in the general climate of health consciousness in the United

---

36   Between 1932 and 1972 syphilis experiments were conducted at the Tuskegee Institute by Public Health Services. African Americans were lured under the disguise of free health care into being guinea pigs in tests to study the progression of untreated syphilis. Not only were they not informed, they also did not receive treatment after it became available. The study ended because of the whistleblower Peter Buxtum. In 1972 the revelations of the Tuskegee syphilis experiments on African Americans showed that the abuse of power and corruption of science was not only a problem of the past nor of evil regimes. However, the crimes were discursively contained as "well-intentioned but misguided" science (Brandt 27). The proper guidelines had "not yet" been put in place, which would guarantee medical research and practice to fulfill its true self: to be serving truth and security. The revelations triggered major changes in clinical studies introducing informed consent, communication of diagnosis, and the foundation of the Office for Human Research Protection (Brandt).

37   Similar discussions were led in 2015 about the development of CRISPR, a new gene editing tool that seemed to promise a new revolution of scientific research (Kahn).

38   "Health is a state of complete physical, mental, and social well-being and not merely the absence of disease or infirmity" (WHO, "Basic" 1).

States. Robert Crawford describes how "prevention of illness becomes a more pervasive standard by which behaviors [sic] – eating, drinking, working, leisure activities – are judged" (Crawford 370). Normal everyday activities become security performances aiming at maintaining good health, which "has become a paradigm for good living" (Crawford 380). The health practices carry the ideology, concepts, and logics of medical security into private lives and the most private living spaces. He asserts that in the late 70s "[t]he concern with personal health has become a national preoccupation" (Crawford 365).

Medical security practices, initially perceived as a threat to freedom had become fundamental to achieving the American Dream. Health becomes a modern version of "beata vita," the good life, which also represents a biologized reiteration of the "pursuit of happiness." Health has become a value that "subsumes a panoply of values: 'a sense of happiness and purpose,' 'a high level of self-esteem,' 'work satisfaction,' 'ability to engage in creative expression'" (Crawford 380). Inflected by a biologized sense of security this good life and happiness can be measured, analyzed and regulated. The good life is thus conditioned on the reiterative performance of security practices that are prescribed by the all-encompassing biological security narratives.[39]

In the U.S. the practice of choice for many it seems, was the consumption of drugs and psychiatric medication. In the 1970s Nixon describes the climate as a "culture of drugs," warning that "[w]e have produced an environment in which people come naturally to expect that they can take a pill for every problem – that they can find satisfaction and health and happiness in a handful of tablets or a few grains of powder" ("Remarks"). Other increasingly important players in the proliferation of medical categories have thus clearly been pharmaceutical companies and their interest in opening new consumer markets for medical goods. The medical fix averting the dangers of the non-normative body and behavior was provided by drugs such as Ritalin against ADHD or hormone replacement therapy for andro- and menopause (Conrad, *Medicalization* 23–31), tranquilizers like Serentil for anxiety, among many others (Metzl, "Crisis"). Security became something consumable through the purchase of medical services or goods in a much more invasive way than for instances the healthcare manuals that Tomes describes for the early 20th century. The new goods of the "medical messiahs" intervene and produce bodily processes according to a norm established in security narratives. And the use of pharmaceuticals was early on a question of both curing disease and maintaining a healthy norm as well as of enhancing performances. Elliott describes how medical interventions represented a possibility to quench the "American obsession of fitting in" and achieving the American Dream (Elliott xv).

---

39   In the 1970s the legitimacy and sole authorship of (bio)medical science as the arbiter of security was challenged by new health movements. However, these movements also further reiterate and reinforce the importance of health to achieve the American Dream and the self-reliance related to its origins. It finds expression in holistic health and self-care (Crawford 366) or homeopathy, movements originally geared against the security narrative that prescribed medical intervention. Crawford shows that though rejecting medical interventionism and seeing the body as a holistic entity, the movements reiterate and increase the medicalization of life. As a message from within, health becomes not only the individual's responsibility but also the individual's fault. With this moralistic perspective "blame is brought front-stage" (Crawford 378). The choice of a particular security practice becomes a profession of faith in the legitimacy of the different security narratives.

The rise of pharmaceuticals foreshadowed the "opioid overdose epidemic" (CDC, "Understanding") in the United States in 2018.[40] Already in 1971 Nixon addressed the American Medical Association House of Delegates with a warning about the dangers of legal drug abuse. He laments that "one-third of all Americans between the ages of 18 and 74 used a psychotropic drug of some sort last year" (Nixon, "Remarks" 766). But Nixon should have better addressed burgeoning pharmaceutical and biomedical companies. Because the doctor, once the hero and narrator of the biological security narrative had become rather a "storefront" for biomedical and biotechnological services, representing the "erosion of medical authority" (Starr 1982 in Conrad "Shifting Engines" 4). This development further increased with the biomedicalization and the rise of big science in the 1980s. The erosion of authoritative autonomy, however, further impelled the deepening stronghold of the messianic narrative of scientific salvation. Elliott, Conrad, as well as Clarke et al. point to the immense power privatized research and pharmaceutical companies represent in the (bio)medicalization of life. Most of these scholars also assert that the rise in diagnosed afflictions might be correlated with the rise of direct-to-consumer marketing that is still practiced in the United States. In many cases these advertisements are both promoting the medication or treatment for disease as well as marketing the disease itself, "selling sickness" as Ray Moyniham and Alan Cassels called it.[41] While Nixon criticized the abuse of the security practice of pharmaceutical medication, he did not question the general security narrative and the legitimacy of pharmaceutical medication as a solution to mental health problems. He did not question the security narrative of scientific salvation as such.

When Richard Nixon signed the Cancer Act in 1971 he proclaimed: "America has long been the wealthiest nation in the world. Now it is time we became the healthiest nation in the world" (State of the Union Address). This Act started what is commonly known as the "war on cancer." It reiterates the militaristic language introduced by bacteriology extending it to non-infectious disease contexts and making the protection from cancer officially part of the American national agenda. In this speech Nixon aligns biomedical research with two other major scientific breakthroughs: "The time has come in America when the same kind of concentrated effort that split the atom and took man to the moon should be turned toward conquering this dread disease. Let us make a total national commitment to achieve this goal" (ibid.). Both scientific accomplishments are impossible to understand without their relation to World War II and the Cold War. By aligning cancer research with the atomic bomb, the arms race and the race to the moon, it becomes an issue of national security.[42] This analogy further enforced the militarized understanding

---

40   In 2018 the extent of the opioid crisis in the United States became apparent as a result of the number of drug overdose deaths. It refers to both the abuse of legally prescribed opioids as well as illegally produced drugs.

41   Their study shows how conditions ranging from high cholesterol, and depression, to social anxiety disorder, or and irritable bowel syndrome became objects of medical marketing that created "potential patients" (inter alia 3) and "potential markets" (inter alia 83).

42   Biomedical research was not only symbolically aligned with national security. Similar to the race to the moon, biomedical research was supposed to guarantee economic and national security (Bud, *Uses* 166). In the "race to human health" as Tobell calls it, biomedical practices became direct object of national security concerns. They were used as foreign policy and public relations tools during the

of biological security and its practices. Not surprisingly then, Nixon describes the major funding effort as "perhaps the largest attack against a single disease in the history of man." In April 1972 Nixon institutes the Cancer Control Month as an additional measure to achieve security and "to control this brutal killer" ("Proclamation").

Nixon's speech reiterates the hope and faith in science that had already marked the beginning of the 20th century. His speech defines bodily security as an absence of suffering that can be provided by scientific research. Knowledge does "not yet" allow for the desired security but the possibility of security from suffering cancer is represented as unquestionable; it is just a question of time. Scientific research is represented as a source of hope. *The New York Times* quotes Nixon declaring "But, we can say this," he added, "that for those who have cancer, and who are looking for success in this field, they at least can have the assurance that everything that can be done by Government . . . in this great, powerful, rich country, now will be done and that will give some hope and we hope those hopes will not be disappointed" (Schmeck). Nixon declares that each afflicted American deserves the hope that everything is done to protect their from suffering. By establishing this hope as a promise to every afflicted American he elevates health to a right of every American. Nixon thus turns non-contagious disease officially into a national concern, which he also expressed in his attempts to establish universal healthcare in his 1974 address to Congress ("Special Message").[43] In the decades following the Cancer Act disease and biological security become more and more closely related to national concerns, leading to the militarization of biological security.

Imagining Total Control: Militarization of Biological Security and the Logic of Pre-emption

While for a long time the successes of bacteriology had fostered the promise of the end of threatening epidemics in the United States, the swine flu outbreak in 1976 dismantled this narrative of security. Despite the small number of infected individuals in the U.S., the "re-emergence" of infectious disease revealed that the security narrative of the successful "'conquest' of infectious disease" (Tomes, "Merchants" 543) was precarious at best. The event produced a rupture between the imaginary of security and the material reality of the disease outbreak. It disproved the "imagined immunity" (Wald, *Contagious*)[44] provided by medical progress. The deferral of security – once again when it seemed graspable – did not lead to a reconsideration of the imaginary of security. Rather the deferral led to a further expansion and militarization of biological security narratives and the rise of catastrophic event scenarios. The "concept of the 'catastrophe risk" (Cooper 81f) was

---

Cold War, as biomedical practices were "exported" to countries that were geopolitically crucial in terms of containment. This initiative was called "Project HOPE" whose objectives were institutionalized with the "Health for Peace Bill" in July 1960 (Tobell 445, 448).

43   Nixon asserted that healthcare costs of Medicare and Medicaid instituted by Johnson's "War on Poverty" had to be confronted with a healthcare reform, which entailed universal healthcare. Not surprisingly, his proposals were rejected in Congress.

44   Priscilla Wald uses this term in the title of the first chapter of her book *Contagious* where she elaborates how "belonging took a biological turn" (30).

adopted from "the language of insurance institutions, capital markets, and environmental politics" (ibid.).

The "return of the microbe" (Collier and Lakoff 9) and the notion of insecurity became ever more urgent when seemingly healthy young people began to suffer and die from AIDS. The circulation of the risks of this contagious disease and the missing knowledge of how to treat it reinstated the pervasive but almost forgotten narratives of the "gospel of germs." After a delayed response, the public reacted with panic to the increasing media representation of AIDS, leading to the fear of public toilet seats and pools. The infected were officially defined as the other by the Center for Disease Control and Prevention (CDC) in the so-called "4-H-List" as " homosexuals, hemophiliacs, heroin addicts, Haitians" (Treichler 20), who were excluded socially and morally as well as being constructed as a menace to the healthy body of the nation.[45] Decades later, in 2000, HIV-AIDS would become the first disease to be declared an international security threat by the UN. The U.S. government nationally affirmed this convergence of security rhetoric and health by declaring the spread of HIV also a "national security threat" (Koblentz, "Biosecurity" 96). Infectious disease thus moved from a public "health threat" to a security threat and a question of national security.[46] In this context disease became a threat to the way of life – to the pursuit of happiness and the American Dream – and not just an obstacle to the accessibility of the American Dream for certain individuals.

In the past decades, biosecurity attained yet a new emphasis and urgency in the United States, which is increasingly focused on the possibility of bioterrorism. This represents a shift from militarized language and metaphors in narrativizing security to a conceptual conflation of biosecurity and war and a "militarization of the concept" of security (Burgess 2). In the United States, the concerns about a possible biological attack on the public had already increased in the 1990s after events such as the car bomb attack on the World Trade Center (Schoch-Spana, "Bioterrorism" 8). With the terrorist attacks of 9/11 and the anthrax letter attack thereafter, biological terrorism and natural contagious outbreaks became almost one conceptual entity in speeches and in news reports as much as in official papers. Cooper cites the 2002 "Public Health Security and Bioterrorism Preparedness and Response Act," which outlines "the same emergency procedures for bioterrorist attacks and epidemics" (Cooper 80). Another such example is the "National Security Strategy" of 2006, in which the government announced the plan "Biodefense of the 21st Century" "incorporating innovative initiatives to protect the United States against bioterrorism" (White House, "Strategy 2006" 19).

With this shift of focus from natural to bioterrorist threats, new logics were introduced to confront the uncertain probabilities posed by such a threat of emergent disease. Within the past three decades, as Andrew Lakoff and other scholars contend, the

---

45   The AIDS crisis is one of the most prominent cases in which medicine, science, and governance "failed" the promised security for all. The delayed response to the epidemic shows that biological security is not distributed evenly. It clearly hierarchized the need to respond and only (re)acted once the center of society was reached by the threat, which is often correlated to the wide public circulation of the disease through the publicity about Rock Hudson's infection.

46   Erin Koch argues that also the "The declaration of a Global Tuberculosis Emergency demonstrates a shift toward the framing of infectious diseases as security threats, rather than merely as threats to public health" (122).

main focus of public health has added the urge of preparedness and pre-emption to the mantra of prevention. This development became especially obvious in 2003, when the national vaccination campaign against smallpox in the U.S. was initiated (Koblentz, "Biosecurity" 128). Though in 1980 the WHO had declared the eradication of smallpox, it was predicted that it could re-emerge triggering the vaccination campaign over 20 years later. "[S]mallpox had appeared as an object of 'potentiality,' of danger in the present by virtue of a series of events and elements suggesting its possible occurrence in the future" (D. Rose 89). George W. Bush's announcement of the vaccination program impressively articulates the pre-emptive logic of security that governed the decision-making process for initiating the vaccination program, which is more commonly associated with the invasion of Iraq.[47] He said: "Our government has no information that a smallpox attack is imminent, but it is prudent to be prepared for the possibility that terrorists . . . would use this disease as weapon" (Bush, "Remarks"). This means that, though there are no known facts about potential bioterrorist attacks in the future, measures have to be taken in the present to avert this potential future. The logic of pre-emption, thus, shifts the horizon of security, this time both deeper into the body as well as forward into the future. And this logic is not only applied to the possibility of bioterrorist attacks but also to naturally occurring contagious diseases. Another articulation of this pre-emptive logic can be found in the Bush administration's response to the avian flu epidemic in 2005: "Scientists and doctors cannot tell us where and when the next pandemic will strike, or how severe it will be, but most agree: at some point we are likely to face another pandemic" (Bush, "Pandemic" 2005). This logic of pre-emption, which was well-established by 2005, legitimized the initiation of a $7.1 billion pandemic preparedness strategy (in 2001 it was "just" $294.8 million), which exemplifies the explosion of perceived risks and the force of pre-emptive logics.[48]

The broad adoption of pre-emptive logics did not replace older practices but led to the expansion of already existing surveillance techniques.[49] But the rise of catastrophic contagious disease scenarios produced the need for additional "ways" of understanding,

---

47   This pre-emptive logic reached its apogee with George W. Bush's speech at the West Point Military Academy and the invasion of Iraq: "If we wait for threats to fully materialize, we will have waited too long — Our security will require . . . all Americans . . . to be ready for pre-emptive action when necessary to defend our liberty and to defend our lives."

48   This fusion of public health and national security has detrimental effects on public health draining funding, time, and attention from health care infrastructures, which are equally important to provide biological security in emergency outbreaks and is inevitable to solving present public health issues.

49   The CDC was founded in 1946 as the Communicable Disease Center. In the 1970s it became the Center for Disease Control, "and Prevention" was added in 1992. Today, its scope has broadened from contagious disease to chronic diseases, mental disease, disabilities, addiction, and more. One of the national initiatives is the BioSense Platform, which is based on syndromic surveillance and has been monitoring irregularities in reported disease symptoms since the 1990s (Fearnley 62). Today, in addition to BioSense, it runs BioWatch, which is an environmental pathogen detector, and BioShield, which is a program focused on pharmaceutical and vaccine production (Fearnley 76). Both help to protect the nation as part of the National Biosurveillance Integration System (NBIS) or National Biosurveillance Integration Center (NBIC). The NBIC was established in 2007 as an amendment to the Homeland Security Act of 2002 (Title III) (qtd. in Alperen 224).

calculating, and communicating security. Preparedness and pre-emption are the predominant practices and logics employed to calculate the (unknowable) future. While prevention works on known threats, preparedness and pre-emptive measures intervene in the field of the unknown. "Prevention operates in an objectively knowable world in which uncertainty is a function of a lack of information, and in which events run a predictable, linear course from cause to effect" (Massumi, "Potential" 2). The security narratives of prevention, based on calculation and controllability, leave, as Ruth Levitas asserts, no room for an uncertain future as it is "unthinkable" ("Discourses" 201) within this framework of securitizing. And though the epistemology of pre-emption is "unabashedly one of uncertainty" (Massumi, "Potential" 3) the logics of preparedness and pre-emption offer a way of domesticating this uncertainty by making the unknown future a "future perfect" (Massumi, "Future Birth" 6). Brian Massumi and Melinda Cooper are among the leading scholars who have studied the logic of pre-emption. Cooper defines pre-emption as describing an act "to counter the unknowable, before it is even realized. In short, the very concept of the catastrophe event seems to suggest that our only possible response to the emergent crisis (of whatever kind – biomedical, environmental, economic) is one of speculative *preemption*" (83). This means that a potential future event has to be foreclosed by actions taken in the present.

In the narrative of pre-emption security is always already lost. The present might seem secure to the layperson, but it is always on "the verge of disaster" (Ben Anderson, "Anticipatory" 4). Furthermore, this "disaster is incubating within the present and can only be discerned through 'early warnings' of danger" (ibid.). Such an understanding eradicates the idea of a natural state of security that has to be protected or can be returned to. Rather it creates a perpetual state of insecurity as the breeding ground for potential threat. Preparedness and pre-emption thus establish a new relationship to the future and to security. "Rather than acting in the present to avoid an occurrence in the future, pre-emption brings the future into the present. It makes present the future consequences of an eventuality that may or may not occur, indifferent to its actual occurrence. The event's consequences precede it, as if it had already occurred" (Massumi, "Future Birth" 8). To facilitate this bringing "the future into the present" new methods have to be created to be able to read the warning signs and to determine a threat before it materializes.

Preparedness and pre-emptive security measures are not only based on past data (such as preventive measures) but also on "imaginative techniques" (Collier and Lakoff 13) and on storytelling. To create the security narrative, threats have to be imagined in the very literal sense of the word. "Calculation occurs through a huge range of techniques: including threat-prints, data mining, impact assessments, trend analysis, and complexity modeling of various forms" (Ben Anderson, "Anticipatory" 8). But they also occur in acts of storytelling and enactment "through which future possibilities and potentials are disclosed, objectified, communicated and rendered mobile (such as scenarios, trends, forecasts, predictions, signals, plans and roadmaps)" (Ben Anderson, "Hope" 158). Preparedness practices take on various forms – from information drives and emergency response drills to scenario and tabletop exercises.

Preparedness practices such as "scenarios, exercises, and analytical models to simulate uncertain future threats" (Collier and Lakoff 13) are used to estimate and prepare for emergent disease such as swine flu, SARS, Nile virus, or H1N1. They are institutionalized methods in which fictive scenarios of epidemic outbreaks are practiced. To give an example, "Dark Winter" was the name of one such table-top exercise enacted in June 2001. It was based on the fictional narrative of a smallpox attack (UPMC "About"). The sequel "Atlantic Storm" was performed in January 2005 and represented a smallpox outbreak within a global context (UPMC, "Atlantic"). But these scenario games do not simply offer daunting stories of contagious catastrophe. This form of preparedness practice is an increasingly common method,[50] which uses "imaginative enactment" (Lakoff, "From Population" 36) to discern threats and prepare for them. In these practices uncertainty is appropriated and temporally displaced by the narrativization of biosecurity.

Similar to the theatricality of the operating theatres of the 19th century, these security practices are theatrical. In these exercises government officials become the actors in a "drama of security." Atlantic Storm for instance involved 16 government officials impersonating the respective national heads of state. They entered into a "what if" scenario set up on a stage performed for an audience of security experts who were seated in the audience space, as well as the audience of the recorded and animated version of the exercise accessing it via the internet (UPMC, "Atlantic"). Like "rehearsals" for a nuclear attack in the 1950s, preparedness practices such as scenario exercises make threats appear as "imaginable, manageable, and most of all, capable of being acted upon" (T. Davis, *Stages* 3). The scenario game represents a scripted performances with a detailed sequence of events. The players interact with a fictive storyline and have very limited freedom of action. The sequence of events is carefully scripted "as it is currently envisioned by biosecurity experts whose aim is to intervene in the present" (Caduff 256). Within the exercise the events are therefore fixed by stage direction.

Both scenarios indicate the unfolding of an apocalyptic disease event which is inescapable. There is no possibility for the actors to successfully intervene in the unfolding events leading to a worldwide catastrophe. Rather than offering a variety of pathways the performances "manifest the apocalyptic 'voice of prophecy,' speaking to an inconvertible future event" (Schoch-Spana, "Bioterrorism" 12). Science as the arbiter of security installs itself as both narrator and hero in its self-legitimizing tale. The only conclusion that can be drawn from the exercise is the need of preparedness and pre-emptive measures that were inscribed in the story as amiss beforehand (in Dark Winter the missing vaccine, in Atlantic Storm the lack of vaccine units and the missing global coordination). In pre-emption and preparedness measures the scientific findings are thus themselves produced by narrative practice.

Using the form of apocalyptic narratives, the exercises appropriate a deeply American genre and its use of fear and hope.[51] While fear and hope played a crucial role in the rise of the biological security narrative, it becomes paramount for preparedness and pre-emption. In the preparedness exercises "fears, hopes and anxieties" (Ben Anderson, "Anticipatory" 7) are mobilized to make the "not yet materialized" threat present and experi-

---

50   According to the Harvard School of Public Health Center for Public Health Preparedness thirty-eight exercises were conducted in the United States in 218 cities and towns involving 5,892 participants (Biddinger et al. 101–102).

51   For the role of the apocalyptic narrative in American cultural history see Bercovitch *The American Jeremiad*.

enceable. Lakoff asserts that one function of the scenario-based exercise is "to generate affect of urgency in the absence of the event itself" ("From Population" 35). The affects facilitate the bridging of present and potential future creating a form of "transtemporality" (Massumi, "Fear" 36) – a blurring of both temporal states.

Furthermore, affective urgency replaces rationality and fact, creating what Massumi has conceptualized as "affective fact" (Massumi, "Future Birth", "Fear", "Autonomy of Affect"). Affects represent in the exercises the only "knowledge" on which decisions can be based. But these affects are not spontaneous reactions to the storyline. As the sequence of events also the affects are intentionally scripted. And like the Puritan predecessor of apocalyptic narratives, the narrative of inevitable doom spreads fear of an unchangeable future as well as formulates hope. While Jeremiads proposed societal change the preparedness practices establish pre-emptive research as the katechontic element,[52] the messiah that can stop the inevitable turmoil of the disease apocalypse. Though focused on the looming risks of imminent destruction the biosecurity narratives are optimistic tales that reinforce and reiterate hope and the belief in absolute security.[53] The narratives formulate hope for change which in turn reinforces the messianic narrative of scientific salvation that had been established in the 20th century.

Pre-emption has become the most prominent paradigm of biosecurity and its contagious apocalyptic scenarios pervade not only governmental institutions concerned with the biosecurity of the nation. The scenario games are available to the public as audience via internet streams, others involve the public as actors and spectators in exercises such as "Sooner Spring" in 2002.[54] But preparedness exercises are just one way for pre-emptive security logics to circulate. Projects such as the PrepareAthon – a virtual community for participants of preparedness activities across the nation (FEMA, "PrepareAthon") – make the logics of biosecurity a more widespread and normal way of understanding security. Also, biosecurity pamphlets, news stories, or travel advice have made fear and perpetual insecurity "now in almost every conceivable sphere of thought and life" (Ben Anderson, "Hope" 158f) a spreading sentiment that finds expression in movements such as the so-called "prepper culture."[55] The growing cultural phenomenon of biosecurity culture is a trending market which includes survival and emergency kits, specialized gear, and information. But it also manifests itself in what Nancy Tomes terms "epidemic entertainments" such as in Steve Soderbergh's thriller *Contagion*, or the growing genre of biosecurity videogames such as *Pandemic*, *CellCraft*, *Plague Inc.*, *Infectonator*, or the *Bioshock* series.

The adoption of pre-emptive logics and the rise of a biosecurity complex have attracted a burgeoning scholarly interest in sociology and the growing subfield of Biosecurity Studies. The paradigm of contagious epidemics and their pre-emption dominates

---

52   'Katechon' is a biblical concept (King James Bible, 2 Thessalonians 2.6-8) referring to the retaining of the antichrist and the apocalypse, or rather the person that delays the coming of the end.

53   Bercovitch asserts this function of hope and optimism as the most fundamental element of the Puritan Jeremiad as well as of its secularized successors.

54   18,000 residents of McAlester, Oklahoma City, "attended one of seven distribution points for 'antibiotics' in the form of jellybeans and fruit punch" (Schoch-Spana "Bioterrorism" 10).

55   Prepping represent a growing movement of people in the U.S. who train and prepare "to survive a world-ending calamity" (Moses n.p.).

biosecurity practices as well as their study. Since biosecurity is predominantly understood as the governmental response to contagious disease, the study of biosecurity is largely reduced to these contexts.[56] However, the logic has been integrated in the understanding of health and security also outside of contagious diseases. The necessity and urgency to pre-empt the emergence of all forms of diseases has become the official mission of NIH in its Report to Congress:

> Our goal at NIH is to provide the scientific evidence base that will usher in an era where medicine is predictive, personalized, pre-emptive, and participatory. This will be a profound transformation from the current model of late-stage "curative" interventions, and one that this Nation must undergo in the coming decades if we are to succeed in providing access to care for all Americans at reasonable costs. (NIH "Biennial" 10)

This shows that the same logics that are applied in military defense also determine how bodily security is understood outside of contagious disease contexts. The way how pre-emptive logics are employed and anticipatory knowledge is produced are also applied to the biological security of individuals. The pre-emptive and preventive security logics enter the way the body is understood and encountered, influencing the understanding of self and identity also on a more individual level. They become the leading paradigm for understanding individual biological security, producing new relations between the individual and their body.

---

56   Nick Bingham and Steve Hinchcliffe, among many others, assert that biosecurity in the U.S. "has come to represent a governmental concern with the – either purposeful or inadvertent – spread of biological agents into the human population" (Bingham and Hinchliffe 173). Also Collier and Lakoff formulate the same focus on biosecurity in their attempt "to map the emerging field of 'biosecurity' interventions'" (8). They propose the field of "infectious disease" (9), "bioterrorism" (10), research on new pathogens (10), and food safety (11).

3. Reading the Signs: The Biosecurity Individual, Biomedicalization, and Biomedical Salvation

> And in the Minutes of the Darkness wherein he lay thus feeble and sore broken, he sometimes let fall expressions of some Fear lest he might after all be Deceived in his Hope of the Future Blessedness.
> *Cotton Mather*

Cotton Mather's report on the dying of his father Increase Mather reveals the stark ambiguity of Puritan attitudes toward security. At the end of his life, which he led as a towering example of Puritan faith, Increase Mather seems to doubt. Salvation and sainthood, the most important pillars of Puritan striving in their pilgrimage through life, represented a never to be attained security that was *always* in doubt. Yet, only in this doubt might have rested the possibility of security as heavenly salvation. The perpetual insecurity represented in this example is not exceptional, but in line with the spiritual and ideological belief of the Puritan faith (Stannard 1316). Life and fate are given by God and preordained, to understand one's fate the individual had to be able to read the signs correctly, creating a hermeneutic reading for experiences of conversion. In the end, spiritual security remained unattainable and was often rather recognized by others, as in Cotton Mather's reading of Increase Mather's dying.[1] The belief in a preordained but unknowable future security created an obsessive focus on risks, and devilish temptations that dominated the Puritan understanding of their living surroundings as manifested for instance in Jeremiads or in Captivity Narratives. The hermeneutic insecurity and obsessive reading of signs that dominated Puritan culture indicates a sense of perpetual insecurity and threat. The reading of signs was for the Puritan faith thus a crucial and unavoidable tool of salvation. The relation to security that this example represents is a crucial analogy to the security produced in biomedical discourses.

Four centuries of medicalization and biomedicalization have changed the understanding of life and the relation to the body radically. Today, security is not to be found in

---

[1]   In contrast to the dying father, his observing son is sure of his salvation, understanding it as a didactic example for the aspired calm death (Mather 208).

the beyond but is fixed in the materiality of the body. But biomedical security narratives are anchored in the excessive reading of signs as a precondition to achieving security. Living in a biosecurity culture, individuals rely on hermeneutic reading of their own body, its surface as well as its biological make up. Also today people feel constantly at risk. The biologically predetermined fate has to be divined and tended to, and only through security practices can the fate and potential of an individual be achieved. But the reading is motivated by a fundamentally different understanding of security than that of the Puritans. The potential of ambiguity and uncertainty of knowing one's preordained fate has been replaced by scientifically provided "certainties." "To live well today is to live in the light of biomedicine" as Nicholas Rose puts it ("Human Sciences" 7). Salvation today is not granted and judged upon by a fierce God but by the possibilities of science, more specifically the field of biomedicine and biotechnology, which holds the normative power over (the understanding of) life, good life, and livability.

The promise of total security in the face of an always precarious normal also defines biomedical studies and research in non-contagious health contexts and makes logics of biosecurity crucial for understanding individual biological security. In this chapter I will focus on the growing complex of biomedicalization to emphasize the new relations it forges between individual and their body and the new biomedicalized identities that are based on professionalized readings and translations of bodily signs. I will explain how the progress of biomedicalization individualizes biosecurity practices giving shape to the imaginary of security as total control. I will then turn to the increasing responsibilization of the individual to emphasize how biological security appears as a question of choice, which makes individual biosecurity a deeply American matter. In a further argumentative step I will show how biomedical security narratives produce realities in *what if* scenarios that define not only bodily security and threat but also the understanding of good life and livability.

The Power of Translation: The Biosecurity Individual and the Vision of Total Control

Clarke et al. define the current developments as a process of biomedicalization – a further development of medicalization – which was facilitated by the rise of the "Biomedical TechnoService Complex, Inc." ("Biomedicalization" 162). The processes of biomedicalization exacerbate many developments already present in medicalization, but they also decisively change many relations between patient and doctor, present and future, and most importantly body and self. According to Clarke et al. biomedicalization is largely marked by technoscientific developments, which shift the focus to risk. They attempt to control as well as to transform the body itself creating new visions of bodily security and new biosecurity identities. Biomedicalization is driven by a further commodification of health and life itself, which has been analyzed as biovalue or biocapital (Cooper, Sunder Rajan). Furthermore, these developments are established through new forms of knowledge production and distribution. (Clarke et al., "Biomedicalization" 163)

The developments of biomedicalization started in the mid 1980s and have increased significantly since the turn of the century. They describe a "shift to highly inventive technoscientific biomedicalization" (Clarke et al., "Charting" 88), which has facilitated, among many other things, the development and proliferation of diagnostic technology. In fact, medical screening technologies have become so common that diagnostic techniques are closely associated with certain conditions, such as ultrasound and pregnancy, or MRI for cancerous tumors (van Dijck, *Transparent* 12). The biotechnological possibilities of visualizing further change the understanding of the body and security shifting the perspective from "clinical gaze" to "molecular gaze" (Clarke et al., "Biomedicalization" 164) as mentioned before. The technologies have not only facilitated the definition of more disease categories but have allowed detecting them earlier and earlier. Today, biomedical technology and research focus on the increasingly early detection and prevention of disease or deviation, such as cancer, diabetes, obesity, depression, or autism, in most cases by focusing on risk markers in the molecular stages of the disease.

Risks rather than diseases themselves have become the focus of research as it is paramount to detect them at "their earliest molecular stages" (NIH "Future" n.p.). This relatively new focus is described as a form of "surveillance biomedicine" (Clarke et al., "Biomedicalization" 166), which comprises securitizing practices originally targeting the population. But it no longer aims at interventions on the level of the population only. Rather, surveillance medicine has extended its reach to individualized practices defining risk groups as well as individuals at risk and their future. Risk analysis geared toward estimating emergent risks on the basis of a population are applied to the analysis of diagnostic assessment (Fosket; Clarke et al.). This means that the individual body has become "a world in which everything is normal and at the same time precariously abnormal" (Armstrong 400). It represents the body as a world that is harboring is own future demise.

> This new Surveillance Medicine involves a fundamental remapping of the spaces of illness. Not only is the relationship between symptom, sign and illness redrawn but the very nature of illness is reconstructed. And illness begins to leave the three dimensional confine of the volume of the human body to inhabit a novel extracorporeal space. (Armstrong 395)

The extracorporeal space that Armstrong emphasizes is the "space of risk." It is extracorporeal because the understanding of risks is produced outside of the body in technoscientifically facilitated risk assessments. It describes a potential for a disease, which itself is not present in the body. Instead of defining and treating disease the biomedical security narrative focuses increasingly on defining, diagnosing, and treating risks. This new form of "clinical gaze" adopted in "surveillance medicine" strives for an ideal of total security.

Health risks therefore no longer designate the difference between healthy and sick, between security and insecurity. This distinction has been blurred and largely suspended by technoscientific developments. The state of insecurity no longer coincides with the traditional status change of a healthy person becoming a patient. It no longer describes a difference between "being healthy" and "being sick," but rather the potential for either. The new medical gaze of surveillance medicine therefore shifts the logics and dynamics of the experience of biological security. Health becomes an ambivalent experiential situation, a "precarious state" (Armstrong 397) which is described in risk categories, most commonly "high risk," "medium risk," and "low risk" (Lupton, *Imperative* 92). Even the healthiest individual is thus still considered "at risk."

These descriptions might seem abstract and remote from everyday life at first sight, reserved for extreme medical cases. However, practices of surveillance biomedicine are a normal and standard procedure in many parts of life from childhood to adolescence, ageing and dying. Notions of biological security have become increasingly important for cultural conceptions of life and livability most explicitly in the example of pregnancy and prenatal testing. I will therefore use this example to illustrate new relations forged by the regimen of "total control." "[I]n the United States alone, more than 80 million ultrasound examinations are performed on women every year and many women have more than one ultrasound during their pregnancy" (Nash 5). This might not be surprising as the use of biosecurity practices seems so natural and intuitive. Why shouldn't one "control" biology and make sure everything is all right if it is so easily accessible? However, Deborah Lupton points out that "[t]here is no evidence that routine ultrasound screening is beneficial to the health of the infant" (*Imperative* 96). Nonetheless, the tests are presented as imperative to secure the health of mother and child and as a prerequisite for a good life – meaning a life free of disabilities.[2]

Pregnancy, childbirth and childhood are early and prime examples of the medicalization and biomedicalization of life (Ariès, *Centuries*; Conrad, *Medicalization*; Elliott). Prenatal testing has existed since the 1970s and became a crucial practice giving information about the development of the fetus.[3] Based on the accumulated data over the decades the different fetal biometric exams yield different calculations in the different trimesters. Their proclaimed beneficial effect is the predictive translation of signs to facilitate informed choice for potential necessary interventions. These security practices are the point where individual and national discourses of biosecurity intersect in the most obvious manner, allowing for biopolitical rule over processes such as population growth.[4] They describe practices of "surveillance medicine" on an individualized level. Prenatal testing assesses the possible future risk indicated in the individual fetus and maternal body. The possibilities of biotechnological interventions have fostered the belief that life should not only be controlled and managed in the present but in its future potential. Security does therefore not describe a present state but a future one, shifting the temporal relation from reaction to anticipation.

The biomedical as well as cultural and social overemphasis on risk produces what Catherine Belling has called in a different context "hypochondriac hermeneutics," which describes an almost compulsive reading of our bodies: "we read our bodies, looking

---

2   This prerogative of prenatal screening, which is evidently researching and working for a future free of disabilities, is opposed by disability rights advocacy groups that critique this practice and discourse in a supposedly "post-eugenic" society.

3   "Besides ultrasound, women can opt for amniocentesis, serum alpha-feto-protein screening, triple tests, a genetic testing for single-gene disorders. Every new test, of course, yields new information, and every additional bit of information may confront the pregnant woman with more options" (van Dijck, *Transparent* 109).

4   Other examples are the availability, as well as structural and educational support of contraception, the question of abortion rights, or fertility treatments.

at them as if from outside ourselves at the same time as we feel them as from within"
(Belling, "Hypochondriac" 376). People – caught between the dread of fear and the desire for security – take on a hermeneutic attitude, reading their bodies as if it was an
assembly of signs: the hiccup could mean that the umbilical cord is wrapped around the
neck, the placenta could move, iron levels could fall too low, one could eat the wrong
food, consume too much caffeine, come into contact with chemicals, or bacteria such as
toxoplasmosis or listeria. The security practices for pregnant women are rigid and start
often with the pre-emptive consumption of supplements such as folic acid and Vitamin
D, which is used by almost 80% of pregnant women in the U.S. either prescribed by a
healthcare provider or as over-the-counter consumer good (Aronsson et al. 2).

But most risks remain experientially inaccessible and uncontrollable for pregnant
women without professionalized help. The gaze of surveillance medicine implicates every individual, no matter of their own feeling of "well-being." Preventive diagnostic practices and treatments are thus represented as an increasingly important and normative
part of pregnancy, necessary to know one's current state of security. If "neither health nor
disease are stable but perpetual becoming" (Armstrong 402) security has to be constantly
re-verified, reproduced, and checked for potentials that are fixed to the different stages
of pregnancy, or the life course in general. Every check-up is thus a performative act producing "security." The performance of security temporally fixes the transient state of security, by presentifying it, offering above else "parental reassurance" (van Dijck, *Transparent* 107). The growing possibilities of technoscientific developments therefore also produce a growing insecurity about people reading their own bodies. Already discoveries
such as "X-ray machines overruled patients' own experience of disease's symptoms. A patient's experience was inherently subjective, and hence unreliable" (van Dijck, *Transparent* 87). This trend is exacerbated by further technoscientific developments, which seem
to eradicate the possibility to know one's own body. This means that the individual can
never be sure of themself being in need of technoscientifically produced "certainty." Ultimately, the biomedical apparatus threatens to strip women of a certain sense of self and
body which is constantly reproduced as at risk and in need of professionalized reading.
Instead of an individual "unmediated" experience of conversion, the biosecurity individual relies on ritualized performances and translation by experts.

In pregnancy, security, thus, does not represent a stable condition, which is then
threatened: in the discursive formation of pre-emption this "condition of security"
appears to be always already precarious. The "tyrannies of nature" – laid out in the
omnipresent biosecurity narratives targeting pregnant women – are hanging like a
Damocles sword over their heads. Continuously medically observed, the pregnant body
is marked by its risks, which start to increase for an otherwise healthy pregnant woman
with her 35th birthday. And women are made acutely aware of this shift. Rachel Adams
describes her first pregnancy with the definition of this "risk identity": "I was thirty-
six, a year beyond the age when the chances of having a baby with Down syndrome
and other genetic conditions start" (98).[5] This quote comes from Adams's book *Raising
Henry* in which she reflects on her experience of becoming mother to a son with Down

---

5   And also her son Henry is predominantly defined by his risks from the biomedical discourses and
     services that ought to help the Adams's family (24,25,76).

syndrome. Her acute awareness of having assumed a risk identity by being pregnant at 36 makes the option of screening and testing an important question. The understanding of security changes the understanding of Adam's corporeal reality. Risk becomes in this context a "disease like state in itself" (Fosket 331) that needs to be treated. The risk identity determines the recommendations for the different screening methods:

> Dr. Lewis, presented us with a full range of options: we could start with a noninvasive test called the "fully integrated screen," a combination of ultrasound and bloodwork to predict the likelihood of genetic abnormalities. The screen can tell you whether your fetus has a one-in-twenty or a one–in–one thousand chance of having a genetic anomaly. But it can't give you a definitive diagnosis. We could also go directly to amnio. Or we could do no testing at all. (R. Adams 99)

In this, as in most representations of medical encounters in the memoir, it seems that the security of a pregnancy, or rather its outcome is determinable by different methods of screening. Biological security is represented as a choice the individual can take by simply picking the proper security practice.

Help Yourself, So Help You Science: The Question of Responsibility and Choice

The choices offered by biomedicine and diagnostic testing are represented as unquestionably liberating, offering and facilitating the freedom to choose and to make one's own fate. Firstly though, biosecurity demands the obligation to choose choice offered by the security practices as Adams shows in the quote above: "Or we could do no testing at all" (99). This dynamic of having to choose indicates a fundamental characteristic of surveillance medicine: the responsibilization[6] of the individual and the need for "technologies of the self" as Foucault defined them in his homonymous lecture. The security narrative of total control exacerbates the responsibilization of the individual for their own body, which had become already central in the security narrative of preventive medicine. If everything is possible, then everything becomes the responsibility of the self-reliant individual. Risks can be assessed in pregnancy early on in the integrated screen between weeks 11–14, which assesses the likelihood of Down syndrome, trisomy 18, or spina bifida. For "more" security people can also opt for pre-implantation genetic diagnosis (PGD) (McCabe and McCabe 203–4), which illustrates the shift from observation of symptoms to the control of the bodily make-up facilitated by technoscientific developments.[7]

Prenatal testing can be interpreted as an early form of a pre-emptive strike, which reflects the new understanding of security. It represents an ideal of total health which requires a continuous self-control of the individual. Individuals thus have to perform

---

6   "Responsibilization" is a term used in sociology to describe the shift of responsibility from one level to another; here it is the shift from a governmental to the individual level.

7   Additionally, newborns are screened for "50 conditions . . . at birth in the United States, most of which are genetic" (Vailley 375).

anticipatory actions to "know" their bodies. Because security measures and practices in current biomedicine are highly individualized and *individualizing*, many scholars try to rethink Foucault's concept of biosecurity, or think beyond Foucault as it is usually called, to encompass current forces of responsibilization of the individual.[8] Nikolas Rose attempts to approximate the *beyond* as "ethopolitics"[9] rather than biopolitics emphasizing the ethical obligation of individualized security practices for oneself and for one's offspring.

Security practices of ultrasound, and further tests if indicated, have become a normative behavioral codex. They represent actions in the present that thwart a potentially diseased future. Nobody is forced to be tested, genetically or otherwise, but the engagement in the "regimes of behavior change" that testing implies is nonetheless represented as an obligation (Shostak 243). The societal compulsion of testing is expressed in every doctor's visit, but also in the representation of parenting books and manuals, in advertisements, or in conversations with friends, as Adams makes clear in her memoir. She describes how she is asked by many different people in different social contexts if she didn't get tested, after her son Henry was born with Down syndrome. The prevalence of such questions indicates how normalized and expected the security practices are. This shows that the "pastoral power [of biosecurity] . . . takes place in a contested field" (Rose, "Politics" 9) and is not simply imposed by the state.

Nonetheless, social expectation is also expressed in legislative changes. "[I]n 1986, California was the first state in the country to pass a law requiring that all pregnant mothers be offered MSAFP (maternal serum alpha-fetoprotein) screening to assess the probability that their fetuses would be affected by Down syndrome, spina bifida, or neural tube defects" (Stern 213). Biosecurity practices – or rather the proper choice for the appropriate security practice – are framed as Constitutional rights and as crucial practices of individual freedom. Regardless of the personal choice and necessity of biosecurity practices the predominant consensus is that the application and use of biosecurity measures is an individual right not to be infringed upon by the government as Elliott points out (xix). If knowledge produces the responsibility to choose and decide, and if that is framed as a right – the right to choose – then ultimately these practices are made to represent practices of freedom and citizenship.[10]

It is thus not only lifestyle and external risks that have to be controlled but the individual biological make-up. Since the body is understood as a fateful given or "preordained fate" that can be optimized and influenced, the individual needs to tend to

---

8   Many scholars attempt to think in this context *Beyond Foucault* (Rabinow and Rose) or *Beyond Biopolitics* (Clough and Willse), which means thinking a concept written for the relation between state and population – since "Discipline is exercised on the bodies of individuals, and security is exercised over a whole population" (Rose, "Politics" 24) – in relation to the individual (without conflating *discipline* with *security*).

9   "If discipline individualizes and normalizes, and biopower collectivized and socializes, ethopolitics concerns itself with the self-techniques by which human beings should judge themselves and act upon themselves to make themselves better than they are" (Rose, "Politics" 18).

10   Melinda Cooper points out that George W. Bush legitimized the research on already available embryonic stem cell lines as well as the unconditional health care for unborn babies with the foundational rights of the United States, "chief among them being the right to life" (Cooper 152).

their biological make up. Knowing represents in this context both an indispensable tool for recovery (Rose and Novas, "Citizenship" 447–448) and a prerequisite for security. For such a structure of responsibilization to work the individual needs what Rose and Novas call "scientific literacy" ("Citizenship" 443). They point out that education enabled people to take responsibility for reproductive choices and their own heredity ("Citizenship" 442). Only with appropriate information and knowledge can one choose the right measures. The American Pregnancy Association for example provides information about the diverse birth defects as "awareness and education are key to preventing birth defects" ("Birth Defects" n.p.). The prerogative of this pregnancy related biosecurity education is thus prevention and pre-emption. The information about biosecurity, however, is provided not only by governmental, scientific, or pharmaceutical institutions, but increasingly also circulated in online self-help forums and social networks. This describes the changed production, distribution, and consumption of biosecurity narratives (Clarke et al., "Biomedicalization" 163). These new forms of distributing a biomedicalized understanding of security represent the shift in authorship of security narratives, which are no longer merely produced by scientific experts. The diversification of knowledge production and distribution is often understood as a democratizing force. Nevertheless, in these "new" forms of distribution the dominant logics of biosecurity are reiterated and restaged and the responsibility and obligation of the individual is further enforced. In either case, the choices for security rely on narratives, fictions of security, to produce the "appeal" of a particular understanding.

Fictions of Security: Biosecurity and Good Life

Prenatal testing mandates decisions or rather choices based on the knowledge tests provide. The choice, however, is more often than not based on a fiction of security. Every screening method and every diagnosed risk represents future scenarios that are formulated in security narratives. Since "[r]isk factors, above all else, are pointers to a potential, yet unformed, eventuality" (Armstrong 402) the narratives established by individualized surveillance medicine are necessarily "fictive." The indication of a risk potential leads, if one chooses to pursue biosecurity, to further screening and diagnostic testing and to the decisions that potentially follow every exam. However, the security practice of the ultrasound exam does not yield certainty. The most immediate information that comes with the consultations about the test is based on statistic averages. They are "what if" scenarios in which the individual is "invited" to think through life with common but also increasingly rare conditions.

The information these scenarios are based on is authored largely by the "Biomedical TechnoService Complex, Inc." (Clarke et al., "Biomedicalization" 162) and therefore comes from the institutions that celebrate the possibilities of surveillance medicine and the possibilities of intervening in life. The authors promote a clear desirability of "total health" that appears accessible – after all, their messianic promise is the eradication of diseases and the vision of total control. However, in many cases the "what if" scenarios do not fulfill the promise of "total security" but lead to the choice between termination or continuation.

> If the ultrasound scan shows a fetus to be normal, parents can relax and enjoy the rest of their pregnancy; if the sonographer detects fetal defects, the woman and her partner can decide to terminate the pregnancy. In both instances, ultrasound is said to offer the parents peace of mind and hence be a desirable practice. (van Dijck, *Transparent* 107)

The security narrative offered in these exams reiterates the prerogative of knowing and defines the limit between "acceptable" and "unbearable" life. Such norms of life and livability are based on averages, which indicate when the acceptable is transgressed and interventions become necessary (and possible). The decision for or against abortion is never a direct suggestion. Rather, counseling informs the individual about the potential future explaining it from a biomedicalized perspective. The implications of the test, however, reiterate the clear desirability of a healthy baby without any recognizable, or rather foreseeable potential "lacks." Though diagnostic technologies represent ever new ways of visualizing the body, these medical practices are never just diagnostic in the same way as diagnostic categories are never simply descriptive. They communicate "a normative ideal" which represents the matrix in which the individual can understand their own body (van Dijck, *Transparent* 15).

Rayna Rapp shows in her study *Testing Women, Testing Fetus* that not all prenatal tests that indicate a possibility of a disease end in diagnosis, implying the high rate of detected risk markers which turn out to be "false positives," but also the many abortions which are based "only" on probabilities of disabilities and disease. Yet furthermore she makes clear that not all prenatal diagnoses, such as the prior knowledge of a present birth defect, end in abortion. The dangers of testing are the focus of bioethics committees and are further expressed in the critique of prenatal testing as a renewal of eugenic methods and thinking expressed by such diverse scholars as Minna Stern, Linda and Edward McCabe, or Jürgen Habermas. The fear is that "if driven solely by market demand, American's tendency to choose the 'best' for their children could eventually translate into two branches of Homo sapiens: a wealthy genetic elite that replicates itself through designer babies and a medically underserved genetic underclass" (Stern 12). Similarly, disability rights groups warn against the widespread routine practice. The biosecurity narratives define good life as well as undesired life, and performatively reiterate this "undesirability" of persons with disability in every security practice with the underlying logic of the eradication of disability. In a way, the practices produce and make visible the disposability of individuals and not only of "disposable populations" (Giroux 186).[11]

The biosecurity practices have pervaded American culture and the understanding of life so deeply that the by now routine application of ultrasound exams to secure the baby's health is not just used as a diagnostic device. Rather "the ultrasound exam of a pregnant woman is concurrently a medical diagnostic checkup, a psychological event, and a photographic ritual" (van Dijck, *Transparent* 101). This medical routine is understood as a crucial practice of bonding with the unborn baby, which the FDA promotes as a beneficial effect (FDA "Ultrasound"). While the "fetus" is monitored and checked for birth defects, it only

---

11   Henry Giroux speaks about a "biopolitics of disposability" (175) in his analysis of hurricane Katrina and the structural racism it made visible.

seems to turn into an "unborn baby," a future person *through this act*. And the visualization of this future can be materially fixed in take-home ultrasound images. These images materially manifest the security of the pregnancy – fixing it temporarily – and therefore represent the promise of a happy future. Ultrasound images exist in color and in black and white, in 2D, 3D, and 4D. The ultrasound is a medical practice as well as a consumer good in its own right. In 4D – a 3D scan in motion – the baby is shown as if the fetus was waving, walking or sucking its thumb, staging it in peaceful acts that embody security and make a not yet existing future (identity) present. This crucial first way of knowing a person normalizes a biomedicalized understanding of identity. These images of biosecurity have become a fixture in life narratives represented in family picture books, and social media, movies, art, and literature. The urge for ultrasound testing has thus produced entirely new consumer markets. Ultrasound diagnostics are a growing market in the U.S. and worldwide. It is estimated to reach $7.2 billion by 2022 with a growth of 5% (MarketWatch). In comparison, the NIH invests approximately $41.7 billion in scientific research annually in total (NIH, "Budget" 2020). Besides the rising healthcare sector of sonography so called "keepsake" sonograms are offered by companies under no proper medical oversight.[12] This trend reflects the increased marketization of health and life.

Clarke et al. emphasize the commodification of the entire health sector – including care and research – as one of the most crucial characteristics of biomedicalization. This shift is also visible in the changes of corporative structures of biotech companies as Bud asserts: "A study of the founders of U.S. biotechnology companies has shown that whereas in the period of 1971–80 almost twice as many had academic as had business origins, by the mid-1980s, two-thirds were from business" (Bud, *Uses* 193). Biocapital not only describes the corporatization of science but the commodification of life itself. Scholars such as Kaushik Sunder Rajan and Melinda Cooper describe how life and bodily matter have been renegotiated as biocapital. Analyzing for instance the market of embryonic stem cells, Cooper asserts that "what is at stake and what is new in the contemporary biosciences is not so much the commodification of biological life . . . but rather its transmutation into speculative surplus value" (Cooper 148). She shows that "the emergence of the biotech industry is inseparable from the rise of neoliberalism as the dominant political philosophy of our time" (Cooper 19).[13] This "surplus life" is part of a growing industry and decisively driven by venture capital and risk investment, which means by future markets and fictions of potential future success.

Similar to Cooper, Sunder Rajan focuses on the market structures dominating the creation of the value of life by analyzing patent laws of genomic material and information (*Biocapital* 7). More so than Cooper he emphasizes the symbolic capital of biomedicine asserting that it is "both material and symbolic" (Sunder Rajan, *Lively* 19). With reference to Marx he emphasizes the "*mythical* and *magical* nature of the commodity" (*Bio-*

---

12   The FDA warns against this non-medical use of ultrasound (American Pregnancy Org., "Keepsake" n.p.).

13   Cooper stresses that the current state of bio-economy relied on the changes of intellectual property rights such as the Bayh-Dole Act in 1980 that permitted the ownership and patenting of government funded research: "the biotech 'revolution' would have been inconceivable without a full scale legislative and political campaign to revolutionize property itself" (Cooper 145).

capital 18). Sunder Rajan specifically highlights the centrality of the "theological character of the commodity" in Marx (*Biocapital* 18). Stressing the influence of ideology in the
question of valuation Sunder Rajan identifies the symbolic capital of biotechnology and
biomedicine as the underlying promise of "being in the business of saving lives" (*Biocapital* 19). This symbolic capital is especially important as biotechnological developments
rely on speculative capitalism. They depend on what Sunder Rajan calls the articulation
of vision and hype as the "grammar of biocapital" (*Biocapital* 111). More important than
the actual monetary gain that is produced by the emphasis on the promised future, his
analysis shows that the messianic narrative of scientific salvation structures the understanding of the practices, services, and goods that surround it. He defines American "biocapital as salvationary" (*Biocapital* 185) representing magical cures, promising a better
future and the security of life, today as much as in the past. The symbolic capital produced by the messianic narrative of scientific salvation encompasses not only biomedical practices and goods as such. Promising security by perpetual and constant control,
surveillance biomedicine has been brought into the home through a wide array of (mostly
digital) devices: in pregnancy it is over-the-counter fetal heartbeat monitoring systems,
pregnancy apps, or milestone calendars. Thriving in a neoliberal "stakeholder society"
(Petersen, "Governmentality") these devices have become a normal part of life and of understanding life.

Similar to ultrasound, other biosecurity practices have left the confines of strictly
medical use and entered the extended market of biotechnological consumer goods, such
as genetic testing. 23andMe is a biotech startup which sells DNA kits over the internet.
For $198 one can obtain the diagnostic analysis of one's DNA for "genetic health risks,"
"inherited conditions," "traits," and "wellness" (23andMe "Find out").[14] The individualized
biosecurity practice echoes the medical self-reliance that was central in the 18th and 19th
century. However, the security narrative that suggests genetic testing seems much closer
to the Puritan hermeneutic insecurity and the belief in a predestined fate, a true self that
has to be revealed – albeit now these revelations are secured in biosecurity narratives.

But 23andMe establishes not only genetic risk, it promises to decipher the genetic
identity of the individual. The gene is described as the key to understanding the human in
regard to the bodily security as well as to identity itself as Nelkin and Lindee have shown
in their analysis of the DNA as a cultural icon. The reports on wellness and traits that
23andMe offer gesture in this direction (23andMe "Advertisement"). More aggressively,
however, their commercials drive this point home. The test provides knowledge that will
help the consumer understand themself better. It thus represents "biological identity

---

14   Initially the test was marketed as a security practice offering the diagnosis of hundreds of genetic
      diseases. This had to be temporally halted following a warning by the FDA in November 2013 to
      discontinue the marketing and sale of the test as a diagnostic tool (Gutierrez 2013). It was rein-
      troduced in 2015 with fewer disease diagnoses. Today, it provides information on 10 "genetic
      health risks" (such as BRCA1/BRCA2 (selected variants), coeliac disease, late-onset Alzheimer's Dis-
      ease, Parkinson's Disease), reports on the individual's status as "a carrier for [40] inherited condi-
      tions," as well as 25 reports on "Traits" (features, taste, smell, hair loss) and 5 reports on wellness
      (23andMe, "Find out").

practices" (Rose, "Politics" 18).[15] Additionally, the test includes the ancestry service which provides information about which population groups are represented in one's DNA. The security practice of genetic testing has thus become a recreational identity practice.[16]

The prime actor in the contemporary drama of biosecurity is the gene and genetic markers. Diagnostic tools that provide a new insight into the body have revolutionized the conceptualization of health, making self-surveillance an integral part of everyday life. Identity and the understanding of the body become therefore more and more intimately entwined with biomedical security practices. They have become common identity practices simulating security based on knowing one's genetic identity, one's past (heritage) as well as one's future (fate).

---

15   Similarly, Sunder Rajan asserts that "In one register, then, Lively Capital . . . refers to the lively affects—the emotions and desires—at play when technologies and research impinge on experiences of embodiment, kinship, identity, disability, citizenship, accumulation, or dispossession" (Sunder Rajan, *Lively* 16).

16   Together with Ancestry DNA, Living DNA, Family Tree DNA, and MyHeritage DNA, 23andMe represents the leading companies for ancestry testing. On its homepage it declares itself to be the biggest ancestry service in the world providing certainty about one's heritage. However, this promised security is nothing but a marketing stunt as these tests are notoriously unreliable. This problem had been raised early on by experts of population genetics and has recently gone viral in social media. In January the story of identical twins who had tried ancestry DNA testing was published on marketplace. They sent their DNA samples to the five biggest companies offering the service, receiving 10 different sets of results of possible genetic heritage.

4. The Biosecurity Individual and the Drama of Biosecurity: Performance, Performativity, and Affect

> The unexamined life is not worth living.
> *Aristotle*

Biomedical knowledge has become increasingly important for the understanding (and study) of identity constructions. But biological determinism is one of the oldest and at the same time most contested conceptualizations and constructions in identity discourses. Theories of identity construction reject essentialism or a biologized understanding of identity. This repudiation was crucial to dismantle and deconstruct what had previously legitimized the oppression of "minorities" (or more broadly the other). Nonetheless, the fluid cultural identities always retained a haunting presence of biology. Both Sarah Ahmed and Iris Young respond to this dilemma in the context of feminism and feminist theory, which deconstructs biologically based identity ascriptions as performativity and constructivism. With this theoretical perspective, however, feminist theory allegedly threatens to diminish the very object/subject of its own discourse. Biology represents here what has to be deconstructed while at the same time, it has to be maintained as the unifying claim of the group feminism claims to speak for.[1]

The notion of biologically determined identity constructions has resurfaced in uncanny ways, especially in its relation to disease, disability, and genetics. Biosecurity has become an additional identity marker, representing a further intersectional identity that influences and is influenced by other markers of difference. The understanding of biosecurity as well as the access to biosecurity are exceedingly determined by race, class, gender, and sexuality. Class in terms of both financial and cultural capital is crucial to access many forms of medical care in the U.S., let alone preventive and pre-emptive measures. The costs of the above mentioned prenatal and perinatal care represent a substantial bud-

---

1   Ahmed calls this supposed dichotomy and incompatibility an "imaginary prohibition" (Ahmed, "Imaginary" 9) and proposes to differentiate between theory and practice as two distinct discourses to maintain the potential for postmodern theories "to the articulation of political choice" ("Beyond" 72). Also Young calls for "pragmatic theorizing" (Young 718) as groups are necessary to counter liberal individualism's denial of reality of groups.

get for the biosecurity pregnancy.[2] Most of the costs are covered by health insurance, or Medicaid for those who are eligible. But a high number of underinsured and uninsured patients have to cover the varying costs for the different screenings themselves.[3] The program of Medicaid has been decisively extended in many states making perinatal care – one of the central mechanisms of (population) biosecurity – more widely available. Already in 2009 Medicaid covered "more than four in ten births nationwide" (Ranji and Salganicoff 1). In other areas, however, "the right to hope" as Nixon put it in the 1970s is a hope for the few.[4] Furthermore, biosecurity decisively influences the position of an individual in terms of class since the costs of treatment for an (unexpected) illness or injury often causes economic problems.[5]

Additionally to income, education and cultural capital determine the "scientific literacy" (Rose and Novas, "Citizenship" 443) of an individual, which is necessary to "properly" use biomedical possibilities. "Scientific literacy" implies the understanding of biological processes, their potential risks and the "appropriate" preventive and pre-emptive security practices as well as an understanding of the diagnosis and result. What do the risk potentials and the absolute potential of a disease really mean? The ability to translate the technoscientifically produced biosecurity knowledge relies on the ability of the individual practitioner and the surrounding culture to provide a pervasive security narrative.

Race and gender further determine biosecurity identities through questions of access, availability, and treatment options as the recent publicity of "Black Birth Matters," an offspring of the Black Lives Matter movement, made strikingly obvious. The movement reveals the systemic pattern of producing racialized risk individuals, which the high death rates of black women after giving birth, as well as the disproportionately high rate of infant mortality make strikingly clear. "In the US, the black infant mortality is double the white infant mortality rate" (Wallace et al. 140). And while pregnancy related death – a death during pregnancy or within a year of giving birth – is rising steadily in the United States in general, black women are more than three times as likely as white women to be affected (CDC, "Pregnancy Mortality"). Serena Williams, the tennis star, and Erica Garner, the Black Lives Matter activist were the prominent individuals who brought this disparity into the limelight of public debate.[6] Such examples show how structural

---

2   The Health Care provider Parasil provides an estimation for the costs insuring each trimester, which depends on the security options an individual chooses and can accumulate to more than $ 10.000 if complications are detected and more invasive screens become "necessary." The delivery in a hospital alone can amount to $30.000. (McFarland n.p.)

3   The introduction and expansion of the Affordable Care Act has halved the number of uninsured individuals in the United States to 8.1% for the total U.S. American population according the U.S. Census Bureau (Berchick et al. 5). However, of the 19–65 years old, 15.5% of Americans were uninsured. Of those insured 28% are underinsured (Collins et al. 1).

4   The widening care gap in the United States is reported almost daily. The problems are so severe that the Boston Globe reports 250.000 GoFundMe requests a year to raise money for health-related treatments (O'Neil n.p.).

5   The Commonwealth Fund emphasizes the increased risk for "medical debt" especially for those underinsured with high deductibles as well as the uninsured (Collins et al. 7).

6   Erica Garner died in December 2017 of cardiovascular problems after giving birth. Serena Williams also suffered complications after giving birth. She was still in hospital when she felt that she was experiencing a pulmonary embolism – blood clots obstructing the arteries of the lung – so she

racism leads to disproportionate health risks a person is exposed to, which reach beyond environmental risks produced by living and working conditions.

Understanding security as performative does not diminish the suffering of the individuals as unreal but emphasizes that security narratives and practices greatly influence the production of varying securities and diverse biosecurity individuals. Biologically inflected security narratives structure U.S. society, marking and making belonging. Scholars in anthropology and sociology such as Rabinow, Rose, and Novas regard the developments and possibilities in biotechnology and biomedicine as producing a new form of identity, such as "biosocial collectivities" or "biological citizenship" (Rabinow and Rose 197). They describe a biologically based understanding of group affiliation expressed in patient advocacy groups for instance.

Though predominantly describing group identities, most of the sociological studies of biomedicalization also emphasize that the "medical gaze" has become a "reflexive gaze" ("Citizenship" 10) as for instance Rose and Novas point out. This "reflexive gaze" not only indicates the ascription of a biologized identity but the appropriation and adoption of biosecurity identities. Biomedical and biotechnological developments have changed the understanding of person, body, life and its lived realities. Rose and Novas assert that biomedical technologies facilitate "the creation of persons with a certain kind of relation to themselves" ("Genetic" 445).

These biosecurity identities that most of these sociological studies aim to describe might not fit the static mechanistic relations described in Foucault's concept of power and security. Rather, power is more fluid, influencing a more existential understanding of being that can be described and analyzed more thoroughly as performance and performativity. With Foucault, Judith Butler understands the subject and its body as a form of obedience or "effect of power." Paraphrasing Foucault, she asserts that "regulatory power produces the subjects it controls, that power is not only imposed externally, but works as the regulatory and normative means by which subjects are formed" (Butler, *Bodies* 22). According to Butler, this formation of the subject focuses on bodily identity and the individual body rather than on the ephemeral power itself. Her theory of performativity is situated at the intersection of body and self, culture and nature, in which the body becomes center stage for the individual. Since biosecurity is an embodied state of being that challenges and determines the identity of an individual, I will turn to how the body and identity of a person are intricately linked and equally constrained through performative acts of biosecurity. I will argue that biosecurity identities are at core performative, both in its deconstructive as well as its theatrical sense. To understand how biosecurity is experienced by the very same body that is defined by biosecurity narratives, I will then turn to affect theory and how the body is "marked by feeling."

---

alerted the nurse and asked for the necessary medical treatments. Only after repeated demands for a CT scan, which can reveal the blood clots, and for an infusion of blood thinners did Williams receive the necessary care (Salam n.p.). Williams was able to insist on her opinion, not letting the nurse and medical staff overrule her feelings, due to her social standing and position of relative power. But only because of her high scientific literacy – she knew about her increased risk for blood clots – was she able to insist on the treatment and screening method she needed.

Speaking Bodies: Biosecurity, Embodied Identities, and the Body as Stage[7]

Butler expanded the concept of performativity established by Austin's speech act and Derrida's theory of deconstruction, applying it to bodily practices and the question of identity and subjectivity. The theory recognizes the body as central in the production and understanding of identities. However, identity is not understood as an expression of an a priori innate truth that resides in the body. By defining the relation of body and identity as "non-referential" she establishes a rigid anti-essentialist critique of a natural "truth." But performativity for Butler is not just non-referentiality translated to the body. She describes how subjects are created in the performance and embodiment of "specific historic scripts" and "possibilities" in a complex "process of appropriation" (Butler, "Performative" 521). She therefore describes the process, temporality and relationality of producing bodily identities that become understood as natural expressions.

Although it is one of the strongest points of critique against Butler, I wish to retain the theatrical aspect of her theory, which she stresses in her early writings. In the 1988 article "Performative Acts and Gender Constitution" Butler emphasizes that the "'performative' itself carries the double meaning of 'dramatic' and 'non-referential'" (522).[8] This theatrical aspect of performativity is highly criticized for reducing identities to acts of putting on a role as one chooses. But the implications of understanding performativity as theatrical are crucial for understanding biological security. The structural analogy to theatrical performances allows for Butler's insistence that gender is "only real when performed" ("Performative" 527), which is fundamental for the understanding of biosecurity. As shown with the example of prenatal testing, biosecurity has to be performed and represented to become tangible. The security practice of testing is performative as it makes security present in a form of visualization such as ultrasound, MRI, colonoscopy, among many others. The biosecurity identity is "made" in the act of the security practice, only "being present" when it is actualized in performances. If identities are constructed by bodily performances and security practices are integral part of everyday life, then these practices are an inevitable part of identity. However, not only the biosecurity practices are highly performative: the body itself becomes stage and actor of the security drama.

In her theoretical approach to gender Butler describes embodiment as central for the constitution of an identity. She thus stresses the importance of the body as a means of being and a means of constructing and communicating identities. The body is therefore understood as a "communicative interjection" (Seale, *Constructing* 2) rather than merely a material object. Understanding the body as language makes it part of a symbolic system in which the body appears as "a historical idea," which Butler derives from Merleau-Ponty's *Phenomenology of Perception*. The body "gains its meaning through a concrete and

---

7   "Speaking Bodies" is a reference to Shoshana Felman *The Scandal of the Speaking Body*.

8   I do not mean to conflate performance as an art form and performance in every day life. I am aware that "[t]he stretch between theatrical and deconstructive meanings of 'performative' seems to span to polarities of, at either extreme, the *extroversion* of the actor, the *introversion* of the signifier" (Parker and Sedgwick 2). Nonetheless, I think that both understandings are crucial for the approach of performativity since also a suppression of acts is a form of staging, or rather not staging and hiding.

historically mediated expression in the world" ("Performative" 521). And this mediated expression is not only determined by race, class, and gender, but significantly by biosecurity narratives that define the healthy and able body, its movements and expressions, and its appearance in public.

Performativity describes identity not as something one simply is, but as an act taken on like a role. The bodily performance that produces social identity is understood as "an act which has been rehearsed, much as a script" (Butler, "Performative" 526). In this argument Butler relies as much on Derrida's notion of reiteration, as on Foucault's notion of discourse. The script refers to the reiterated meaning, which in the case of biosecurity is the readable body established by the rise of science.[9] With Foucault, Butler argues that the scripts for particular roles are not free-floating options to choose from. The theory of performativity focuses on how these bodily identities are produced within a social matrix of norms. Performances are therefore "never fully self-styled, for living styles have a history, and that history conditions and limits possibilities" (Butler, "Performative" 521). Bodily identity is thus a "reiterative and citational practice" (Butler, *Bodies* 2) that is governed by possibility and constraint.[10]

Focused on the restrictive norms of gender performances and the dynamics of gender relations, Butler refers to a "heterosexual matrix" (inter alia *Bodies* xxvii) as the normative cultural narrative which establishes meaning and genders persons. Biosecurity is another part of a greater set of cultural norms and ideals that serve as the comparative blueprint of an intelligible, normal, and valued body. The normative constraint, which compels subjects to embody and cite certain norms, is not restricted to gender performance. When Butler writes "that 'persons' only become intelligible through becoming gendered in conformity with recognizable standards of gender intelligibility" (*Gender Troubles* 22) she not only emphasizes the importance of gendering in our society, but thereby also stresses the significance of the body in general.

Butler defined gender (and gendered identity) as a speech act in which the subject materializes through embodiment. Making the body center stage of the self means also that the self is at risk from its body. Physical ability then becomes another key to the "range of possibilities" that constitute Butler's performatives. In other words, the materiality of the body is a decisive factor of how we (are able to) act and thus, according to Butler, how we perceive ourselves. Individuals are therefore in more than just one way overdetermined and limited by their bodies: discursively as well as biologically the body defines the self in its existence as a skin of constraint in forming an identity. And every "bodily betrayal" represents a potential disruption of an identity. The moment the individual afflicted with Alzheimer's Disease does not remember the way home or their own name for instance, stands paradigmatically for the injury the body can "inflict" on the

---

9   "The body is not passively scripted with cultural codes, as if it were a lifeless recipient of wholly pre-given cultural relations. But neither do embodied selves pre-exist the cultural conventions which essentially signify bodies" (Butler, "Performative" 526).

10   "The 'I' that is its body is, of necessity, a mode of embodying, and the 'what' that it embodies is possibilities. But here again the grammar of the formulation misleads, for the possibilities that are embodied are not fundamentally exterior or antecedent to the process of embodying itself" (Butler, "Performative" 521).

"self." The diagnosis of a disease often represents a performative shift in the identity of the afflicted individual, who has to renegotiate their identity, as represented famously in illness narratives. An equally important moment of rupture represents, however, the moment the body impedes us from performing our "normal" identities. It is not only the body that can be injured by disease, disability, accidents, and so forth. The body as central to performing one's identity represents at the same time its gravest enemy.

With the insistence on reiteration Butler explains how norms govern bodily performances, but most importantly she describes how performances hide their embeddedness in discourse producing "the illusion of an abiding gendered self" (Butler, "Performative" 519). Performances thus describe "a signifying practice that seeks to conceal its own working and to naturalize its effect" (*Gender Troubles* 184). This appearance as natural is one of the most important effects of biosecurity performances "that create the effect of the natural, the original, the inevitable" (Butler, *Gender Troubles* 23). This means, however, that identity is confined by cultural narratives that compel us to enact certain attributions as if they were unquestionable, given facts.

In this understanding of the constitutive constraint the subject and its behavior appear determined by discourse, "in no way . . . a locus of agency" (Butler, "Performative" 519). The subject appears almost tricked into following the script, or as otherwise oblivious to their being an accomplice to power discourses. Various scholars criticize that this element of constitutive constrain would foreclose the possibility of agency and therefore produce a limited subject. But Butler is careful to open up a space of possible resistance. She emphasizes the synchronic structure of performance as capable of challenging and opposing the diachronically established iterability of the body and its meaning. The performative scripts are thus "historically revisable criteria of intelligibility which produce and vanquish bodies that matter" (Butler, *Bodies* 14). Butler finds the possibility of transformation "in the arbitrary relation between such acts, in the possibility of a different sort of repeating" ("Performative" 520).[11]

To open up this possibility of resistance, bodily identity has to be understood as "an active process of embodying" (Butler, "Performative" 521). Embodying an identity is thus an act of taking up a position within a narrative frame, which Butler describes as essentially dramatic. As actors on the stage, individuals follow or transgress social scripts – establishing social identities. "One is not simply a body, but, in some very key sense, one does one's body" (ibid.). Doing one's body in the context of biosecurity not only refers to appearance and behavior in public, or the exclusion of the sick and disabled from public space. It describes the actual doing of one's body following different health regimens, such as surveillance medicine. To become a biosecurity individual is thus to "take up a position" in relation to previously established biosecurity narratives.[12] This positioning is most superficially the use of biosecurity practices to maintain and protect the bodily appearance, for instance by covering up signs of aging. However, biosecurity not only describes willingly performed acts and embodied identities. Also in the context of uncon-

---

11   Nonetheless, in such a resistance to the performative, the normative meaning is cited as that which is opposed, and thereby the cultural matrix is to a certain extend re-produced and re-enforced.

12   To explain the taking up of a position Butler relies on Lacan's positioning in a symbolic order.

trollable bodily appearances a staging and hiding of "conditions" must be understood as inherently performative.

Though biosecurity is broadly represented as "choice," in opting for practices that have a beneficial effect of protecting and improving life and quality of life, the biosecurity identity is also clearly an ascription. Biosecurity narratives position people and make them position themselves in determined relations to objects of security as well as to other people. They influence life and identity construction on an individual as well as a collective level. This "taking up a position" describes both a willed position, as well as an inescapable matrix in which the individual understands themself and others. Butler describes how gender is the most pervasive way of understanding a person, an almost inescapable compulsive categorization. She uses the example of naming a child: "naming is at once the setting of a boundary, and also the repeated inculcation of a norm" (Butler, *Bodies* 7). Similarly, biosecurity also seems to be one of the most common and pervasive ways of understanding a person.

Today the position of the biosecurity self, like the gendered self, precedes birth and an autonomous subject position, representing the first way how a potential human is understood. Biosecurity practices allow for the determination of gender before the fetus is born and therefore precede it. Considering the example of individual biosecurity and prenatal testing, biosecurity becomes the prime and prior category of understanding human life, the one that allows for the understanding of an identity in the first place. The ultrasound serves initially to assess the security state of the pregnancy; if no red flags are raised the technology can be used predominantly as a proleptic identity practice. The technoscientific practice stages a biosecurity identity on screen, looked at by the attending doctor and the expectant parent(s). This biosecurity identity is the deciding humanizing factor which allows for intelligibility and recognition – the formation of an identity. The biosecurity individual is in that sense indeed "a phenomenon [that] is named into being" (Butler, *Bodies* 13) by the performance of biosecurity practices.

Understanding identity as performative and procedural, means that an identity made in time is "in no way a stable identity" (Butler, "Performativity" 519). Identity in Butler is not just "in flux" as Stuart Hall puts it, but is literally becoming in the moment of the performative act in a "constant state of againness" (Taylor 21). In biosecurity this instability is part of the normative matrix that defines the identities. The biosecurity identity has to be constantly stabilized as the materiality itself is defined by change. This instability, representing a feared future, is the most forceful constitutive constraint producing biosecurity identities.

Biosecurity as an identity marker is not only something one is born with. It does not represent a fixed quality but rather a moving target like class identity, which can change throughout the life course. Rita Felski describes the distinction between race and class in "Nothing to Declare" as the difference between the "identity inescapable" (38) and the "contingency" (ibid.) produced by the permeability of class. The porous boundaries between different biosecurity positions are central elements of biosecurity. In the pre-emptive biosecurity discourse this permeability is the constituting logic of understanding the body and the self. But unlike class, biosecurity is marked by an inevitable "downward spiral" since health risks increase with age, and all life inescapably ends in dying and death. Similar to the concept of age, biosecurity changes with time. Rüdiger Kunow points out that, age is "a difference that time makes" ("Coming of Age" 295), or that comes with time.[13] Biosecurity identities, which include the ageing body, follow a similar inescapable temporality. They represent a construct by which people are understood, not in terms of a fixed identity marker but one that is in a constant process of becoming (or coming with time). Especially since biosecurity narratives today are focused on disease markers and susceptibilities that make bodily security often only appear in abstraction or in form of anticipation, performativity becomes ever more central.

For instance, the separation of identity from materiality challenges our notion of a biologically determined life course with its different phases (rise, climax, decline). The importance of performativity is especially prevalent during transitional phases.

> Models of the "life course" cannot . . . be seen to stand in any unmediated relationship with the materiality of the body. Rather, they present particular, often politicized, positions, which mobilize moral, legal, emotional and biological evidence and so lay rhetorical claim to the "real." (Draper and Hockey 43)

The transitions between distinct stages of life are ostensibly caused by biological processes of the body, which seem to naturally determine a person's changed identity as for instance in ageing. The implications for the identity of such a changed bodily existence, however, are based on cultural norms. Such transitions often rely on "performative shifts" that mark a rite of passage at a precise moment in time. They represent crucial stepping stones marking the biosecurity individual in their normative position in life and progression through life. These "performative shifts" a person realizes throughout the life span are often disguised as natural bodily transitions. Most of these physical transitions, which change the social status of a person, are accompanied by rituals. Biosecurity practices are an important part of these rites of passage today. This is most obvious in cases where the transition from security to insecurity is imperceivable for the individual.

However, biosecurity is not a construct that could be resolved by removing discriminatory practices, stereotypes and oppressions. A sick body does not necessarily become healthy by removing the negative cultural associations with a non-normative body. The corporeality itself thus seems to resist its absorption into discourse, at least initially.[14]

Bodily Matters: Biosecurity, Intangible Materiality, and the Body as Actor

The performativity of identity in general is easily plausible as identity traits and behavior rely on enactment to be recognizable. However, to understand biosecurity as performative implies not only the scriptedness of bodily behavior, as in willed acts prescribed by security narratives such as exercising, dieting, or the explicit transgression by resisting

---

13   Age itself is represented as lack by the biosecurity narrative, a process that has to be slowed down and prevented for as long as possible.

14   There are bodily facts that are undeniable and inevitable. "Surely there must be some kind of necessity that accompanies these primary and irrefutable experiences. And surely there is. But their irrefutability in no way implies what it might mean to affirm them and through what discursive means" (Butler, *Bodies* xi).

the normative script of biosecurity. Rather, it describes, according to Butler's theory of performativity, the relation to the body itself, to its very corporeality. When Butler claims that gender is performative she argues much more than that outward behavior relies on performative scripts. She asserts that "the body is not self-identical or merely factic materiality" ("Performatives" 521). This means that not only the identity is essentially performative, but also the materiality of the body itself (on which the identity relies). If the body is essentially "a process of materialization that stabilizes over time to produce the effect of boundary, fixity, and surface we call matter" (Butler, *Bodies* 9) then the security recognized in and embodied by the body should similarly be understood as a process of materialization. Biosecurity thus represents a "regulatory ideal" (Butler, *Bodies* 1) or a security imaginary that subjects are motivated to aim for, or to maintain. This is crucial in respect to biological security narratives that largely define and categorize this materiality in abled and disabled, healthy and sick, or at risk. Like sex, biosecurity does not represent neutral scientific descriptions but "regulatory norms" (Butler, *Bodies* 2) which materialize through and in the corporeality of the individual.

A body free of disability and disease can thus not be understood as a "natural" state but rather represents a norm or construction, which is today predominantly conceptualized in security terms. The construction of the body has been recognized in various fields of theory, most importantly in Disability Studies, and Aging Studies. There is the attempt in Disability Studies to solve the problem with the distinction between construction and materiality introducing the distinction between impairment, as the supposed "neutral," and disability, as the social and cultural construction.[15] Similarly, the separation of disease and illness attempts to distinguish medical definition from individual experience. However, this distinction seems to avoid the paradoxes of bodily being, a being that is always in society, always both private and public. The easy division between value laden construction and neutral materiality seems to obliterate that materiality appears always already within a construction. The distinction of disability and impairment seems to risk producing a further way of concealing a construction as natural. Shelley Tremain argues that impairment also has to be understood as a construction and "effect of power" (188), since materiality cannot be understood as distinct of its construction. In Butler's own words, "the fixity of the body, its contours, its movements, will be fully material, but materiality will be rethought as the effect of power, as power's most productive effect" (Butler, *Bodies* 2).

But how can the insistence of "corporeal style" (Butler, "Performative" 521) and "forced materialization" persist when applied to biological vulnerabilities in terms of a cancer affliction or genetic diseases? In this context performativity has to be rethought in terms of the relation between the agentic subject and the materiality as passive. As performativity understands the body in terms of communication, this communication cannot be reduced to "conscious enactments" but also accounts for "uncontrollable" bodily appear-

---

15   For the social construction of disability see Simi Linton "What is Disability Studies" or Tom Shakespeare "The Social Model of Disability" for the British context. For the cultural construction of disability see Anne Waldschmidt "Disability goes Cultural" and Lennard Davis "Visualizing the Disabled Body."

ances.[16] The structure of the dramatic is helpful to understand the relation between self and corporeality in such acts that are out of the subject's control. Butler claims that the body is "a materiality that bears meaning, if nothing else, and the manner of this bearing is fundamentally dramatic" (Butler, "Performative" 521). The individual represents in many constellations of biosecurity not a willingly performing actor but the audience of the performance of the body. The body is thus not only stage but also actor of the drama of biosecurity. Since a performance is constituted by the interaction of actor and audience though, the individual is not passive, but rather active in decoding the bodily performance, which is overdetermined by security narratives. This is not a radicalization of Butler's theory but essential in the theoretical frame of performativity, in which the materiality of the body can only become intelligible according to prior conceptualizations. The performative scripts and stage directions for this drama of security are provided by biomedical discourses: any deviation from the course that "ought" to be followed by the actor/body is eyed suspiciously and corrected if possible.

Today in academic discourse it hardly seems radical to deny the natural connection between sex and gender, it is indisputable that the distinction between masculinity and femininity is a cultural construction. Nonetheless the complete negation of a "natural" that somehow manifests itself in our acts – that is thus expressive and not performative – remains a heavily critiqued aspect of the theory of performativity. The theory is criticized primarily because it is understood to dissolve the body – its suffering, feeling, experience, authenticity – into discourse and language. But especially in a field of scientifically defined security with a forceful truth claim to the objective description of biological states and processes it is important to insist on studying security as performative. Science, as I have shown, does not establish neutral categories of security, but represents an ableist and healthist security discourse that is deeply influenced by social and cultural bias. In regard to gender, Tremain shows how even the naming of molecules in the study of hormones, is deeply engrained by "prevailing cultural ideas" (191) thus producing sexed materialities.[17] Biosecurity practices simulate a stable relation of material sign and knowable fact, representing the body as readable text. "[T]he relationships are not self-evident, however, but instead make visible use of the body to create complex bodily associations or connections which are highly *mediated*" (Draper and Hockey 51) by cultural narratives.

Furthermore, Butler's insistence on the constructedness of bodily matter does not deny the material existence, but the possibility "to know" ("Performative" 524) the body in its neutral (not culturally predetermined) materiality. "[T]he existence and the facticity of the material or natural dimension of the body are not denied, but reconceived as

---

16   Butler asserts that "the *appearance of substance* is precisely that, a constructed identity, a performative accomplishment which the mundane social audience, including the actors themselves, come to believe and to perform in the mode of belief" (Butler, "Performative" 520).

17   With reference to Anne Fausto-Sterling's *Sexing the Body* she explains "with each choice these scientists and researchers made about how to measure and name the molecules they studied, they naturalized prevailing cultural ideas about gender. In short, the emergence of scientific accounts about sex in particular and human beings in general can be understood only if scientific discourses and social discourses are seen as inextricable elements of a cultural matrix of ideas and practices" (Tremain 191).

distinct from the process by which the body comes to bear cultural meaning" (Butler, "Performative" 520). Butler thus questions the accessibility of the prelinguistic or natural "pure body" (*Bodies* 10), as the materiality appears to us always already absorbed in its construction. In the reading of biologic ascriptions, definitions, categorizations, and negotiations of the biosecurity, the understanding of the body as something that "bears meaning" ("Performative" 521) is therefore a valuable analytic tool.

Biosecurity narratives claim the body and its materiality as a prelinguistic site and undeniable "truth." Similarly as the category of sex, biosecurity becomes "something like a fiction, perhaps a fantasy, retroactively installed at a prelinguistic site to which there is no direct access" (Butler, *Bodies* 5). Security narratives that describe the body, its life, its potentials, represent the norm against which the individual can understand their own corporeality. Instead of purely objective descriptions the biosecurity narratives represent "necessary fictions" to use Butler's own words (*Gender Troubles* 98), that claim the prelinguistic site of the body, rather than merely describing it. This means more bluntly that biologically inflected security narratives with their claim to "the natural" create the meaning of the very body they are describing. Apart from that, "natural" processes are hard to find in the biosecurity culture of the U.S. that had started the race to the inside of the body already in the 1950s. With Butler I would like to suggest that "[t]he point of such an exposition is . . . to show that to invoke matter is to invoke a sedimented history" (Butler, *Bodies* 49). It thus offers the possibility to understand how biosecuritized bodies materialize.

To materialize the norm and make it pervasive biosecurity narratives rely on the formation of the other, which Butler understands as both the abject that is needed to constitute the self and the spectator or witness. Biosecurity narratives establish what Butler calls an "exclusionary matrix" (Butler, *Bodies* 3). They describe not only the ideal (of a biosecurity individual) but also a "domain of abject beings, [...] those 'unlivable' and 'uninhabitable' zones of social life that are nevertheless densely populated" (ibid.). The abject in biosecurity is most frequently attached to the very materiality of those bodies that are not "normatively human" (Butler, *Precarious* xv). These non-normative corporealities serve to form and understand the norm. The self is thus also here understood "contrapunctually" (Said 52), in opposition to its supposed other. "The subject is constituted through the force of exclusion and abjection (Butler, *Bodies* 3). In biosecurity, the other is the non-normative body – the impaired, sick, old, depressed – contrasting the healthy, young, and productive body. The other is in Butler's theory necessary for the self as "the 'constitutive outside' against which the accepted subject may be understood and defined" (Armour and St. Ville 7). However, in the context of biosecurity abject and desired, or "the prohibited and permitted" as Foucault put it (*Security* 20), no longer exist purely as binaries of normative and non-normative materiality, as I have shown before. In biosecurity terms the abject is at the same time inside and outside of the self in a literal sense, since the potential to become the abject comes from within and forms a constant potential. This should not only be understood in a psychoanalytical way, but is rather represented as a (possibly) inescapable future scenario. The abject defines "failed matter," which in biosecurity narratives turns into a continuously "failing matter." In biosecurity narratives the abject serves to make the risk recognized in the body tangible, and make their meaning felt.

Bodily matter is disciplined according to an able norm, and the appearance of "failed matter" is confronted by social sanctions and constraints which are not subtle but rather obvious in the social, cultural, and economic repercussions that follow if we do not do our bodies "properly." What Butler describes as the punishing for transgressive gender performances, which are important in compelling people to "do their gender right" (Butler, "Performative" 522) is easily translatable to biosecurity identities. For instance, the individual who does not comply with security scripts is punished institutionally through loss of healthcare coverage or higher deductibles. Furthermore, people who do not conform with the biosecurity standard, because of an increased risk, a preexisting condition, or other corporeal differences, are punished in similar ways. Additionally, individuals are sanctioned socially through isolation which affects the disabled, sick and elderly. Similarly, social judgment is cast in reaction to certain risk identities such as Type 2 diabetes which is deemed a "lifestyle disease," or in response to disabilities that are defined as "preventable" by prenatal testing. The shame and blame projected onto the diseased or disabled body shows that the body, also in its inevitable materiality, is "a social phenomenon in the public sphere" (Butler, *Precarious* 26).

However, the other is not just understood as an arm of panoptical power.[18] The other is a necessary part of performativity. To claim that "[a]lthough we struggle for rights over our own bodies, the very bodies for which we struggle are not quite ever only our own" (Butler, *Precarious* 26) indicates that performativity is a "symbolizing practice." It therefore needs the other, the "interlocutor" as Austin called it. The position of the witness is essential for the performative process to work since the body requires a watching or witnessing, a reading and accepting or refusing to accept what it signifies. When Butler claims that "my body is and is not mine" (Butler, *Precarious* 26)[19] the other does therefore not only appear as constitutive constraint but as a necessary constituent of recognition. By understanding the self as "invariably in community, impressed upon by others, impinging upon them as well, and in ways that are not fully in my control" (*Precarious* 27), Butler is considering the ethical claim the other makes, thereby emphasizing the deeply relational structure of performativity. As indicated before, a speech act is deeply relational, depending on and being constituted by the interaction of actor and audience. As audience I also understand the subject itself, which turns into a "compulsory witness" of their own body's performance. Such a bodily performance has to be recognizable to be "successful" and to produce an intelligible self.

But the claim of the other, as Butler argues, has its social and cultural limits. She opens a possible space in which the performative fails to produce its abiding effect. "[T]he failure to mark that which resists symbolization" (*Bodies* 21) becomes visible and important in the precariousness of human existence. In *Precarious Life* Butler turns to Levinas's "face" to describe the human suffering that might exceed its embeddedness in construc-

---

18   "Panopticism" is one of Foucault's techniques of power based on the prison architecture of Bentham's Panopticon, which he used to define how individuals are disciplined (*Discipline* 195–228).

19   In genetics the body is indeed literally mine and not mine as we do not hold ownership of our DNA. Once submitted it becomes a free for all, meaning companies hold it.

tion.[20] "For representation to convey the human, then, representation must not only fail, but it must show its failure. There is something unrepresentable that we nevertheless seek to represent, and that paradox must be retained in the representation we give" (Butler, *Precarious* 144). But regardless of this possible unrepresentability in suffering that could potentially reveal the human, it nonetheless has to be recognized and therefore understood through discourse and language. Though pain and suffering are the most prominent tropes of unrepresentability,[21] in biosecurity practices they are routinely assessed, qualified and quantified to facilitate their treatment. Butler herself also concedes: "if vulnerability is one precondition for humanization, and humanization takes place differently through variable norms of recognition, then it follows that vulnerability is fundamentally dependent on existing norms of recognition if it is to be attributed to any human subject" (Butler, *Precarious* 39).

Biosecurity discourses define precisely these norms and delimit what is understood as "a life that qualifies for recognition" (Butler, *Precarious* 24). Studying "common corporeal vulnerability" in the context of grievability, Butler describes dehumanization as a form of "derealization" (Butler, *Precarious* 34) which manifests in the ungrievability of certain deaths. This discursive "derealization" translates easily to failed bodies that do not meet the standards of acceptable life. It applies to all those lives that are deemed unlivable, and disposable because "certain lives are not considered lives at all, they cannot be humanized" (Butler, *Precarious* 34). The discursive exclusion from the "we" or "I" "then gives rise to a physical violence that in some sense delivers the message of dehumanization that is already at work in culture" (ibid.). In the drama of biosecurity directed by a discourse that seeks to prevent and preempt disease and disability this question of good life is defined in future scenarios, it defines what will become livable or unlivable life. The abject which motivates the biosecurity practices "through the regulation of phantasmatic identification" (Butler, *Bodies* 97) is thus more often than not represented as a matter of good life or precarious existence, of life or death. It is deeply felt and determined by fear, anxiety, and shame, but also hope, relief, and happiness. The body is thus not only understood rationally but is marked by feeling.

Marked by Feelings: Biosecurity and the Force of Affect

The pervasiveness of biosecurity narratives seems to eradicate the possibility of experience outside of normative scripts. To deny the possibility of perceiving the body as a natural entity apart from rational thought influenced by the prescriptive biosecurity narratives appears to deny other ways of knowing the body, "such as affectively and experientially" as Julia Walker argues (166). But biosecurity identities are highly affective and

---

20   Levinas describes the "face" of the other as an ethical claim of the priority of the other's mortality over mine: "In that relation with the face, in a direct relation with the death of the other, you probably discover that the death of the other has priority over yours, and over your life" (Levinas, *Alterity* 164).

21   In the study of suffering it is asserted that suffering "comes unsharably into our midst" (Scarry 4) and that it is "inaccessible to language" (Scarry 5).

intensely felt. In fact, it is often a feeling, pain, and suffering associated with the failing body that make biosecurity identities become relevant and central to the individual in the first place. Quoting Drew Leder's *The Absent Body*, Ahmed asserts that "the body tends to disappear when functioning unproblematically" (4 qtd. in Ahmed, *Politics* 26) and that its dysfunctioning and "[t]he intensity of feelings like pain recalls us to our body surfaces: pain seizes me back to my body" (ibid.). It resembles a moment of "crisis" that interrupts the "silence of the organs" (Canguilhem, *Writing* 43). To live with constant pain due to rheumatism, the fear and pain felt when the body does not retain its fluids as it is supposed to, when it cannot perform daily tasks, these intimate feelings are central to how an identity can be performed and understood. The physiological pain and discomfort that accompanies many stages and shades of bodily existence makes affects essential for understanding biosecurity.

However, to presuppose that these feelings are more "truthful" or "authentic" insights into the human seems to miss that also this most intimate knowledge depends on the mediation through the symbolic, as Eve Kosofsky Sedgwick shows with regard to shame (*Touching Feeling* 35–66). On the one hand, feelings and affects are experienced with and through the body, which then becomes determined by this experience.[22] On the other hand, the objects that cause experience and affect are themselves positioned inside the symbolic. Hair loss, for instance, is a vastly different experience for men than for women, for young than for old. Bodily processes and their affective meaning do not only appear as present events but are anticipated within determined contextual frames. This anticipation of an incident largely influences our experience, or even the capacity to experience, as for example "the placebo effect" demonstrates.[23] The fact that a "fictive" object can cause change in a body shows how important knowledge, or rather thought and belief are to the very working of the body and the way it feels. Similarly, the anticipatory feeling toward pain proves to greatly influence the experience of pain itself. It matters significantly if pain is a temporary state on the way to recovery, or a potential life long presence. Seale names for example the pain of childbirth, which "under certain circumstances, is psychologically and culturally shaped into an expression of personal growth, so that it may even be welcomed, and attempts at anesthesia scorned as leading to 'inauthentic' experience" (Seale, *Constructing* 42). The feeling of pain and suffering is thus greatly influenced by the cultural context in which it occurs.[24] The understanding of "positive" pain in childbirth represents a radical departure from the security narrative of painless childbirth dominating the understanding of security for most of the 20th century as previously discussed. This shows that performativity must allow for change as radical as the complete reversal

---

22   The body is so central for certain emotions that "qualities of excitement, joy, fear, sadness, shame, and anger cannot be further described if one is missing the necessary effector and receptor apparatus" (Sedgwick, *Touching Feeling* 20).

23   The placebo effect has been tested showing in "animal and human experiments in which the 'expectation' of certain effects led to measurable physiological changes in the subjects" (Schleifer 128).

24   Ahmed asserts that "the experience of pain does not cut off the body in the present, but attaches this body to the world of other bodies, an attachment that is contingent on elements that are absent in the lived experience of pain" (Ahmed, *Politics* 28).

of the understanding of the feeling of a natural process.[25] The pains of childbirth are of course not unreal, artificial, or nonexistent, but their experience is decisively shaped by biosecurity narratives that create the *mode* of anticipating.

Pain thus has an invariably social side to it and does not only appear as "unsharable," or as a de- or re-centering of the self. "So while the experience of pain may be solitary, it is never private" (Ahmed, *Politics* 29). Ahmed emphasizes the performativity of pain by pointing out the importance of recognizing and witnessing to "authenticate its [pain's] existence" (*Politics* 31). This is important when regarding biosecurity, which is dedicated to pain management and control as I have previously pointed out. However, the "Biomedical TechnoService Complex, Inc." (Clarke et al., "Biomedicalization" 162) does not tend only to physiological pain. Emotions are tightly managed and controlled since the messianic narrative of scientific salvation has expanded to nearly all processes of life. Especially in crisis moments of biosecurity a complementary pharmaceutical treatment helps to manage the – predominantly negative – feelings that arise when the body dysfunctions. As biomedicalized bodily processes, emotions are treated with antidepressants and tranquilizers to keep the patient in the proper "mindset" to pursue biosecurity and fight the battle against nature's mistakes with the weapons of technoscientific biosecurity.[26] I will therefore not turn to affects as an "alternative knowledge" about the body, the human, or the self (Thrift).[27] Rather than focusing on the feeling body trying to find the moment "the human" reveals itself and its "common vulnerability" in the failure of narrative and construction I will argue that biosecurity narratives produce bodies that are marked by feeling.[28]

Both, pain and affects leave their imprints on the body in form of a memory or scar tissue, but affects mark bodies also in their performative, temporally transient dimension. As explained earlier with Butler, the abject or the other to the normative ideal is centrally marked by affects, especially fear, shame, and disgust. The failing and failed corporeality is stigmatized as already Ervin Goffman has argued. In biological terms such a stigma is most commonly recognized in the body as a missing limb, a malignant melanoma, or a missing chromosome, which are perceived as signs coming from the

---

25   The concept of suffering is complicated as a consensus is continuously challenged by the interplay of corporeality and mental processes, questioning "how much is about the physical body, how much is 'perceptual,' psychological or even cultural and political" (Kellehear 388). For a more detailed discussion see Eric Cassel's *Nature of Suffering*, Elaine Scarry's *The Body in Pain*, or Ronald Schleifer's *Intangible Materialism*.

26   This practice is especially prevalent in the "old old," who are frequently treated for geriatric depression to prevent a premature psychological process of dying (Kellehear 389).

27   The considerations and renegotiations of the biological and cultural sides of affect can already be found in William James's (1884) "What is an Emotion" from a psychological perspective and is continued in diverse fields of research today. Brian Nigel Thrift, Eric Shouse, or William Connolly respond to the supposed problem of the privileged position of rationality in critical theory by turning to biologized forms of explanations stressing scholars such as Ekman and evolution, recovering Tomkins in the case of Sedgwick, or using Damasio in the case of Massumi. Ruth Leys argues that this turn to biology is more than precarious first and foremost because she accuses e.g. Massumi of misusing the results for the benefit of his argument. What lies at the heart of these considerations is the problem of agency and determinacy of human action and reaction.

28   I will use the terms emotion and affect synonymously.

body creating a seemingly natural reaction to the bodily materiality. Affects thus mark the body and individual in their positionality within the security narrative.

Like class belonging, biosecurity "belonging" is marked "as a structure of feeling, a complex psychological matrix acquired in childhood" (Felski 39).[29] As indicated before, biosecurity identities are "becoming in time" a bodily reality that is marked by change, which is more often than not encountered in a shameful manner. Shame describes, according to Felski, "a range of experiences of dislocation including those of class" (39). The shame and stigma associated with shifts in biosecurity are similar forms of "dislocating." Shame is an affect that literally marks the skin, making the person blush, stutter, or sweat. "[S]hame impresses upon the skin, as an intense feeling of the subject 'being against itself'" (Ahmed, "Politics" 75). It triggers the desire for concealment (ibid.) and decisively increases physiological pain or discomfort produced by the failing body, as studies of psychology show (Cohen and Pressman). What is shameful, however, is unquestionably influenced by cultural narratives. Shame "comprises a painful experience of self-consciousness, resulting from a sudden recognition of a discrepancy between one's behavior and that of one's peer" (Felski 39), a discrepancy between the "ought to" and the "reality."[30]

In the context of biosecurity, shame does not come only from within the individual but is attached to the bodily matter in a process Ahmed calls "passionate attachments" ("Affective" 118).[31] She explains in her theory how affect "shapes the surfaces of bodies and worlds" ("Affective" 121). Taking the "surfacing of bodies" ("Affective" 117) a bit more literal than in Ahmed's own use, I suggest that the affects used and produced by biosecurity narratives codetermine the meaning of the body surface proper. In describing an ideal of health the narratives attach certain bodies with affects, which marks them and determines the meaning of the materiality of those bodies. Biosecurity narratives thus establish and reiterate affective relations to the body as object, to biosecurity and its practices that "define" the body, as well as to other people. The largely anticipatory biosecurity focuses on future states and risk, rather than only on a present bodily state, producing seemingly stable affective attachments that are crucial for the performativity of biosecurity to be successful in the Austinean sense. Especially fear, anxiety and hope become central if not the only forms of relating to the future and are therefore central to understanding and experiencing biosecurity. In preventive and pre-emptive biosecurity practices, this affective relation to a future is especially crucial for the understanding of

---

29   Rita Felski asserts in her study of the lower middle class that class belonging relies on a structure of feeling paraphrasing Carolyn Steedman's *Landscape for a Good Woman*.

30   This is not an inescapable experience, as I have shown with the patient and disability rights movement, which struggled for a re-evaluation and renegotiation of these ascription, representing a position of empowerment: "we can only be ashamed by somebody whose 'look' matters to me. . . . If we feel shame, we feel shame because we have failed to approximate 'an ideal' that has been given to us" (Ahmed, "Politics" 76).

31   Ahmed uses Marxist theory of accumulation to understand the effect of circulation of affective attachments. She describes the "accumulation of affective value over time" within an affective economy (ibid.) The circulation of affects that produce a kind of "truth" effect that simulates an inherent connection between object and affects ("Affective" 120).

biosecurity. The affectivity produced in the performance of biosecurity practices represents often the only form of relating to the techno-scientifically produced futures. These anticipatory affects make a future state tangible "as if" it was present, as I have shown with the example of the biosecurity pregnancy.

Rather than necessarily fearing a particular disease, however, biosecurity today adds a constant insecurity, an affective relation of self and body that can be described similarly to class anxiety of the lower middle class. Felski writes that "because of its acute anxiety about status, it is hypersensitive to the most minute signs of class distinction" (40). Class anxiety translates into biosecurity anxiety of a subject that can never be sure of itself. However, the biosecurity individual has to rely on techno-scientifically facilitated evidence, results, diagnosis – or in the best case no diagnosis, to know "the most minute signs" of potential difference. In a perpetual state of becoming the biosecurity individual seems suspended in the ambiguity of feeling secure, healthy, and hopeful, and the fear, anxiety and shame associated with the "defect" bodily matter.

But biosecurity narratives cannot be reduced to fearful doomsday visions that haunt the individual and produce negative affective relations to the body. Rather, as I have emphasized before, biosecurity represents a forceful messianic narrative of scientific salvation. The negative emotions are contrasted by the hope attached to biosecurity practices and biomedical knowledge production, which promise to offer relief and another attempt at happiness. "What is at stake in these stories is not just survival, or getting better, but living life to the full, again" (Sunder Rajan, *Biocapital* 187). As in the apocalyptic security narratives of national biosecurity, science represents the katechontic element which can avert the inevitable demise.

Part II: Fictions of Biosecurity

The time, has come, it may be said,
To dream of many things;
Of genes – and life – and human cells –
Of Medicine – and Kings.
Edward Tatum

These lines, which Edward Tatum offered at the inauguration of the Merck Sharp and Dohme laboratories in 1966 represent genetic research as the harbinger of future security. His poem celebrates the coming of genetics and its push for research in genetic engineering. It reiterates the messianic narrative of scientific salvation that was established by the biological revolution of the early to mid 20th century and stands paradigmatically for the hopes invested in genetic research. The age of the gene heralded in these lines has appeared graspable, an imminent coming of genetic science, fulfilling the messianic promise of science. Over half a decade later, the poem has become an almost staple reference and citation for scientific projects promoting their relevance and promises to this day.[1] But these lines do not just represent the fervent belief in science as the arbiter of security and herald of the messianic hope for humanity. They also indicate how much biosecurity relies on cultural forms of narrativizing, and on cultural imageries that are part of a cultural archive. Tatum articulates his vision for genetic engineering not in scientific explanations but in the traditional stanza form of the ballad with an alternating iambic tetrameter and iambic trimester. He uses this familiar poetic and artistic form to convey and enforce the message this verse is meant to express: a promise of future security.[2] In doing so he formulates a fictive narrative of a future (security), a "necessary fiction" (Butler, *Gender Troubles* 98) to construct and make pervasive the promise of security, which science is to represent. As argued before, security only becomes present and

---

1   Such as NIH review on CRISPR-Cas technology and Stem Cells (Waddington et al. 9).
2   Tatum uses the poem to "paraphrase" ("Molecular Biology" 31) the tenor of his opening speech. He further cites and adapts Lewis Carroll's 1871 poem "The Walrus and the Carpenter" from *Through the Looking Glass*.

pervasive in the stories we tell ourselves and others about it. In part II I will therefore turn to these necessary fictions by reading cultural representations of individual(ized) biosecurity.

In part I have shown that biosecurity narratives formulate projections of a future, and represent therefore a narrative act of making a future present. The security narratives and the promises established by biomedicine and biotechnology thereby create a close relation to the narrative form of fiction.[3] This association is often used to dismiss either utopian or dystopian visions of a promised biological future. Both critics and supporters of biomedical progress use this label "as a way of trivializing the position of the other, while proclaiming that the research they cite is on the verge of transforming human nature and that the future scenarios they describe are plausible and impending" (Clayton, "Ridicule" 318). But the relation of biosecurity narratives and fiction is closer than such an accusatory rhetoric would like to admit. Not only are narratives necessary to justify security practices, such as costly research, medical interventions, or medical surveillance, but the rhetoric and articulations of research goals or new discoveries bear close resemblance to fictional narratives.[4]

The claim of the "fiction of biosecurity" has two lines of argument. On the one hand, it implies the performative understanding as something non-referential that is "made up," less in a purely imaginative way but in a productive sense of "creating," which I have discussed in the first part of this book. On the other hand, it gestures at the similarities between fiction (as a literary/artistic genre) and security narratives (be they fiction or not). The narrative construction is essential in "making present" the "cultural imaginary" (Iser, Fluck) of security. The claim of fictionality therefore serves to shed light on the production and reproduction of (bio)security narratives as well as the narrative construction used to establish the master-narrative of biosecurity.

These biosecurity fictions circulate in various different forms and pervade society and culture at every turn, shaping the material realities of a "biosecurity culture." However, they not only describe a collective future security but suffuse the individual and intimate narratives of the self, becoming part of individual lives and life narratives. They heavily influence the understanding of the self, and identity formation on a collective as well as individual level. As cultural forms, these narratives represent not only fictions of biosecurity but represent necessary fictions as stories "we tell ourselves . . . in order to live" (Didion).[5] I chose, therefore, to analyze different forms of life writing as expres-

---

3   In fact, both fiction and science always had a very interdependent relationship. Clayton especially emphasizes how "discourses surrounding genetic enhancement is inflected with the 'science-fictional habit of mind'" ("Ridicule" 320), and also other scholars such as Collin Milburn and Eugene Thacker have suggested similar interrelations. Similarly, Latour points out that outside of the laboratory science is almost always represented "as the mirror image of the world" ("The More Manipulation, the Better" 349).

4   Jay Clayton even asserts that science statements of bioethics bear a striking similarity to the genre of Science Fiction (of the 1950s). He exemplifies this with an array of almost indistinguishable quotes from both fiction and science concerning the nearing (posthuman) future ("Ridicule").

5   In Time and Narrative Paul Ricoeur has suggested that narratives are necessary to make time and human existence meaningful (52). Similarly, cognitive studies have increasingly suggested that life is lived and made meaningful in narrative form, reiterating Ricoeur's early concept of "narrative

sions of what I have called the biosecurity individual. These expressions of self, which I do not restrict to non-fiction nor to written texts, represent a promising vantage point on how security narrative are constructed and how they change our relation to the body and impact our understanding of individual life and self.

In the analysis of the biosecurity narratives I will attempt to avoid the pitfalls of both "security realism" (Völz, "Aestheticizing" 619) which reads texts for proof of political and sociological concepts, as well as overwriting the violence and oppressions of security practices by prioritizing aesthetic concepts as if they were apolitical (D. Watson, "Beautiful Walls"). Committed to a performative approach, the aesthetic and the political can hardly be seen as divisible entities, nor can they be fully understandable without one another. The narrative construction of security and its aesthetic qualities are thus important for a more thorough understanding of the material effects produced by these narrative practices. I will emphasize the narrative construction and aesthetics of the text to make clear how security becomes pervasive motivating individuals to act. Similar to Völz I wish to focus on how security narratives "appeal" to people (Foucault, *Security* 21). While Völz seeks to investigate the "appeal" of the concept of security by analyzing the narratives provided in literary fiction, my own approach focuses on diverse discursive forms emphasizing the antagonisms, commonalities, and reciprocities of the different forms of biosecurity narratives. I chose different discursive formations to argue that fictions of biosecurity and its intertextual dependence on a messianic narrative of scientific salvation are not restricted to fictional renderings. I will therefore turn to the genre of life writing and Huntington's Disease; I will read diverse forms of testimony as activism and performance in the context of breast cancer; I will focus on documentary and testimony in the process of dying, and I will analyze fictional narratives. The discursive formations of the security narratives – all with their own specific claims to "truth" – are crucial for the understanding of security and identity represented by these narratives.

Understanding narratives as the most crucial way in which humans understand themselves and their surroundings logically implies that these narratives take on a variety of different forms and, thus, cannot be restricted to specific genres, nor to the traditional understanding of a text as a written document. Nonetheless, in the analysis of the cultural representation of biosecurity, narratives will be analyzed in Literary Studies terms. I will analyze the biosecurity narratives provided in these different discursive formations like fictional narratives, regarding them as constructed. They represent a constructed story through the "artistic construction of incidents" (Aristotle, 1450, 29–32), though not necessarily following the Aristotelian ideal model of beginning, middle and end established in the *Poetics*. Narratives are thus defined by temporally organized incidents which are instigated by a change or obstacle as the plot generator. In the selected narratives, "security" represents the organizing principle establishing the causal relation that gives meaning to the story, to paraphrase E.M. Forster's famous definition of the plot. It is thus important to distinguish between story (histoire) and discourse as established by Gerard Genette's narrative theory. The discursive formation chosen, as well as the way the "text" is assembled are crucial for understanding security

---

identity" ("Narrative"), while scholars such as Jerome Bruner suggest that life is constructed in the act of writing (and reading) an autobiographical text.

as something decisively influenced by voice, perspective, choice of protagonists, and narrative frame, as also Annick T. R. Wibben stresses in her analysis of security narratives regarding 9/11. The narrative construction of expressing the story (histoire) in discourse thus also defines the meaning of security.

In all four examples, security, its maintenance or recovery, represents the motor of those stories and their overt teleology. The security narratives are therefore often end-directed narratives. The closure that many security narratives provide are based, however, on promises of (a) future, which stands in contrast to and in constant struggle with threats. "An ideal typical security narrative," Völz asserts, "opposes the present with two different futures" ("A Nation" n.p.). He defines this tension between security and insecurity competing for the future as a conjunction or interplay of utopian and dystopian narrative. He asserts that the mutual dependence between dystopian and utopian narrative elements "prevents" either from "becoming proper dystopias or utopias" (Völz, "A Nation" n.p.). Especially in the context of biosecurity this competition between hope and fear is crucial to give shape to a pervasive and convincing security narrative.

Utopian and dystopian narratives in the context of scientific progress and medicine as gatekeeper of security have a long tradition, and have pervaded cultures in diverse ways. Literary history is filled with representations, negotiations, and aestheticizations of the messianic narrative of scientific salvation and its all-encompassing security promise, as well as with its downsides and potential dangers. These fictional renderings range from classics such as Mary Shelley's *Frankenstein; or, The Modern Prometheus* (1818), and H.G. Wells' *The Island of Doctor Moreau* (1898), to Theodor Sturgeon's *More than Human* (1953), and Kazuo Ishiguro's *Never Let Me Go* (2005). But also less overtly fictional discourses in the context of biomedical and biotechnological advances have a long tradition of either "utopian" visions of scientific developments such as Donna J. Haraway's "Cyborg Manifesto" or warnings about possible biotechnologically facilitated dystopias, such as the warnings of an engineered and "purified" society in Francis Fukuyama's *Our Posthuman Future*. Similarly, science journalism has followed these two narrative frames in an at times precarious way.[6] In fact, the fields of utopian and dystopian writing could be understood as a form of what Hayden White calls "emplotment" (*Metahistory* 12).

Biosecurity narratives, however, do not provide a narrative frame for historical events only, but rather for a future. While the narratives of medical and scientific progress could probably be categorized in what White defines as "Romance" (*Metahistory* 135–162), more importantly biosecurity narratives shift to a different temporal frame.[7] In "Progress Ver-

---

6   The relation of science journalism and the public has been studied (and criticized) widely (Nelkin, *Selling Science*; Conrad, "Use of Expertise") pointing toward the simplified and sensationalized representation of scientific studies. And since "science journalists become gatekeepers for the infusion of scientific information into the public sphere" (Conrad, "Use of Expertise" 285) these utopian promises of cures and new knowledges or dystopian headlines on newly discovered threats play a crucial role in how science in understood in public discourse.

7   History as romance expresses, according to White, the continual progress toward improvement, very much expressing a teleological idea of history. Romance was "the narrative form to be used to make sense out of the historical process conceived as a struggle of essential virtue against a virulent, but ultimately transitory, vice" (*Metahistory* 150). The other forms are comedy, tragedy, and satire.

sus Utopia" Frederic Jameson asserts that the birth of science fiction represented a new understanding of reality. In accordance to Lukacs's theory of the historical novel Jameson asserts that the shift to utopian narratives expresses a different consciousness to that of the historical novel. "Capitalism demands in this sense a different experience of temporality" (149), one that he recognizes in Science Fiction. Though not focusing on Science Fiction texts, the future represented in biosecurity narratives similarly reflects the present rather than the particular vision of a represented future only, as Jameson asserts. Especially in *Seeds of Time* he makes clear that utopia is always ideology expressing and reflecting the present rather than the future. In the same manner the biosecurity narratives I will analyze represent a present ideology, and are at the same time intervening in this present.

Biosecurity narratives and their "ideal typical" (Völz, "A Nation" n.p.) form of utopian and dystopian narrative elements take on a particular American narrative turn, which further emphasizes this temporal relationality of present and future. The drama of biological security is frequently rendered in apocalyptic narratives lamenting the status quo that would lead to doom and destruction, as in the discussions of the grey doom, or the obesity crisis among many others.[8] Jay Clayton even recognizes a specific form of "scientific jeremiads" ("Ridicule" 334), which functions as a "spiritual renewal" by creating a threatening scenario to "motivate people to act in history – to resist a feared future" (Clayton, "Ridicule" 335), similar to the Puritan predecessor.

Jeremiads are often read and understood as lamentations about the status quo in the contemporary time they were written in, representing doomsday visions of the nearing end. Sacvan Bercovitch asserts in his seminal study on the American Jeremiad that

> its distinctiveness, however, lies not in the vehemence of its complaint but in precisely the reverse. The essence of the sermon form that the first native-born American Puritans inherited from their fathers, and then "developed, amplified, and standardized," is its unshakable optimism. In explicit opposition to the traditional mode, it inverts the doctrine of vengeance into a promise of ultimate success, affirming to the world, and despite the world, the inviolability of the colonial cause. (6–7)

Though the threat and the apocalyptic visions are crucial constituents of Jeremiads, the most important observation that Bercovitch formulates in this quote is the transformation of the threat into a promise. The threat and danger of an impending apocalypse form the horizon for the image of the future that is marked by "unshakable optimism." In that sense the warnings expressed in Jeremiads are rather a narrative element of the optimist's tale that forms the center of the Puritan sermons as much as of today's (bio)security narratives. Examples such as Haldane's or Tatum's speeches, which I have discussed previously, represent precisely this structure of utopian promise struggling against the otherwise inescapable future doom of society. Though biosecurity narratives are neither

---

8   The elderly and the expansion of longevity has been conceptualized as a risk for the nation within decisively apocalyptic tones (Kunow, *Material* 250–252). Similarly, the problem of obesity is framed in an apocalyptic rhetoric forming an "obesity panic" (Campos et al. 58).

purely dystopian nor purely utopian but a confluence of both, they represent a "promis-
ing-machine" (Buchanan 22),[9] as something that orients and motivates individuals, providing a form of a "secular providentialism." With the analysis of the individual(ized)
biosecurity narratives I will show how this collective narrative is applied to individual
life.

Biosecurity narratives pervade the more intimate spaces of individual experience
and individual expressions. They structure the individual and individualizing biosecurity narratives. I will show that the confluence of utopian and dystopian narrative elements expresses more than just the imminent threat and ever encroaching ways in which
humans are controlled and overdetermined by the master-narrative of biosecurity. I will
therefore focus on the way the security narratives are constructed to represent, challenge
and change the understanding of security produced by a given material as well as discursive "injury" to the body. I will explore the role of narrative in the context of the biosecurity.

With my reading of Alice Wexler's Huntington's memoir in chapter 5 I will explore
how the scientific security narratives influenced the understanding of the self, at a time
when the security practice of genetic testing was just emerging. In chapter 6 I will turn
to the contemporary moment, when genetic testing is not only possible but an ethical
imperative for a responsible biosecurity individual. I will analyze the creation of the previvor who stands paradigmatically for the contemporary biosecurity individual and the
messianic promise of scientific salvation. From the epitome of the biosecurity individual
I will turn to the possibility of escaping biosecurity in chapter 7. I will read the documentary "How to Die in Oregon," which advocates physician assisted dying and the possibility
of resistance to the normative biosecurity narratives. In chapter 8 I will then turn the end
of the biomedical utopia represented by Nathaniel Hawthorne and Gary Shteyngart.

---

9   Ian Buchanan develops this term of a "promising machine" in reference to Jameson's text on utopia
and his dialectic of hope.

5. Writing Life – Writing Security: Alice Wexler's *Mapping Faith* and the Emerging Biosecurity Individual

> The primary meaning of existentiality is the future.
> *Martin Heidegger*

"Know your risks" is one of the dominant refrains of our culture today. Like a mantra it reverberates through the most diverse parts of life and seems the unquestionable wisdom of our times. But especially in terms of biosecurity this knowledge is difficult to come by. Biosecurity practices predicting and narrativizing the future are crucial to establish, protect, and maintain (a sense of) security. In this context, genetic testing has become a hallmark security practice, promising to provide knowledge that facilitates security. But what if knowing one's risks does not and cannot lead to security, as in the case of incurable genetic diseases such as Huntington's Disease? What if the mechanisms and technologies developed to calculate risk do not keep their promise and facilitate life, liberty, and the pursuit of happiness? Alice Wexler has dedicated her memoir *Mapping Fate* to precisely this circumstance at a time when genetic testing was just being developed and the era of the gene was still in its infancy. Her memoir with the subtitle "of family, risk, and genetic research" exemplifies both the necessity of narrative to construct a pervasive understanding of security and risk, as well as the inescapable influences of biotechnological developments and their security narratives on life and identity.

Mapping Fate tells the medical history of Huntington's Disease alongside the history of Alice Wexler's family coping with this hereditary disease. Her text explores her mother's suffering from the disease as well as the breach in life which this familial affliction represents for her and her sister Nancy. With the mother's diagnosis the siblings become individuals at risk[1] and need to find strategies to cope with the 50:50 chance of carrying the gene responsible for Huntington's. As such, the text is part of the growing genre of illness narratives, which have attracted a large body of scholarly interest since the AIDS

---

[1]   Wexler's story does not primarily deal with the development of this identity in terms of a "risk society" as it is not the newly emerging risk of a Beckean risk society that challenges the individual and produces this risk identity.

crisis in the late 1980s and early 1990s.[2] Spearheaded by intellectuals and academics who have fallen ill, such as Audre Lorde, Susan Sontag, and Arthur Frank the genre and its critical discussion have proliferated. These texts highlight the vulnerability of the individual put at risk by their own corporeality, and the ways that these individuals "become storytellers in order to recover the voices that illness and its treatment often take away" (Frank xii). They exemplify that illness is not merely a biological matter, but is positioned at the intersection of biology and culture, as various scholars have pointed out (Sontag, Davis and Morris, T. Cole, Charon). Although Alice Wexler's text is decisively different from traditional illness narratives since her memoir "is really less about an illness than about the possibility of an illness" (A. Wexler, *Mapping* xxii), she engages in the same discursive space as these narratives. By representing a story of risk and insecurity Wexler also narrativizes security, which is inseparable from the representation of risk and essential for a sense of self for the biosecurity individual. I will therefore focus on the negotiation of what biological security means and how the biologized understanding of security influences the conception of a "good life" and of identity itself.

With Wexler's memoir I will turn to the most traditional form of autobiographical writing and therefore the discursive formation most clearly regarded to be the "genre of the self." What began in eighteenth century Romanticism as a search for origin has become an icon of subjectivity and individualism (Folkenflik, "Introduction" 8) and the epitome of "western" culture. The genre underwent radical changes, especially during the twentieth and twenty-first century, with a thorough theoretical reconceptualization of the genre in the 1980s. But the representations of life have attained their exemplary and didactic purpose already found in Saint Augustine's *Confessions* as much as in *The Education of Henry Adams*. The changing aesthetics of life writing, however, express and expose changes in the perception and understanding of the self, which is a central question of this chapter. Alice Wexler's memoir therefore represents a promising vantage point to study how security is constructed and the ways in which biosecurity narratives influence the understanding of life and self for the growing group of risk individuals.

I will not read Alice Wexler's memoir with regard to its truthfulness or to authenticate the representation of a life *as* an example of a risk identity. This would be what Völz called a "security realism" (Völz, "Aestheticizing" 619) which ignores that literature is much more than a mirror to an extradiegetic reality. I rather perceive the text as a writing of a life and time that is significantly created in its "final" meaning by the text itself and can therefore never claim to be mimetically mirroring a pre-existing truth or reality. Nonetheless, the claim of authenticity, which resonates in this discursive formation,[3] is crucial for the book's reception and for the construction of the security narrative that defines this risk

---

2   The sociologist Arthur Frank defined illness narratives in *The Wounded Storyteller* as narratives of individuals, who are suffering from an illness and have to therefore renegotiate their life and identity. With the concept of the ill person as a storyteller he assigned the individuals an active role in understanding and negotiating their illness (xi). He categorizes three main types which he terms restitution, chaos, and quest. In contrast, scholars such as Arthur Kleinman and Rita Charon have emphasized the role of the "wounded healer" and the importance of narrative to empathize and bond with the ill person.

3   Paul John Eakin dedicates a whole book to *The Ethics of Life Writing* dealing with the "truthfulness" of the genre and the representative responsibility of the author.

identity. In this chapter I will therefore focus on how this story of a biologically inflected security is told as a "necessary fiction" indispensable to fully understand the self.

Wexler's text is especially interesting because she is representing a changing understanding of security in the context of Huntington's disease based on biotechnological developments. Though Huntington's was known, diagnosable, and incurable, similar to today, the understanding of the disease, the treatment, and the time of the diagnosis have changed due to the development of genetic testing. The text is not only an example of how biomedical and biotechnological advances have changed our relation to body and self today, but depicts the time leading up to and the anticipation of these changes. While Alice Wexler neither gets tested in the storyline of the memoir nor reveals if she is going to, she negotiates the different possibilities of knowing provided by this security practice. She therefore establishes a relationship to security, which represents the historic moment when the relation to the future and the urge to pre-emptively "do something" is just emerging, appearing as a promise of security; a security that is a seemingly natural desire for many people today, when testing has become a more commonplace practice and a prerequisite for biological security.

Published in 1995, two years after the discovery of the Huntington's gene, her memoir was written amidst extensive discourse on genetic testing and at the beginning of the era of the gene. At that time, the benefits and threats of "new genetics" were frequently debated in the public sphere. *Mapping Fate* represents a negotiation of the utopian and dystopian voices dominating public discussions of the potential benefits and perils of genetic testing.[4] In rendering her identity as a risk individual Wexler makes the act of writing a crucial element of her sense of security and her most crucial security practice. In doing so, she offers a variety of multilayered security narratives that influence and at time contrast and contradict each other, competing over the definition of what security really means for her and how to achieve it. In this exploration emotions play a crucial role to establish the necessary narrative of security and to define her identity as a biosecurity individual. I will therefore highlight the function of affects in those narratives, specifically anxiety and hope. To facilitate a better understanding of these competing narratives I will first offer a very brief introduction to the history of Huntington's disease. I will then show how Wexler renders her risk identity as both an ascription as well as affecting her identity on a more intimate level. I will argue that Wexler re-constructs her identity based on the temporality and logic of an always already precarious normality in which certainty becomes a desired object that stands in for security.

Threatened by Nature and Culture: A Short History of Huntington's Disease

Huntington's disease (HD) is a late-onset neurodegenerative disease, which means that the disease affects the brain and leads to its progressive deterioration. The disease's most characteristic symptoms are involuntary body movements and twitches, which make the affliction highly visible. Because of these movements HD used to be called Huntington's

---

4   For a thorough analysis of this opposition between proponents and opponents of genetic testing see Shakespeare.

Chorea "on account of the dancing propensities of those who are affected" (Huntington 110), and popularly it had been referred to as St. Vitus Dance.[5] However, symptoms of the disease are more diverse and range from depression and slurred speech to the loss of balance and the ability to control muscle functions. Ultimately the disease leads invariably to the loss of all mental and physical abilities. The disease usually manifests rather late in life, with the first symptoms emerging during the patient's thirties or forties. Only in the more severe form of Juvenile Huntington's disease do symptoms set in before middle age.

HD is caused by a genetic defect on Chromosome 4 and is described as a dominant mono-genetic disease,[6] which means that it is inherited dominantly on just one gene (De Melo). Children of an afflicted parent therefore have a 50:50 chance of inheriting the disease. These individuals are regarded as risk individuals. For a long time the disease could only be recognized once it materialized in outwardly recognizable symptoms. Only the discovery of the genetic marker "G8" in 1986 made it possible to test for HD before the onset of the disease. The discovery of the gene "IT 15" in 1993 further facilitated pre-symptomatic and prenatal testing (National Institute of Neurological Disorders and Stroke). Though presymptomatic testing has made the diagnosis of the disease possible before its onset, Huntington's remains incurable and always fatal. In contrast to other degenerative diseases there are very few possibilities of treating the symptoms and no approved ways of slowing down the degenerative progression of the disease.

Though the condition had been known for a long time, George Huntington wrote the first scientific description of the disease in 1872 and is credited with its "discovery." His famous article "On Chorea" described the disease as a brain disease (110) and already explained its genetic transmission as a dominantly inherited trait, which never "skips a generation" (Huntington 112). He identified the main characteristics that would remain the standard understanding of the disease until the era of the gene initiated the search for the exact gene and genetic location responsible for the condition. Besides the hereditary nature and the late onset George Huntington emphasized the "tendency to insanity and suicide" (Huntington 111) as a recognizable pattern that can be correlated with the disease. In highlighting this aspect, he stresses the burden that the disease represents for those afflicted as well as for their entire families, for "the poor patient presents a spectacle which is anything but pleasing to witness" (Huntington 112). Already this early description thus emphasizes the social implications of the disease alongside its biological description. Huntington seems to recognize that the disease is not only mentally and physically painful but socially stigmatizing. The bodily performance turned patients into social outcasts. The performative aspect of the disease increases the shame that has been associated with the social and physical difference Huntington's disease produces.

---

5   Saint Vitus dance, or dancing mania, is a phenomenon that occurred in various places in Europe between the 13th and 17th century, and which to date has no conclusive explanation. Huntington's disease is not describing the medicalized version of this phenomenon but was named after it, for the likening to the dance movements (Esterianna).

6   This represents a decisive difference from most other genetic diseases that are caused by multiple factors and not just one gene (De Melo).

While Huntington stressed that "hereditary chorea" affected "few families . . . almost exclusively in the east end of Long Island" (Huntington 111) and was therefore probably of little interest, eugenicists made the disease one of the flagships to promote their programs of "breeding control" to improve and protect the future of society. While the correlation of mental illness, physical symptoms, and genetics were still difficult and intangible during the 1910s and 1920s, often more a pseudo science than anything else, Huntington's represented "the one clear case of neuropathic entity" (Davenport 283). Davenport explained the urgent need to control the reproduction of HD individuals with his findings that most cases "can be traced back to some half dozen individuals, including three (probable) brothers who migrated to America during the 17th century" (Davenport 283–4). To protect the national body from this form of "contamination" and therefore – in the understanding of eugenicists – to protect national security, Davenport suggested the forced sterilization of afflicted people, as well as of those at risk (A. Wexler "Eugenics" 140).

Patients suffering from the disease were thus recast as a threat themselves – to their fellow citizens and the nation. Both, nation and sick individual, were narrativized as in need of medical protection. Davenport argued, as did most of his colleagues and followers, that measures such as forced sterilization were not just crucial to improve society, but to save the afflicted individuals and their future suffering offspring from this harmful fate. The program is thus not only protecting the healthy nation but the potential future afflicted. The HD individual was thus suffering from a triple injury: that of their disease, that of social stigmatization, and that of state enforced security practices. Such programs of non-consensual and not-informed sterilization continued far beyond the eugenic movement as mentioned before. And according to Alice Wexler's paper on eugenics and Huntington's, the eugenic mindset and their security narrative influenced "the priorities of HD research. Even in the 1960s some of the most knowledgeable geneticists and neurologists seemed to give a higher priority to research on 'early detection' for eugenic purposes than to research on therapies and improved care" (A. Wexler, "Eugenics" 140).

The understanding of unlivable life, or dehumanizing life, which underlies the eugenic mindset is still recognizable in the more contemporary understanding of the disease. This evaluation of the disease as the understanding of what the disease "does" to those suffering from it also emphasizes that illnesses are always both biological and cultural. Threatened by their own corporeality HD individuals face another threat. Since the disease dissolves part of the brain tissue, those affected lose their mental ability and ultimately their ability to remember their past and "who they are," they can no longer tell their story. By losing the ability to know themselves and their "healthy" identities they lose what has culturally been made to represent the essence of humanness.[7] Hunting-

---

7   The ability to tell one's own life story (and identity) also represents the touchstone of subjectivity and identity and the normative structure which defines us as human subjects. In that sense, the practice of narrating the self is much more than a deliberate act. In a precarious way, this cultural idea of "the narrative self" excludes a large group of persons that are not able to story their life and identity, such as Alzheimer patients who are often described as "socially dead" (Rhodes and Vedder 4).

ton's is therefore understood to not only rob people of their life but of their humanness, similarly to the understanding of Alzheimer's disease. This represents an additionally threatening prospect adding to the threat of a "premature" death due to the disease.

Not surprisingly then, Huntington's represented a silenced family heritage often hidden away and not talked about; a characteristic already Huntington had described in his observations on the disease (111). Also after the era of eugenics people afflicted with the disease suffered from stigmatization and social exclusion. As in the case of Wexler's family, secrecy and the eventual move into a care facility are common features of a HD family story. The collective silence represents an additional burden for the afflicted. Woody Guthrie, probably the most famous person who suffered from Huntington's disease, is a prime example for the material repercussions caused by this silence. Due to misdiagnosis and social misconception the singer spent much of his life branded as an alcoholic and was admitted to various mental institutions before "the cause" of his behavior was recognized as Huntington's disease (National Institute of Neurological Disorders and Stroke).

The late 1960s saw a change in public awareness of Huntington's disease. During that time Alice Wexler's father founded the Hereditary Disease Foundation and other affected families, such as Guthrie's wife also started major funding efforts to combat the disease. Furthermore, Woody Guthrie's death in 1967 brought national attention to the disease. This was achieved in part by Guthrie himself who already "gave a voice" to the illness in his "Huntington's Chorea Blues" during his lifetime (qdt. in Maloney 133), as well as memorial tributes by artists such as Bob Dylan with his "Song to Woody," and the more explicit poem "Last Thoughts on Guthrie." These representations in the public sphere, though still few and far between, changed the perception of individuals afflicted with Huntington's, explaining their "deviant" behavior within a medicalized context and expressing the suffering implied in the behavior. By making HD visible and known, such representations challenged the social stigma that had been attached to the disease for centuries. In a similar way, Wexler's memoir is also part of this "giving a voice" to HD, making it visible and known.

Since the publication of Wexler's memoir, and in response to the genetic test in 1993, literary and cultural production relating to Huntington's has continued to proliferate. Though the disease might remain comparatively little known to the general public, its evocations in discourse about genetic testing have made it more and more present in public space. Today, representations of the disease can be found in many parts of culture, probably most prominently in the many bio-documentaries that flood entertainment culture and the internet. It is represented in documentaries, via the radio, fiction, autobiographies, and film.[8] In the same way as media coverage of medical surgeries represents

---

8   Documentaries: *Do you really want to know* (2013) by John Zaritsky; CBS Network "Fighting Huntington's Disease" (2010); radio features and podcasts: "What are you doing for the test of your life?", *This American Life:* "It Says So Right Here" Oct 25, 2013 and "Dr. Gilmer and Mr. Hyde"; *WNYC:* "DNA Secrets: The Antidote"; *ABC Health Report:* "Huntington's Disease"; Fiction: Jacqueline Susann (1966) *Valley of the Dolls*; Kurt Vonnegut (1985) *Galapagos*; Nancy Werlin (2000) *Double Helix*; Barbara Vine *The House of Stairs* (1989); Robert Sawyer *Frameshift* (1997); Life Writing: Steven T. Seagal's graphic novel *It's a Bird*; Film *Alice's Restaurant* (1969) by Arlo Guthrie. For a critical reading of biological, or scientific documentaries in entertainment as a succession from the freak show see van Dijck's "The Operation Film as a Mediated Freak Show" in *The Transparent Body* (20–40).

a "normalization of the medical gaze" (van Dijck, *Transparent* 38) these stories represent a normalization of the biologized understanding of security. While earlier representations were often giving a voice to suffering, newer representations seem more focused on the portrayal and evaluation of the medical possibilities granted by genetic testing. Wexler also references this in the title of her memoir. In that sense, many of these representations disseminate biologically inflected security narratives of potential medical salvation. However, this salvation does not take the form of a therapeutic practice – it neither prevents nor cures HD – but offers only hope through a genetic test, predicting either a healthy or a sick future.

Biosecurity, Huntington's Disease, and the Individual at Risk: From a Number to an Identity

Genetic heritage is one of the oldest and at the same time most contested conceptualizations in identity discourses. In the last decades the notion of geneticized identity constructions has resurfaced and gained prominence.[9] In the negotiation of her risk identity Wexler's memoir emphasizes this growing importance of genetic heritage. But she not only highlights the importance of a genetic identity construction and biologized understanding of fate, which she references in her title. She also reveals how this biologically defined identity makes biosecurity and the positioning to biosecurity one of the most important constituents determining her identity. I will therefore consider the implications of her repositioning toward security based on this biologically determined identity, which Wexler renders as ascription as well as self-identification.

Wexler foregrounds the shift in her identity that is caused by her mother's diagnosis with Huntington's. She thus describes her identity in relation to a changed understanding of biological security, which is based on the knowledge regarding her possible genetic make-up. The rupture and plot generator of her life writing text is thus the moment when she and her sister are informed about their 50% chance of having inherited their mother's disease, which they learn about in 1968 in their late twenties. By making this shift the central event of her memoir she emphasizes how central corporeality and biological integrity are to the sense of self and the construction of identity. She renegotiates her mother's identity after she had been diagnosed with Huntington's Disease as well as her own coming to terms with her risk identity. She thus describes her mother's shift from healthy to sick, while she negotiates her own position caught in a transitional zone in which she is marked as "at risk," a transition that does not describe a material reality or intimate experience of a corporeality but a repositioning toward a biological security. It is the moment of consciously becoming a biosecurity individual.

This risk identity is first and foremost a numerical reality and a statistical fact – a biosecurity ascription that Wexler represents as becoming the center piece of her understanding of self and identity. Her narrative establishes clear relations between the

---

9   The importance of genetics as the basis for identity formation has become so prevalent that Priscilla Wald asserts that "no contemporary discussion of identity can afford to ignore it" ("Future Perfect" 682).

official narrative of Huntington's and her understanding of self and identity, introducing risk as equally consequential as actual disease. Being ascribed this risk identity she becomes part of a group which is defined by genetic belonging and, more importantly, by the positioning toward security implied by this belonging. This emphasis on a genetic and scientifically determined understanding of identity opposes the individualism that is so crucial in U.S. American culture. Identity based on biological security narratives seems to therefore contrast the historic and cultural notions of self-reliance and the American Dream. This "new" biological component deconstructs the upheld ideal that no matter where you are coming from you can "make yourself" and that everybody forges one's own destiny. It ties individuals to groups and collectives: their family as well as other individuals with the same "markers." Wexler's insistence on biosecurity and her risk identity seems to therefore produce first and foremost a collective identity that seems deeply un-American. Wexler's text shows that becoming a biosecurity individual is initially rather a passive form of belonging than an active relational process of positioning and identifying.[10]

This ascribed risk identity is determined by biomedical security narratives and research which heavily influences the understanding of body and self. Wexler accentuates this interconnection with the narrative structure of her text. She tells her family history and her negotiation of being at risk alongside the story of HD research and genetics, which radically changes over the course of her life with the identification of the responsible gene "IT 15" and the development of a presymptomatic test. Her memoir forms a traditional life writing text that portrays her family history embedded in historic context focused on the medical history of Huntington's. Formally the different narratives – medical history and family history – are depicted in separate sections. The text is divided in four parts and every part is preceded by a "title page" featuring an image with an explanatory caption which seem to indicate the general theme of the following chapters. While the first part "The Body in Question" represents the most traditional part of autobiographical writing, part two "Chorea Stories" is more concerned with the social story of the disease. In part three "Maps for Misreading" Wexler focuses on research and part four "Genetic Destinations," the shortest of the sections, tells the story of the discovery of the genetic marker in 1984 and of the responsible gene in 1993. These formal subdivisions, however, rather simulate the possibility of distinguishing medical history as ascribed identity from a more intimate understanding of the self because the narrative deconstructs and diminishes these clear cut divisions. In the text personal memoir and medical history are intertwined, constructing an inseparable strand of illness narrative and disease narrative, a "double helix" as Wexler describes it herself ("Mapping Lives" 166). She thus constructs a hybrid text in which medical history and family history are the two pillars on which she constructs her personal life narrative. The text thus echoes structurally the linkage between science, life, identity, and self that are impossible to separate into entities that can be clearly distinguished.

---

10   Iris Young has described such a dynamic as a serial identity construction, which exists alongside and in relation to the active identity. In her article "Gender Seriality" she elaborates on Sartre's concept of seriality applying it to the possibility of understanding the group formation of "women" without having to fall back on essentialist ascriptions.

Wexler further emphasizes this interconnectedness with the narrative tone used to represent both the medical history and the illness experience. Both storylines are filled with intellectual and academic reflections on race and gender binaries, and all textual passages are interlaced with endnotes with further explanations and bibliographic references to the sources used for the "history of HD." The text and endnotes are followed by additional explanations on her sources and interviews, as well as by suggestions for further information. The legitimacy and authority the text gains as a historical document by these explanations are mirrored in the personal narrative sections. Here it is quotes of other people, as well as citations from letters and her diaries that provide the authenticity, or rather "proof of truth" for the story told. The life narrative is thus represented in an almost scientific fashion, further underlining the impossibility to fully distinguish between an ascription based on a scientifically defined trait and the self identification which we usually refer to when talking about individual identities.

Wexler portrays the scientific and numerical definition as crucial introducing and defining the sisters mainly by their belonging to the "risk group" and therefore as numbers in a statistical table. The re-positioning towards security based on the statistical numbers is reiterated throughout the memoir interlacing and preparing the personal story with numerical facts about the general population. Already in the introduction numbers, most importantly the 50:50 chance of carrying the gene, set the stage for individual identity formation. Before this statistical and therefore collective identity is individualized by Wexler's narrative, she thus elaborates on her belonging to the group and being ascribed an identity based on her biological security status. She informs the reader that her family belongs to a very "limited population" affected by Huntington's, namely "30,000 in the United States, with another 150,000 at risk" (A. Wexler, *Mapping* xxiv). Without the need to recognize one another, without even knowing one another, the logic of genetic security makes them a group. Their identity as biosecurity subjects is thus primarily forged within the dominant public discourse and public sphere, in which HD individuals and individuals at risk circulate as a series of cases. Accordingly, Wexler describes them as a chain of people "that all come to resemble one another" (A. Wexler, *Mapping* xi). While biological security seems to represent the possibility of individual and unique pathways, biological insecurity makes people appear "the same:" the same bodily expressions and the same fate. They are thus clustered together by their "common" fate that appears to strip them of their individuality as people.

In Wexler's elaborations on the history of Huntington's research she makes this group identity even more central and obvious when representing afflicted individuals in their relation to research. She highlights that the individuals are often marked as objects of research in which they serve as (ex)samples of genetics. The overarching and connecting link that the gene forms between individuals who would not necessarily ever associate with one another is especially poignant when Wexler describes a HD "neighborhood" in Venezuela. This is the world's largest HD community, which offered the necessary genetic material to find the genetic marker and gene. Though Wexler represents the community members as individuals citing individual stories and describing their living conditions, the commonality of belonging to one group is only based on their genetic information, as "vials of blood" (A. Wexler, *Mapping* 196). It is their common biological material, more so than their fate, that defines their belonging. The different individuals are connected as a group because the genetic test for HD, which will eventually become available towards the end of the memoir, is developed based on the knowledge gained by the study of this community. In fact, most of the current molecular genetic research is still based on the HD community in Venezuela.

The generalized biosecurity ascription of risk individuals defines the group identity of these diverse people and experiences. The example of the Maracaibo community shows that the genetic identity marks a group which transgresses cultural, gender, class, and national borders. Wexler does not, however, describe this belonging in the sense of a community of common suffering – as a common precariousness – but rather in terms of practices of security such as testing. The individual identity at risk is thus most overtly produced in relation to the Foucauldian "mechanisms of security" (*Security* 16). The generalized statistical knowledge that defines these individuals produces, pace Foucault, a series of individuals who are only relevant in relation to the security of the population. It thus describes biosecurity individuals who seem to count only in their multiplicity.

However, Wexler shows that in terms of biosecurity the knowledge is at the same time generalizing *and* individualizing.

> The suffering associated with the disease and with living at risk is intensified by the lack of resources available in our privatized, for-profit medical system. Nearly all of the families with HD who testified before the 1977 Congressional Commission spoke of the limitations of health insurance and lack of access to services. (A. Wexler, *Mapping* xxiii)

In the Congressional hearing individuals diagnosed with Huntington's and those at risk are all represented as one group in relation to the nation. Though individual experiences and testimonies are heard and recognized, in this hearing they represent a group in need of protection not only from the disease but from social and cultural repercussions that follow the biosecurity ascription and group membership. It is thus not the experience of risk and disease that makes them all part of one collective, much less an active association. Rather, Wexler makes clear that the group exists on another basis, namely as insurance cases.

The material effects of the "apparatus (dispositif) of security" (Foucault, *Security* 20) based on probabilities and statistics therefore influence individual lives in a more intimate way, though the individual fate is not the object of that form of security narrative. Though the risk identity is largely defined as a group identity, it cannot be reduced to that. Rather, it is deeply felt on an individual level as well.

> The other day I got a copy of my medical records from my new gynecologist. "Patient has a high probability of developing Huntington's disease," he wrote on the record he submitted to the insurance company. I was furious and called him to protest. . . . Doesn't he know that risk for Huntington's is one of the conditions, along with sickle-cell anemia, muscular dystrophy, insulin dependent diabetes, AIDS, for which insurance companies unconditionally deny medical coverage? (A. Wexler, *Mapping* 231)

The involuntary and passive ascription of officially belonging to a group based on the individual's security status turns into a marker of difference, that is reminiscent of

Hawthorne's *The Scarlet Letter*. The "invisible" potential turns into an actual mark that the individual carries in lieu of an actual physical marker. This visible mark, which Wexler is forced to "wear," positions her in relation to biological security on a social scale and makes her a biosecurity individual, if she wants to or not. HD becomes an outward sign similar to the iconic scarlet letter marking the "sin of flesh" in a genetic sense. Though the mark is carried on her insurance paper and not on her breast, Wexler's "scarlet letter" is as heart-felt as Hester Prynne's in Hawthorne's story. As in the novel, the mark of being a risk individual produces material repercussions and represents exclusion that causes an affective reaction. But in contrast to Hester stitching her own scarlet letter, Wexler is hesitant to accept her marker of difference as it makes her "furious." She rather holds on to the rationalizations she has come to believe in, which is the reduction of her risk to 25% due to her increasing age. Regardless, Wexler will have to bear the repercussions of this mark as the material proof of her potential corporeal deviance and belonging to a risk group.

The biologized or genetic identity that is produced by the knowledge of one's risk is thus of course not just a passive "being positioned toward" identity. Besides the passive and inevitable becoming a number in a statistical table defined by an abstract emotionless probability, Wexler highlights that such a belonging is affectively charged. Statistics, as read by Foucault, are an important tool and mechanism of biosecurity in which the general population is targeted rather than the individual. The use of statistical knowledge in Wexler's representation, however, takes on a decisively different form. While the statistic still represents the belonging to a group that is at risk, it becomes a cipher for the individual. Kathleen Woodward has written about the affective and individual ramifications of probability for the individual in "Statistical Panic," highlighting the importance of statistics in our culture, "where bodies are composed of – and harrowingly decomposed by – statistics" (195). She exemplifies this by her reading of Wexler's memoir showing that statistics are not merely objective and emotionless descriptions of anonymous numbers but deeply felt by individuals. This affectivity expands beyond the repercussions caused by genetic discrimination and represents a crucial bridge between ascription and identification. The affects represent the force that individualizes biosecurity narratives and mechanisms. Wexler's representation thus indicates how the understanding of biological security individualizes, forging biosecurity identities rather than merely "describing a multiplicity." The affectivity forces the individuals to position and recognize themselves as biosecurity individuals based on the active negotiation of their risk identity. "I began really to think about being at risk, admitting to myself that perhaps 'I was trying completely to deny the whole thing by pretending it wasn't there.' I knew I had to come to terms with the illness" (A. Wexler, *Mapping* 71). The life narrative therefore becomes a process of understanding and coming to terms with the meaning of being at risk.

With her memoir Wexler clearly declares her own belonging to the Huntington's community and makes her family an example of this community. Her combination of medical history and abstract fact with her personal life writing represents a transition from passive ascription to an act of identification. In this form of active "positioning" by establishing her individual security narrative, Wexler makes her unwanted mark turn into a truly "self stitched" scarlet letter that she comes to wear, like Hester, as a token of pride. But though "self stitched," Wexler nonetheless makes clear how heavily her understanding of risk and security are influenced by biosecurity narratives and the affective attachments they create.

In Wexler's rendering affects are therefore the most crucial element in individual-izing the biosecurity narrative which defines the intangible experience of being at risk. The "statistical panic" caused by the probabilities of 50:50 frame the narrative of Wexler's memoir and play a dominant role in marking and making her own security narrative. Fear as one of the dominant sentiments defining risk and security offer in Wexler's narrative "both a sense of imperiling intensity that is the sensation of statistical panic and complex emotional reflections of that experience" (Woodward, *Statistical Panic* 208). But though most commonly read as the representation of risk or threat, or in Woodward's analysis the trigger of panic and confusion, at the same time these statistics also harbor hope. On the one hand the 50:50 chance of being a carrier of the gene that triggers Huntington's made Wexler "scared to death" (A. Wexler, *Mapping* 43), on the other hand it still leaves room for hope. This dyad of despair and hope represent competing narrative elements which determine Wexler's memoir and her understanding of being at risk. To fully come to terms with and understand her new identity Wexler therefore constructs her individual security narrative which determines the meaning of this abstract risk.

Precarious Normality and Troubled Happiness: Defining Security and Risk

The constellation of security and risk in the face of a fatal disease might seem self-evident: health versus pathology, or more radically, life versus death. However, Wexler shows that for the individual at risk this is more complicated since the threat is never fully absent, nor fully present. Her memoir therefore emphasizes the importance of nar-ratives for the construction of what security and risk really mean for the individual, first and foremost on an affective level. In negotiating what being at risk from Huntington's means, Wexler highlights how much this diagnosed risk influences her understanding of self, basing her identity decisively on a biologized understanding of self *and* security.

In her negotiation of her "new" risk identity Wexler makes clear that the risk of the genetic disease does not just appear at some point in life. Nonetheless, she emphasizes how much the knowledge of potentially having Huntington's changes her understanding of her life. For Wexler being at risk does not describe a perceivable physical state but an ambivalent experiential situation marked by a shift in understanding. The moment of knowing is therefore crucial for the presence of being at risk. For the life under the sword of Damocles only becomes a life of constant anxiety when the individual knows about the thin thread that divides their life from death, or rather security and insecurity. The moment of knowledge, which is narrated as a form of discovery or revelation, is therefore crucial in the construction of the security narrative. It represents the instigator of the active re-positioning and re-interpretation of Wexler's identity as well as a structuring element of the narrative.

Wexler portrays the new experiential situation first and foremost as an emotional ex-perience marked by uncertainty and fear. The risk identity triggers in Wexler a "crisis of self confidence" (A. Wexler, *Mapping* 56) and the loss of a happy unburdened life. In her narrative the experience of this performative shift is marked by depression which comes to dominate her otherwise "normal," rather secure middle-class life. The thoughts and emotions prompted by knowing her risk haunt the narrative as "the question of probability haunted our lives" (A. Wexler, *Mapping* 39). The fears that represent the experience of risk are described as creeping up in moments and intercepting her "normal" life. In many instances Wexler renders these disruptions as dream episodes that interrupt the narrative and become more frequent as the story progresses.

By the constant evocation of fear and anxiety Wexler's life narrative becomes marked by the oscillating absence and presence of security, narratively recreating the precarious normality that marks her life. Happiness and despair are the dominating and alternating characteristics that Wexler uses to demarcate this alternation of a feeling of security and risk. While freshly in love, she "was often seized with an overwhelming anxiety, as if something terrible was about to happen" (A. Wexler, *Mapping* 58). At the same time "Huntington's simply did not enter into the conscious emotional landscape of our lives" (A. Wexler, *Mapping* 60), for both sisters *"tried at first to live life as if nothing had changed"* (ibid., emphasis orig.). The possibility of being at risk of carrying the Huntington's Disease gene is marked by a conditional "as if," by a sense of indeterminability. And as the experience of risk remains indeterminable in Wexler's narrative, also the crucial moment of becoming a risk individual is called into question. Her own uncertainty of being at risk is translated into the uncertainty of a determinable beginning, an onset that would demarcate security from risk; an uncertainty which Wexler seeks to resolve by re-reading the past.

In narrating her mother's illness experience, Wexler shows what the risk of having Huntington's disease implies. The mother's suffering from HD and her pathway from diagnosis in 1968 to dying in 1979 when "[w]eak and emaciated, she thrashed about uncontrollably, her arms and legs flailing against the rails the nurses raised at the side of her bed" (A. Wexler, *Mapping* 154) makes the risk of carrying the genetic marker experientially present. Her mother's corporeality, described as a performance watched by her daughter, make the possible future tangible, giving the fear of an HD future a material and knowable basis. Knowing what could lie ahead – with a probability of 50:50 – is a decisive part of the experience of being at risk and the fear associated with this risk. Wexler's narrative of the past thus functions primarily as a way of knowing and representing the potential future. The past provides a form of script, not to actively follow as performance (only) but as a way to understand the body that "is and is not mine" (Butler, *Precarious* 26). Like a dystopian narrative it provides a mirror into the potential future. With this image of Huntington's death, Wexler introduces the disease as "the most diabolic affliction man is heir to" (A. Wexler, *Mapping* 87). In the preface she states explicitly that Huntington's is incurable and only "death relieves them [the afflicted] of their suffering" (A. Wexler, *Mapping* xii) configuring security in her family history through its absence. She foregrounds the threat of the HD affliction, which negatively defines the horizon of security in the context of this hereditary disease, prior to introducing her own and her family's story. The disease and its risks thus frame the narrative, effectively eradicating any possibility of security from the family story.

But security is not only absent from Wexler's life, it is also absent from the narrative as something that is "always already" gone. The memoir starts long before the mother's diagnosis, with Wexler's childhood, with her parents' and grandparents' history. Descriptions of her kin mirror the prototypical nuclear "American family," the icon of the American Dream of the Fifties. But the depicted memories of the suburban life and the success story of an affluent society fail to "live up" to the images of happiness they convey. The "pursuit of happiness" never reaches the projected future as the stories are both tainted and haunted by the *knowledge* of HD. Wexler constructs the "precarious normality" retrospectively, narratively creating a temporal relation that implies the "always already" presence of a failed future. She thus juxtaposes narrative time and time of narration to emphasize this temporal conundrum of a geneticized understanding of life and precarious normality of health. Good life and happiness are made impossible by the specter of HD, which Wexler conjures by repeatedly foreshadowing the tragedy which is yet to come.

Wexler makes this temporal logic of the "always already" but "not yet" known disease affliction the guiding rationality of her life narrative. She encapsulates it with the anecdote "fish dream," which introduces her memoir:

> Gasping on the rear floor lay a tremendous carp, ancient and ravaged. This carp had apparently survived many years hidden in the murky shallows of a pond in Topeka. No one had imagined the presence there of anything more substantial than small goldfish until Bill, practicing his casting, hauled up this monster.
> . . . After Dad told us the facts of our family history, this carp swam back into my dreams.
> (A. Wexler, *Mapping* 3)

As the leitmotif of the memoir this anecdote represents the logic of "always already" existing but "not yet" discovered fish. It represents a structural analogy to the presence of the disease in the absence of the event that will reveal it. This temporal logic dominates her desperate search for traces of her mother's "HD-ness" that would allow her to define the onset of HD and thereby to truly understand who her mother was. As the overarching logic of Wexler re-reading her past this temporality therefore defines the moments of security that represented "normal" family problems at the time. She portrays her mother as a highly educated housewife with a background in genetics who showed signs of depression similarly to so many of her female contemporaries living in the "golden cage" of the Fifties, as Betty Friedan has described it in *Feminine Mystique*. But in the case of Wexler's mother the goldfish, symbolizing the "normal" problem of gender inequality, has to be re-evaluated because it might have been a tremendous carp all along. Through the prism of Huntington's in the family any recollection of the past becomes an image of biological insecurity and of the threat that is always already present even while absent in a temporal and ontological sense: lost happiness.

Wexler's memoir is therefore not just a retrospective writing and therefore re-writing and re-interpretation of a life, like most other life writing texts. It is a retrospective search and rewriting for what had been unknown and what became knowable and understandable only with knowledge acquired much later. It is a search for the hidden disease and a re-reading, re-writing, and re-interpretation of life with HD. A similar turning point can also be found in early conversion narratives like Saint Augustine's where life is divided into the time before and after conversion and the moment of revelation. Similarly, traditional illness narratives describe this turning point or "biographical disruption" as Michael Bury calls it, in which the diagnosis leads to a re-evaluation and re-negotiation of meaning in and of life. While this turning point is also contained in Wexler's narrative, the transition referenced here is rather a re-reading of the past on the basis that it is *now* a HD past, while when it was lived it was not and could not have been read or understood as such. It is not the creation of the self as other, as Robert Folkenflik describes it, but the construction of the "new" other replacing the "old."[11] The discovery of the disease thus creates a new identity that extends into the past. Accordingly, the images of the symptom-free mother become descriptions of Huntington's disease, blurring the distinction between pathological and normal, between secure and insecure. With this narrative perspective the memoir reiterates the dominant logic of a genetic security and applies it to identity. Similarly indicated in the title, the genetic defect of Huntington's marks fate, echoing an understanding of the gene as the code of life (van Dijck, *Imagenation*, Nelkin and Lindee), which is always already there and at the same time lies ahead in the future.

The narrative perspective of retrospectivity – the not yet – omits the existential uncertainty of being at risk, which marked the mother's life. More importantly, the logic of "always already" constructed in her mother's past as "pre-symptomatically ill" (Clarke et al., "Biomedicalization") also applies to Alice Wexler, her sister Nancy and their respective risk identity. Not only does the risk of having inherited the Huntington's gene mark their life and health as "precarious" but the logic and narrative structure implies that there is no life prior to HD if a person carries the HD gene. The manifestation of the disease might be absent, but the disease as such is always already present. HD is not something that emerges in the future, though the feared symptoms and proof of HD might or might not, it is always already there. It is therefore knowledge that represents the dividing line "to a 100% certainty that one will or will not develop the disease..." (Wexler, *Mapping* 227) and not the onset of the disease and the presence of disease symptoms. In the absence of such a certainty the knowledge of one's risk replaces the disruption usually associated with the onset of the disease symptoms.

In the absence of a clear demarcation between security/insecurity Wexler searches for "traces of the avalanche that had come crashing into our mother's future" (A. Wexler, *Mapping* 24). In reading her mother's past she is searching for emotions as indicators for the loss of security. "I have no memory, nor does Nancy, of any emotional scene at the time, nor any recollection of Mom's shock or grief" (ibid.). In the absence of her mother's emotional response Wexler seems unable to define the security breach in her mother's life. Flashbacks revealed in comments such as "[y]ears later, Dad would tell us" (A. Wexler, *Mapping* 28) and "could we have known" intersect the reading of the past, which seems to resist to fully express the precariousness Wexler seeks to discover in it. She is therefore never sure of this past she is narrating, never sure when the goldfish turned into a carp; and neither does she seem certain of her own present. She therefore also revisits her own performative shift of becoming a risk individual, in search for any kind of certainty.

For Wexler herself, the knowledge of potentially having HD "melts in [her] memory" with "Russian tanks smashing into Prague, Martin Luther King Jr., dead of a bullet in

---

11   It does not represent the division of "once I was healthy but now I am sick," but of "once I thought I was healthy though now I know I have always been sick."

Memphis, Robert Kennedy, shot in Los Angeles" (A. Wexler, *Mapping* 42). By using the most affective moments of 1968 as metaphors she approximates her inexpressible pain with expression that belongs to the collective memory of the nation. These metaphors attribute the pain to an outside agent, as a "perceived intrusion" (*Cultural Politics* 27) as Sara Ahmed calls it elsewhere, rather than coming from within. But most importantly, Wexler chooses metaphors that are "events" with immediate material as well as affective impact, all of which represent the loss of a future.

Though the moment of knowing for Wexler is marked and singled out in the representation of these historic events, it does not define a moment of onset, a tangible event. It rather remains a moment of shock that, though felt affectively and physically, remains elusive.

> Words are spoken, but I no longer remember them. I recall the whiteness of that apartment, our three frozen forms like a George Segal sculpture, my sister and I sitting with our arms around each other staring at my father's ten-foot high Mike Olodort painting of a huge upside-down Humpty-Dumpty with tiny arms and legs waving in the air and an enormous, sinister smile on his face. There are no tears, no welling floods of grief or anger, but for me only a numb, anesthetized feeling, like being shot full of novocaine. In an instant I shut out my father's words, which I have never been able to remember, as if denial could undo the event. (A. Wexler, *Mapping* 43)

As in many traumatizing moments, the rational mind seems overruled, leaving the situation vague and almost unreal. Rather than describing a direct emotional response Wexler transfers the confusion and disorientation prompted by the information into the descriptions of the surroundings. Wexler and her sister are described as Segal sculptures, which are life-size plaster figures. She represents the moment of shock as a moment when the self becomes other and is looked upon from the outside, described as something detached and foreign. This image is completed by the painting of Humpty-Dumpty hanging opposite the sisters, perfectly symbolizing the moment in which something fragile is irreparably broken. The experience of the event of learning about the mother's disease and their own risk identity is expressed by using the comparison to being anesthetized. Wexler appropriates medical language to describe her memories of that moment and the lack of emotions she associates with it. The memory of her performative shift becoming a biosecurity individual and the beginning of her risk identity, remains caught in an undeterminable space, as "if we had been experiencing fallout from some unseen bomb for all these years" (A. Wexler, *Mapping* 75). The only material effect, which Wexler can find and hold on to, defining the moment when she was told about her risk is that she "marked a new notebook 'Vol.1, No.1'" (A. Wexler, *Mapping* 57). Rather than a material shift and a determinable change, Wexler has to acknowledge that her risk identity and the insecurity associated with it are emotional states.

By representing risk and insecurity as emotional states and the dominating factors in her life, Wexler also narrativizes that which is absent from her and her family's life, namely security. While the rupture triggered by knowing one's risk is represented by fear and shock, security and what is "always already" lost is the possibility of an unburdened life, of happiness. Wexler visualizes this most clearly with the images that introduce the different sections of the memoir, which are conventional images of a family picture book. They represent images of happiness: one depicts her parents as a young couple in the 1940s, another shows the sisters at Alice Wexler's high school graduation in 1963. Both photographs represent times when none of the people depicted knew about the disease in their family, thus "happy times." It represents the normal as the horizon of security. Though the photographs represent what Sara Ahmed calls "happy object,"[12] the established temporality makes it impossible to read this image of the happy family without considering the future to come: the mother's struggle and long process of dying, as well as the risk that looms ahead for the Wexler sisters. The images therefore become at once signifier for the precarious normality as well as for the desired happiness that stands in as a symbol for security.

Defining security in negative terms, so as the opposite of "the drama of families with Huntington's disease . . . played out with minor variations on stages around the world" (A. Wexler, *Mapping* xi), Wexler draws a picture of what is lost. Since being at risk is neither being sick nor being healthy, what is lost first and foremost is the happiness associated with an unburdened life. While Wexler describes her own life at risk as marked by clinical depression, she also keeps reading her mother's life for traces of lost happiness. In her search for her mother's "true self" she tries "to reconstruct the history of her illness, to date the onset of her symptoms" and asks "what in Mom's behavior was due to chorea? What to character?" (A. Wexler, *Mapping* 69). Her mother's submissiveness and "depressive" episodes take center stage in this distinction: In 6th grade "I wondered in my diary if she was very intelligent, because 'she never says much during more profound conversations, nor has any ideas'" (A. Wexler, *Mapping* 27). Her sister's memories also provide traces of the "always already" lost. As a child and long before the sisters knew about the disease Nancy "had started 'sobbing and shaking in despair, crying that I no longer had a mother, that my mother had escaped somewhere and left a shell, that I didn't want only my father's voice, my father and a shadow, but I wanted two parents'" (A. Wexler, *Mapping* 32). The re-reading of her and her sister's childhood memories are defined by the unhappiness of the situations, which are read as potential indicators for the presence of HD. Her re-reading of her family's history and the search for the moment of knowing the risk in the past are readings of family happiness intercepted by the disease.

The happiness that Wexler represents as being amiss is attached to surprisingly conservative ideals. The potential loss of a future, which Wexler describes as a central characteristic of being at risk, becomes attached to the normatively mandated "purpose" of life, its "reproductive futurity" (Edelman 21). In fact, most of her explicit reflections on "sorrows for myself and for my sister, for our blighted future, for the children we would never have" (A. Wexler, *Mapping* 69) center around the question of reproduction. In this quote, as in many other similar comments Wexler emphasizes the loss of happiness of a heterosexual normative nuclear family life – the normative image of security. The normative script is so forceful, that Wexler, who will come to embrace her homosexuality, is burdened by yet another transgression of norms. Expressing the double burden of being a woman and at risk she is overdetermined and marked as other twice by the biological

---

12   The photograph represents a happy family as "both an object (something that affects us, something we are directed toward) and circulates through objects" (Ahmed, *Promise* 45).

make-up of her body. Being at risk made her feel "less like a woman" because she is not supposed to have children, and when she does try to conceive (in a relationship with a man) anyway and discovers her infertility she "feel[s] like a diver who can't come up for air" (A. Wexler, *Mapping* 231). Describing her feelings as suffocation, she reveals a further injury to the body that is again both biological and cultural at the same time. She highlights the restrictiveness of social norms, that she has internalized despite her homosexuality – a normativity of the gendered life course in which "'no children' signifies the loss of a fantasy of the future as that which can compensate me for my suffering" (Ahmed, *Promise* 183).

With the construction of healthy happiness vs. disease despair Wexler establishes a rigid and clearly defined binary opposition that undercuts the blurry lines of being at risk. And though the possibility of being at risk by anything else but HD is not absent from Wexler's life writing, other risks disappear behind the intangible threat of HD. Wexler re-reads her parents' failed marriage and divorce on the basis of her mother's changes "from the lively, witty, vivacious woman" to a silent and silenced housewife "obsessed with household chores and domestic routines" (A. Wexler, *Mapping* 28). And though she wonders how much of this is due to the oppressive social norms of the time or her mother's character, Wexler's re-evaluation always falls back onto the distinction between having HD and not having HD. Every problem is always only seen through the lens of HD or completely disappears behind it. This is most revealing, and shocking, when Wexler narrates how her mother, still free of symptoms, is gang raped in Mexico City in 1963 while visiting Nancy. The shocking scene of sexualized violence and female vulnerability, when they "drove her high into the Lomas de Chapultepec, where they dragged her out onto the ground, beat her severely, and raped her, each one sitting on her head while another took his turn" (A. Wexler, *Mapping* 39) breaks with the general narrative of illness. But though this scene exemplifies the biggest risk for women,[13] in the memoir it remains comparatively uncommented and therefore appears rather inconsequential for the mother's as well as the daughter's lives and psyche. In contrast to the ongoing and never ending worries and negotiations of HD and being at risk, this rape scene is marked by its passing character. In contrast to the disease it remains narratively contained to this one scene, an episode that though gruesome is defined by its limits: being kidnapped and raped, being recovered and brought back to the U.S., suffering anxiety attacks for a while, and overcoming the event. With the inclusion of this violent rape of her mother, Wexler highlights that life, and especially for women, is constantly at risk from many things *besides* HD. Yet, differently from the self contained narrative of rape, the risk of having Huntington's Disease is emphasized as something that cannot be overcome. The lack of an "event" in its performative and therefore temporary character represents it as uncontainable.

The indeterminable characteristic of risk and uncertainty, as the lack of a proper event that one can face up to and "come to terms with" further emphasizes the need and desire for certainty, which is the "place holder" for the potential event in the future – the diagnosis or onset of the disease. Knowledge is therefore an object of desire that de-

---

13   According to the CDC one in three women experiences sexualized violence in her life, while one in five women falls victim to rape or attempted rape during their life ("Sexual Violence").

termines one's being in the world. While Wexler represents uncertainty as the loss of a future, certainty comes to represent security and the possibility of a future.

Reading the Body – Translating Certainty: Performativity and Security

Certainty as "the object of desire" seems unquestionable in light of the suffering which Wexler attaches to the biosecurity identity of being at risk and the uncertainty she foregrounds as "an unbearable tension" (A. Wexler, *Mapping* 81). However, such a certainty as a supposed key to security is not without its problems in the context of Huntington's disease. Rather, it has to be constructed as an object of desire by making it promise security.

The importance of certainty and the need to know in this complex constellation of uncertainty reverberate throughout the text. Knowledge structures the narrative and the notion of knowing and discovery are leitmotifs of the memoir. As the story of the disease and the genetic marker, the exposition of the different family members learning about HD is also structured by the secrets of HD and their discoveries. Wexler introduces her mother's family as surrounded by "mystery" (A. Wexler, *Mapping* 8) and the grandfather's death is described with the same words: "Abraham developed a mysterious illness and died at the age of fifty-two" (A. Wexler, *Mapping* 9). This enigma, which the reader knows to be HD, has to be revealed and discovered, both accidentally and secretly by the different family members. The mother picked up the name at her father's funeral, "words that had sent her off to the library to discover that Abraham's sickness, Huntington's chorea, was inherited, but that only men could get it. At least that is what she told us later, after she herself fell ill" (A. Wexler, *Mapping* 10). Though always present in the body, HD seems to be in need of discovery. Focused on this "naming into being" (Butler, *Bodies* 13) every person's encounter with HD is related and reconstructed in great detail.

Wexler constructs this moment as the revelation of a true identity, as argued before. She describes this moment in her mother's life as "that day in 1968 when our mother's body spoke that (death) sentence. This book, in part, is my translation" (A. Wexler, *Mapping* xix). Explicit in this quote is that this form of certainty can hardly be qualified as security and exemplifies how complicated it is to speak about a form of security in the context of a degenerative genetic and fatal disease. Nonetheless, this example of knowing, and resolving the existential ambiguity of uncertainty by trading it in against what Wexler calls "the death sentence" is represented as a form of security. By making herself the translator and the body the cipher that needs translation she turns herself into a "native informant" for the reader. She is representing certainty as something that though already exposed has to be revealed, and is in need of translation to be understood (properly) as security. By making the body speak an unknown language she emphasizes the performative character of body, biology, and security. She thereby creates a vision of the body, and for genetic identity, that is there and is readable as a text of another language.

Since Huntington's is mostly known by the incontrollable body movements it triggers, certainty relies on performativity, so a physical performance and a witnessing audience. Wexler highlights the performative characteristic of the moment of discovery in her description of her mother's first perceived symptoms. It is not the self that recognizes the first signs of the disease but rather an outsider who perceives the symptoms as deviant behavior. Her mother is described as crossing the street one morning being addressed by a stranger: "'Hey lady,' he called out, 'aren't you ashamed of being drunk so early in the morning?' But she had not been drinking – in fact, she drank very little – and she must have known instantly what the words really meant" (A. Wexler, *Mapping* 44–5). The other is represented as the witnessing and judging audience while the afflicted self is described as a shameful spectacle. The body as spectacle emphasizes the sociality of the body "impressed upon by others, impinging upon them as well" (Butler, *Precarious* 27).

While other disease symptoms might trigger insecurity and anxiety about their meaning and ramifications, HD symptoms are usually well known to those afflicted. As a hereditary disease most have seen family members display the same twitches or other symptoms. This intimate understanding of the diseased corporeality plays an important role in Wexler's construction of security. The individual at risk is able to read and understand the bodily performance in contrast to the outsider witness who misreads the mother's physical difference as social deviance. The understanding of the performativity of the body that just has to be read properly, as well as the experience of being exposed by the betrayal of the body leads Wexler to a form of compulsive self-surveillance: "I watched myself for signs and symptoms. Sitting in the library or playing piano, I would inspect my fingers for jerks and twitches" (A. Wexler, *Mapping* 64). In an attempt to control the uncertainty she reads her body almost obsessively for the disease as well as for certainty, which she so urgently longs for.

However, despite the intimate knowledge of the corporeality of the disease the lay reading of one's own body seems not to be able to provide certainty. Rather the body is in need of a professional reading for a translation of the body and its security status which ultimately lies beyond the individual's understanding. The Wexlers know HD symptoms well. The mother's father, as well as all three brothers had died of the disease by the time the mother shows the first symptoms; the familiarity with the corporeality of HD once it sets in is emphasized repeatedly throughout the book. Nonetheless, Wexler's narrative emphasizes that the intimate and private knowledge is never enough but has to be verified by a professional expert: the doctor as arbiter of security. The ultimate verification of the intimate reading of the bodily performance is therefore relegated to the doctor. His diagnosis is based on nothing more than what the Wexlers know themselves, namely the family history as a disease genealogy and the outward signs of Huntington's that the mother embodies. Nonetheless, the medical reading of the body represents a different form of authority and thereby a different form of certainty. "After seeing her and hearing the family history, the neurologist knew at once. There was never any doubt" (A. Wexler, *Mapping* 45). Though the professional diagnosis neither provides new insights for the family, nor a different possibility or access to security – the disease is present and is going to end fatally – it is considered essential.

The reaction of the Wexler sisters to this diagnosis reveals another crucial element of the security narrative in the context of HD and certainty as something that comes too late. The sisters are hesitant and afraid to talk to their mother about her diagnosis. First of all, it is the sisters and the divorced husband who receive the fatal diagnosis instead of the afflicted mother, who is thereby turned into a disempowered and incapacitated passive patient. Along side the loss of a possibility to return to a healthy and secure life, the mother is initially stripped of her subjectivity and autonomy in an attempt to protect her and to provide at least the appearance of being safe. This withholding the certainty of a fatal diagnosis was common practice during the "regime of silence" that dominated at the time.[14] The sister's hesitation to inform their mother is thus based on an alternative understanding of security which makes clear that the certainty attained by reading the outward signs of the body is insufficient. Though their mother "accepted the information bravely" (A. Wexler, *Mapping* 55) once they told her, the sisters feared that informing her would cause panic and despair. In this instance, as in many others throughout the story, Wexler points out that once the disease starts it is a slow and relentless decline until death. The knowledge and certainty of this deterioration thus cannot provide any possibility of achieving security in terms of health.

The certainty provided by the diagnosis also comes too late in another sense. The outwardly perceivable symptoms of Huntington's are the first signs the individual can perceive, and were for a long time defined as the onset of the disease. Today, however, it is agreed that "[s]ubtle personality changes sometimes precede the involuntary choreic movements by many years, so much so that doctors now refer to a zone of onset rather than an age of onset" (A. Wexler, *Mapping* 48). The understanding of the performativity of security thus has to be extended from corporeality to the performance of self. It is not only the body that is at risk of becoming uncontrollable but initially the self. With this explanation Wexler makes clear that the body as sign and cipher for the truth within, is an unreliable text. The onset of the disease represented by corporeal outward signs comes after the disease has already set in, and after the disease has already started to "alter" the true self. The certainty of the onset of the disease, which lies beyond the experiential realm of a layperson therefore becomes the justification why testing is viable and necessary as a step toward security. Wexler thus constructs a security narrative in which the possibility of testing is represented as a desirable practice of security, though she herself will not make use of it. The certainty obtained by testing is stripped bare of the threatening notion of "too lateness."

While certainty consisting in the knowledge of having HD plays a fundamental role in Wexler's construction of security, she also shows the ambiguity of the construct. In the case of Huntington's certainty represents both, the onset of inevitable and fatal decline, as well as the only gateway to security as knowing one's fate. Wexler does not completely silence this ambiguity but rather reveals the necessity of narrative to make an understanding of security tangible and pervasive. She reiterates the dominant biosecurity narrative and the seemingly unquestionable urge to gain certainty with a diagnosis as early as possible by dramatizing the quest of developing a test. Her representation of the coming of the test, which is by now routinely offered, therefore highlights the variability of meaning of security in different conceptual contexts. Though the test does not represent the possibility of a cure, so the "return" to the security it promises those at risk "to escape the oppressive uncertainty" (A. Wexler, *Mapping* 236) and "painful ambiguity of their lives" (A. Wexler, *Mapping* 237) and is therefore perceived as a crucial security practice.

---

14   During this so-called "regime of silence," "it was unquestionably clear that the primary duty of the family and the doctors is to conceal the seriousness of his condition from the person who died" (Aries, "Reversal" 138).

Early knowledge and certainty of one's security status is thus represented as something desirable. As a stand in for security proper, this form of certainty promises manageability and controllability of nature's mistakes:

> The issue of control loomed large. Knowledge one way or the other appeared to give a measure of control, or at least of choice, over how one lived one's life: at the very least, knowledge of one's future in relation to Huntington's seemed to increase the terrain on which one could knowledgeably make decisions. Some people wanted to take the test in order to make decisions about having children or, more often, to inform the children they already had about their own risk, particularly if those children were themselves approaching childbearing age. Many people emphasized the extent to which testing involved everyone in the family, not just those who actually got tested. (A. Wexler, *Mapping* 236)

This form of anticipatory knowledge offered by pre-symptomatic testing, represents essentially not a different form of knowledge than the onset of the disease – it is still "this death sentence" the body speaks, as Wexler puts it. However, it is not understood as a loss of future anymore, but turned into the promise of having a future. It offers the possibility of self reliance based on the responsibility of a biosecurity individual. The looming possibility of the test represents a fiction of security that is culturally and narratively produced, rather than a reality. Based on the security narrative of an always already existing precarious normality that simply has "not yet" been apparent to the individual, the diagnosis by onset is marked as insecure, as too late. This narrative, which is based on biological data and scientific findings configures a fiction of security, which motivates individuals to (re)act. The promise of security attached to presymptomatic testing which Wexler represents in her memoir thus reveals that the security narrative has material effects impacting the life choices of individuals.

This importance of knowing and therefore the understanding of certainty as security is further enhanced by Wexler's incessant search for the reasons why her parents kept her potential risk status and HD affliction in the family a secret. Though she is informed about her risk in 1968 when her family attains the certainty with her mother's diagnosis, her parents must have known about the risk already when Alice Wexler's uncles on the maternal side of the family fell ill and died. The secret that curtailed Alice Wexler's "real identity" from her makes her "furious," further emphasizing the urge and importance of knowing the truth. As her search for the motivations and details of this secret becomes another driving force of the narrative, propelling it backwards into her past, providing knowledge becomes defined as a responsibility. And the failure to inform potentially implicated people is represented as an infringement of their right to know. The security practice of getting tested and the security practice of informing anyone potentially affected are both marked as responsibility. The certainty provided by the test eradicates the "too lateness" of the diagnosis as onset, so that individuals can know before passing it on to the next generation.

Though Wexler represents the dominant biosecurity narrative of certainty as security, which can only be provided by a biomedical reading of the body in form of a pre-symptomatic test, she does not represent it as the almighty and unquestionable narrative of security. The first version of the genetic test was anticipated and celebrated at the time but she does not depict it without its paradoxes. Wexler's memoir makes clear that she herself has reservations about the promises attached to the test. Furthermore, she shows that even the science community itself was "weary of offering the test" (A. Wexler, *Mapping* 224) because of the risk of suicide in those tested positive. She asserts that "[t]here is no question that the worst part about being told you have the gene is the watching and the waiting" (A. Wexler, *Mapping* 237). Wexler's reflections on the test exemplify the disparities between the test embodying the cultural imaginary of security while at the same time providing a "death sentence." Nonetheless, the test offers the possibility of knowing and therefore legitimizes the demand for the security practice, which Wexler reiterates as a necessity and responsibility. The reproachful undertones of her incessant questions whether her parents knowingly put her and her sister at risk mark uncertainty not only as unbearable but represent it as irresponsible. Wexler's narrative exemplifies that "biological identity generates biological responsibility" (Rose, "Politics" 19). Her depiction of this form of "ethopolitics" (Rose, "Politics" 18) as a crucial part of creating responsibility and the urge for biosecurity by transplanting governmentality into the individual ethical choice and practice stresses the importance of affects. The affects invested into the security practice, especially hope, are fundamental to make people feel responsible as well as to shape the understanding of the security practice.

Promising Knowledge and Scientific Salvation

The security narrative of certainty as key to security relies on a broader security narrative of scientific salvation and of hope which is attached to scientific progress. Not surprisingly then, Wexler's memoir establishes a close and obvious association between security and scientific research. She constructs a security narrative in which science and scientists represent the clear arbiters of security and scientific progress embodies the seemingly only source of hope. To make science the main actor that can performatively produce security, she establishes a narrative that negates the ambiguities of the text's introduction. There she mentions the "volatile space" (A. Wexler, *Mapping* xxiii) that genetics inhabit, making clear that genetic research is a "multibillion-dollar industry" (A. Wexler, *Mapping* xiii) and not a philanthropic endeavor. Further, she comments on the implications of the normative power of this "new genetics" and that the geneticized understanding of identity should be watched carefully by society. However, this ambiguity is largely restricted to the introduction and for large parts of the narrative dissolved almost entirely.

More prominently than this explicit critique is the narrative of hope invested in scientific research. Shortly after having informed the sisters about their mother's affliction, "Dad is already full of plans for fighting this illness . . . . The genetic revolution has begun, he says, and everything is possible. Nancy catches his enthusiasm and excitement. They are like two kids spinning out fantastic proposals, already on a crusade" (A. Wexler, *Mapping* 44). While fear and despair dominate the narration and Wexler's experience of being at risk, her father and sister quickly turn to hope as their way of dealing with the situation. The object of their hope is, not surprisingly, science. Wexler constructs a narrative of a biologized security that is potentially attainable. It is therefore the expectation of security, largely communicated as promise and hope, which influences the life narrative. These "passionate attachments" ("Affective" 118) as Ahmed calls them, form the "desired object" that comes to represent the possibility of security, marking security as defined by emotions. Although Wexler herself does not unconditionally share this hope, or the faith in science, it is represented as the only way out. Both the sisters will pass this affective attachment to scientific security on, though on different levels, contributing to the circulation of this security narrative. Together, they will use it as consolation when telling their mother about her HD diagnosis, Nancy Wexler becomes a leading force in scientific research and Alice Wexler writes a memoir on the disease.

The promise of scientific salvation has a long tradition in "western" cultures, representing mastery, control, and security, as I have argued earlier. In relation to the body, it not only represents the ultimate dream of control, but the promise of seeing "the truth" (Foucault, *Birth* 155) as modern medicine challenged the "space in which the bodies and eyes meet" (Foucault, *Birth* xi). Wexler herself warns that the history of science and scientific research is not simply a factual history of re-presentation but a story rendered as perpetually progressing steps of discoveries; she cautions that scientific knowledge is merely represented as naturalized knowledge. Nonetheless, when Wexler explains research findings, such as the discovery of the disease by George Huntington, she echoes the logic and teleology of scientific progress toward controlling nature's mistake and managing biological security. In fact, the promise of science and the hopes invested in its progress dominate the hopeful, almost utopian narrative strand of her memoir.

She traces the dominant narrative of approximating security with the progress of science showing how the scientific "discovery" of Huntington's and its recognition as a biologically caused disease affords afflicted individuals more security. She asserts that the establishing of the disease category provides them with an explanation for their suffering from a "definite illness" (A. Wexler, *Mapping* 46). Though not changing the "Otherness" that was socially and culturally attached to the disease this shift reframed the non-normative behavior and the social reaction to it from revulsion to compassion. Suffering all the same, the medicalization of HD meant the eradication of an epistemological deficiency that puts the individuals at risk of being "queer rather than sick, and affected individuals as mean and malicious rather than ill" (A. Wexler, *Mapping* 46). However, the alienation of families suffering from this neurodegenerative disease did not end with the insertion of the disease into neatly framed knowledge categories of modern medicine.

In following the messianic narrative of medical salvation, Wexler even highlights the research of the eugenics movement as progress toward security, though for other reasons than their original claims and methods. As explained before, Huntington's was Charles Davenport's prime example and favorite research object. Though Davenport's studies were clearly putting afflicted individuals at risk instead of providing security for them, Wexler stresses that his research also "helped [to] call attention to" the disease, instigating scientific research. His studies represent "powerful testimony to the emotional horrors of the disease, as well as the resilience and courage some people mustered in dealing with it" (A. Wexler, *Mapping* 49). The dark past of genetic research, which Wexler does not hide, is not represented as a weakening of "the promise of science" and its incessant progress toward security. She thus reiterates the image of "new genetics" vs. "old genetics,"[15] as I have discussed previously, rendering this past scientific activity as science used and produced for the wrong reasons, as an unfortunate aberration from the proper path toward security. The knowledge produced by this "science gone wrong," however, is still represented as a valuable stepping stone toward security.

Wexler reiterates the narrative of continuous scientific progress that is approximating a security which is just not reachable *yet*. This temporality represents a necessary utopian narrative element to establish and maintain the hope that this time scientific salvation could be within reach. Her father expresses this hope as follows: "[I]n certain respects, the timing of Mom's diagnosis was fortuitous in that it coincided both with a revolutionary expansion on molecular biology and with an awakening of interest and activism focused on the disease" (A. Wexler, *Mapping* 87). What Wexler's father describes as fortuitous is not better treatment or a cure at the time but a promise which is based on faith and hope rather than facts. Scientific progress as an approximation of security is thus established as an "affective fact" (Massumi, "Future Birth" 34). It is represented as a belief that "offered him [the father] hope at a moment when he feared his family might be obliterated" (A. Wexler, *Mapping* 96). This hope is, though narratively present "directed at an object that is not yet present" (Ahmed, *Promise* 181) – a cure, a test, a treatment – and therefore becomes first and foremost an instigator of action. Within the dyad of hope and fear Huntington's turns into a challenge that one has to take on, rather than a fate one has to accept and surrender to.

While the experience of suffering from HD and the unbearable uncertainty of being at risk represent the first part of Wexler's translation of the "language of the HD body" (xix) – the fearful and threatening narrative strand– the competing narrative of hope is represented as the second part of her translation: the translation of science. Since scientific knowledge is highly specialized and not immediately intelligible or self evident, one "had to learn some basic science" (A. Wexler, *Mapping* 88) to understand risk but also to share and partake in hope. She introduces the reader to a new vocabulary necessary to gain access to biosecurity. She explains hereditary rules of recessive and dominant genetic elements, the difference of phenotypes and genotypes, what independent assortment of heritage means, the discovery of the DNA structure as a double helix, and the working of recombinant DNA. In representing her father's genetic education and becoming a bioliterate subject, she educates the reader, establishing the necessary bioliteracy to understand the importance of genetic discoveries. These explanations are crucial for understanding her later representation of more complex genetic research such as discovery of the Huntington's gene IT15 (A. Wexler, *Mapping* 258–259) as a quest for security. Each step and each discovery is contextualized by the possibilities it offered and therefore represented as an approximation of future security.

By explaining the working and meaning of science Wexler partly overcomes the difficulty of presenting genetic research as unequivocally beneficial and an "object of hope." In contrast to the eugenic past, the ambiguities and fears these developments caused at

---

15   "Some invoke eugenics to distinguish the present from the past: thus contemporary molecular geneticists usually argue that their discipline, in common with the rest of medicine, has decisively rejected eugenics in favour [sic] of individualized, voluntary, informed, ethical, preventive medicine organized around the pursuit of health" (Rose, "Politics" 3).

their respective time remain comparatively unrepresented and hidden.[16] By using figures and animations of science books, she not only educates the reader but makes "the mystery" of genetics more tangible and therefore less threatening. Her representation embodies the scientific knowledge of the time, emulating the increasing visualization techniques that represented major stepping stones in genetic research. She highlights that initially "there was no way to look directly at genes at all. No one knew what a gene was. All measurements of linkage were based on the observation of identifiable traits" (A. Wexler, *Mapping* 91). By doing so she reiterates the link between seeing and knowing (Foucault) and the paradigmatic metaphor of the language of the gene that merely has to be decoded by an able translator, which was championed and circulated widely with the initiation of the Genome Project. With her explanations and the use of these images she does not only translate this "genetic language" but narrativizes it as an increasing approximation of security in a teleological structure of scientific progress.

Wexler further increases this seemingly inherent connection of scientific research as the arbiter of security by the repetitive description of the visualization of genes as a looking at the "actual molecules" representing it as mere observation. She describes this gaze as a descriptive act, rather than an intervention and changing of the "object" that is looked at (van Dijck, *Transparent* 6). This harmlessness of "just looking at," which Wexler depicts in these descriptions has two important sides. On the one hand it portrays research as only trying to understand what is at hand, merely finding new and better ways of imaging and thereby knowing. On the other hand, visualization also represents a form of circulation and the normalization of scientific findings in the public sphere. She traces the improvement of imaging that is so crucial, not only for scientific progress but for generating public understanding of genetics as a practice of security. The portrayal of scientific knowledge and research in Wexler's narrative therefore represents scientific progress while at the same time circulating hope and faith in scientific knowledge.

Wexler emphasizes the importance of this affective attachment and its circulation, which makes the connection of genetic research and security seem all the more natural and unquestionable. By foregrounding her father's and sister's activism in advancing genetic research she retells the enthusiasm of the 1950s and 1960s when "a golden age of biology had just begun" (A. Wexler, *Mapping* 96) and she recreates a "new sense of excitement" (A. Wexler, *Mapping* 187) about each additional development. The narrative chronicles the hypotheses of GABA research (A. Wexler, *Mapping* 126–27) followed by the assumption that Huntington's could be an autoimmune disease (A. Wexler, *Mapping* 128–29), as well as the suggestion that it was caused by a slow acting virus (A. Wexler, *Mapping* 132–33), and other promising but erroneous approaches. Wexler portrays the different discoveries as part of an "affective economy" (Ahmed) in which even the erroneous findings and disappointing approaches contribute to a further circulation of hope. She shows how everything seems to have "generated new hope" (A. Wexler, *Mapping* 97). As such, every report from the different workshops and centennial symposiums, as well as the different scientific hypotheses can be seen as further manifestation and normalization of the link between science and security. Wexler thus reiterates a narrative of sci-

---

16   For a detailed description of the criticism of genetic research see Bud's chapter "Wedding with Genetics," as well as Shakespeare, and De Melo.

entific salvation and shows how the scientific findings become more and more forceful and stable, for "the more they circulate, the more affective they become, and the more they appear to contain affect" (Ahmed, "Affective Economy" 120).

Wexler further recreates the enthusiasm and affective attachment by rendering the scientific research as a quest which is spearheaded by her sister Nancy. In the narration of discoveries, the overarching logic is the development of a cure, or as Wexler puts it, "an end of Huntington's." The "discovery" of the Huntington's community in the Lake Maracaibo communities in Venezuela therefore represents a watershed event for "they might offer the crucial key" (A. Wexler, Mapping 182) to the secrets of Huntington's disease, and therefore to security. The project, which is headed by her sister Nancy receives "glowing report" and had "'high priority'" (A. Wexler, Mapping 189). The affective vocabulary that is used to describe her sister's project is intriguing in two ways. It reveals the importance of an "enthusiastic supporter [Carl Leventhal], helping Nancy negotiate the hurdles toward long-term, regular funding" (A. Wexler, Mapping 190). Wexler therefore exemplifies how important it is to narrativize scientific research within a security narrative to receive financial support. But the choice of words also exposes that science is not an objective emotionless discipline but a highly affectively loaded and subjective process.

This importance of affects in defining scientific research as progress toward security is further enhanced in Wexler's description of the community in Venezuela. The image of the Laguneta community, which is used to introduce section three "Maps for Misreading," reveals the polyvocality of security narratives, and the colonial perspective that underlies discourses of biosecurity and the bias they create. Individuals born into this community carry the highest risk of having inherited HD in the world and live under one of the worst conditions for HD afflicted people in terms of health care. At the same time, the community embodies the anticipated and needed clue in the hunt to discover the secret of Huntington's precisely because of this high number of afflicted individuals. Wexler renders an image of Laguneta which combines absolute insecurity –the biggest HD community living in absolute poverty – with the shining hope of finding a cure and the genetic marker of Huntington's, so the origin of a possible solution and the recovery of security. Only a large family with many infected individuals could offer the possibility of finding the genetic trace of the disease and "they did indeed meet a large family in which both parents had the disease. Some of their fourteen children had a good chance of inheriting two Huntington's genes. . . . Nancy on the other hand, found the whole experience exhilarating" (A. Wexler, Mapping 186). Nancy's professional "exhilaration" about the existence of this family stands in stark contrast to the description of the despair associated with HD "at home." To "stand a good chance" is a decisively different emotional expression from the unbearable tension that defines the life of both of the Wexler sisters in the memoir. While the entire memoir is dedicated to the struggles of two sisters at risk in the United States, the possibility of 14 children with two afflicted parents carrying the disease is described as a victory and a crucial step towards achieving security, or rather a further approximation of security.

While the promise of security in form of a cure remains unattainable throughout the memoir receding with every approximation, the possibility of testing replaces this goal. Over the course of the memoir the possibility of testing becomes more and more possible as the marker for the genetic disease is identified in 1983. Wexler shows how the "coming of the test" represents a further circulation of the security narrative of medical salvation in the public space. She describes how media reports and research panels amplify the narrative of hope and salvation to a broader public. Wexler shows how the development of a reliable test began to also dominate the public imaginary of biosecurity, mainly driven by newspapers and magazine publications that celebrated the discoveries as major milestones of science. "The paper 'A Polymorphic DNA Marker Genetically Linked to Huntington's Disease,' appeared in the November 17, 1983 issue of the prestigious British science journal *Nature*, accompanied by two enthusiastic editorials. *The New York Times*, *The Wall Street Journal*, the *Los Angeles Times*, *The Boston Globe*, and *The Washington Post* ran the story on the front page" (A. Wexler, *Mapping* 219). And also Wexler's narrative places these discoveries in a climactic narrative, which represents both big discoveries in the history of Huntington's – the G8 marker and the IT15 gene – as providing the long anticipated and desired key to security.

Nonetheless, Wexler's narrative does not obliterate the disparity between the promised security as cure and the developed test. But while the initial development of the test "opened an abyss in all our lives, a vast space between prediction and prevention" (A. Wexler, *Mapping* 221), its deferral, so the disappointment and failure to provide the promised security seems to heighten the affective investment in its potential. Especially for the discovery of the gene in 1993 Wexler shows how forceful the affective attachment to the narrative of scientific salvation is. She reports how "[t]oday the newspapers all carried the story of finding the gene. They call it 'the longest and most frustrating search in the annals of molecular biology'" (A. Wexler, *Mapping* 258). The hope invested in research is so forceful that when the long anticipated knowledge is found "it didn't seem real" (ibid.). "And Marcy and MacDonald told me, 'When we called people their first reaction was relief – thank God it's over! – and the second reaction was pure joy'" (ibid.). The reactions of these scientists show how pervasive the narrative scientific salvation is, for "it" – the quest for the promised security – is "over" already before it really is. To this day a cure for HD has not been found. But rather than a failure Wexler shows that it is perceived by those involved as a moment of relief. The hopes and desires attached to the narrative of scientific salvation establish the created possibility of testing as the objects of desire and crucial key to achieving security.

Science in Wexler's story is never quite there yet. With the discovery of the gene security further receded, remaining almost in reach but not yet attainable. And also retrospectively Wexler reflects on the discovery as a crucial further approximation of security. Narratively, the discovery of the gene is turned into a necessary approximation because it allows scientists to "explore how those extra CAG repeats interfere with the normal functioning of the gene" (A. Wexler, *Mapping* 260). And though testing does not bring the promised security for the individual she makes clear that it is nonetheless a crucial security practice: "[w]hatever the risks of presymptomatic testing, there was no question that a reliable test indicating which individuals carried the gene could offer scientists valuable data about the early pathology of the illness" (A. Wexler, *Mapping* 222). Despite the insufficiency of the test, and the "not yet" of a cure for Huntington's, science is represented as the unquestionable arbiter of security and only harbinger of hope. Echoing a messianic narrative of scientific salvations, the trials and tribulations on the way to this security are to be endured until science will come and bring security to those afflicted.

And though Wexler does not tell a success story she shows how the scientific findings embedded in this pervasive security narrative create faith: "what has changed is the psychological landscape, the wider horizons of hope before us" (A. Wexler, *Mapping* 261).

In Wexler's narrative this creation and proliferation of faith and hope become the success of the climactic and end directed narrative toward security. The last section of her memoir, "Genetic Destinations" (A. Wexler, *Mapping* 241), is preceded by a group photo of the Huntington's Disease Collaborative Research Group with the caption listing the names of all the participants. The people researching HD in the different fields and disciplines personify the promise of security, which is not unambiguously there at the end of the book. Nonetheless, the image and their scientific achievement – the development of a genetic test – represents the end of a successful mission, "the completion of the operation proper" (*Transparent* 32) as van Dijck reads those images in the analysis of medical documentaries. This form of representation hides the further deferral of the anticipated and promised event.

Wexler's narrative is far from being a simplistic salvation narrative of the messianic "coming of science" though it has close affinities to it. Though her narrative construction follows the formulaic structure of this discourse Wexler is able to maintain a critical stance, reintroducing ambiguities into the text. The main subversion that Wexler offers within this narrative of scientific salvation is her own emotional detachment from the dominant circulation of hope, excitement and anticipation. Initially she cannot share her father's and sister's excitement, and later she quotes emotions of others. It is her father's enthusiasm for new genetics and her sister's enthusiasm for the discoveries in research that she *reports about*. Only when she describes her search for "Venezuela's patient zero" does she actually narrate her own excitement and passion. "We found the Spanish sailor! I remember thinking as a I showed the page to Fidela that I would never again feel such a thrill of discovery" (A. Wexler, *Mapping* 201). In contrast, her personal encounter with research findings, particularly of the genetic marker, are rather framed by fear and anxiety. As mentioned previously, Wexler herself does not get tested and neither does she reveal in her memoir if her sister Nancy is going to get tested.[17] In constructing her individual security narrative she emphasizes different actors and ways of making security, which I will turn to in the concluding section. The story of the research progress leading to the discovery of the gene[18] is told alongside and intersects with the story of the personal life, making them an inseparable part of each other. Discursively they thus establish a "mock" semantic and logical relation of the two success stories: discovering Huntington's, and successfully coping and living at risk. The story presents the coming of age story of science and of the self, which offers a possible subversion of the narrative of scientific salvation.

---

17   Nancy Wexler revealed in 2020 after 40 years of researching the gene and heading the most prestigious genetic counseling institutions that she herself had tested positive for Huntington's. The New York Times article was fittingly titled "Haunted by a Gene" (Grady).

18   Wexler does not follow the "traditional" plotting of science stories as van Dijck describes it: "Popular science stories usually present scientific events as a teleological structure: experiments resulting in a discovery. In gene narratives, the order of telling is a reconstruction of the logic of argument, never an account of experimentation" (van Dijck, *Imagenation* 19).

Making Security – Writing Life

I have argued that the security narrative which Wexler offers depicts inescapable despair caused not only by the onset of the disease but the risk identity she and her sister are ascribed, as well as the hope attached to science as the arbiter of biosecurity. Wexler thereby depicts the dominant discourse of scientific salvation, a utopia that is continuously deferred as it does not culminate in a cure but only in further hope for better treatment and a certainty that would resolve the unbearable risk. She makes clear that the dream of control and manageability looms large over the life and identity formation of the biosecurity individual at risk. But her security narrative does not render science as an almighty source of security.

By combining the narratives of her family's activism for and in the Huntington's community as one story with the medical history of HD, Wexler produces an image of making security that goes beyond science as the only harbinger of hope and security. Rather she emphasizes a formation which I would describe as "biosocial security." The term "biosociality" was coined by the anthropologist Paul Rabinow and describes the social relations forged by developments in the field of genetics (*Essays* inter alia 99) as well as the sociality formed on the basis of biology by activism or self-help groups (Rabinow and Rose 197, Rose and Novas 6). The term has been widely adopted and modified, coming to embody a more general field of identity formation. However, I would like to use the term in its more traditional meaning to portray the specific social identity formed in activism, which is crucial for the biosecurity individual and the act of making security.

Wexler's memoir shows that disease activism is a crucial part of "the Huntington's world" and their struggle for security. She stresses that just as her father had done, "several other people with the illness in their family had begun major fundraising initiatives" (A. Wexler, *Mapping* 87). By narrativizing the ongoing struggle and formative influence of her family in the scientific process and progress Wexler makes their actions part and parcel of the security narrative. In that respect it is crucial that she not only tells the story of her sister becoming one of the leading scientists in the Huntington's community and working on the project in Venezuela which offers the "single most important piece of information" (A. Wexler, *Mapping* 253) to solve the Huntington's secret. At the same time, she foregrounds her father's activism in funding and organizing workshops, which she represents as equally important in the discovery of the gene. His activism brings about structures that facilitate the interdisciplinary work, which was formative for this field of research. With the hybridized narrative form of life writing and disease history she manifests the interconnectedness and interdependence of these supposedly distinct forms of making security traditionally recognized in activism and scientific research.[19] By representing the network of different people, institutions, and disciplines involved in the Huntington's community, making security is rendered as a group effort.

While Wexler represents the mutual importance of different actors for reaching security, she also makes clear that the biosocial community and its ideas of security are not homogeneous. The private engagement of people like Woody Guthrie's wife, and the

---

19   In 2012 Nancy Wexler, at that time a leading geneticist and bioethicist, emphasized the importance of "advocacy driving science" in the eponymous article which highlights precisely these networks.

Wexlers reinforces the narrative of science as salvation, for all stress the importance of research. However, her explanations of their activisms also signal toward different approaches of how to best advance toward security, within this frame of biomedically procured security. They embody a "distinct set of priorities: direct versus indirect support of science and funding of basic research almost exclusively versus diversified spending on science, public education, and patient services" (A. Wexler, *Mapping* 123). These different tactics reveal different interpretations of security. While direct funding leaves no room for other sources of security but biomedicine, the latter emphasizes the importance of educating and mobilizing the public as another roadmap to security. However, since Wexler's father's Hereditary Disease Foundation stands for the former, and it is Alice Wexler's father's and sister's experiences that structure the narration of illness and the history of research, this approach dominates Wexler's narrative. She therefore reiterates and reinforces the dominant security narrative of biomedical salvation.

Above all, the story of "making security" shows that the biosociality does not only exist on an activist basis that stands in opposition to the scientific community. Rather it exemplifies the interdependence of both activism and scientific research. Wexler points out that on the one hand HD afflicted families need the structures of biosociality, such as self-help groups where "hearing other people at risk talk about Huntington's made it feel less like her individual burden" (A. Wexler, *Mapping* 116). On the other hand, their stories function as a motivation for research:

> Each workshop began by introducing to the group a person with Huntington's disease, sometimes accompanied by an entire family . . . . A simple neurological exam followed, showing how the disease affected one's ability to count, to recall, to walk across the room or hold one's arms straight out in front. Often spouses or siblings would tell their own stories, giving a powerful portrait of how the disease affected an entire family. The emotional representations were always very moving and sometimes shocking to the scientists, who often had no clinical experience and had never seen a person with Huntington's. (A. Wexler, *Mapping* 111)

The HD afflicted families are at the same time depicted in their serial as well as their biosocial implication. While they clearly function as examples of a bigger group of people, they are at the same time objects of science that are being studied and looked at. More importantly though, their suffering is used as an example to connect the highly specialized research on the molecular level with the impact and implication they have for the lived experience of individuals. It makes the researchers part of the biosocial HD community. This structure emphasizes the importance of narrative for a comprehensive understanding of biosecurity and self. In these cases, the narrative act of telling the life story becomes an important part of making security. In the same way as self help groups and research actively engage in forming a HD community, they are deeply entrenched in the circulation of hope. As an "affective community" (Ahmed) that is unified by the affects attached to certain objects, in this case hope attached to science, they represent and further circulate hope. They are not represented as a distinct group that reacts to and redefines itself on the basis of biosecurity, but rather as part of its narrative construction.

The biosocial identity embodied by the father's as well as the sister's activism is represented as their way of fighting the disease, not only literally in the form of research, but emotionally as a way of coping. "All this activism helped ease the pain of watching Mom's decline, but it could not stop the inexorable progression of disease" (A. Wexler, *Mapping* 63). Though neither form of engagement could ultimately save the mother from Huntington's disease it represents the production of hope for future security. While biosocial activism evidently engenders a hopeful discourse for the greater community of HD, it does so also for the people that are actors within this dynamic of "making security." "As she [Nancy] grew active in the small Huntington's community in Detroit, she began to speak more openly in Ann Arbor about her work, as well as about being at risk" (A. Wexler, *Mapping* 115). Not only does it advance research, it allows for an active way of confronting the disease which stands in stark contrast to the passivity traditionally associated with "being afflicted" and becoming a patient.[20] Despite the beneficial role of the hope attached to scientific salvation in the memoir, at the same time it represents a normative discourse of what is expected. When revealing that, "[f]or a long time I felt ashamed that I was not as active as my father or my sister" (A. Wexler, *Mapping* 71) Wexler expresses a sense of guilt. Similarly to the urge of testing as a moral/ethic imperative and normativity in "surveillance medicine," the engagement in activism seems another one. It represents the imperative of actively facing one's fate and making it one's own.

Wexler's appropriation of her risk identity in the narrative act, so by the writing of her memoir, also represents an act of activism that is aimed at making security. By representing her family's activism and way of coping with the risk identity she herself engages in the very same form of activism. Rose and Novas have attested the importance of "scientific literacy" ("Citizenship" 443) for the formation of a biosocial identity. The memoir with its clear didactic purpose and educational mission embodies precisely that. The extensive representation of genetic and HD research educates the implied reader and embodies this need for knowledge. However, she also raises awareness of the biological as well as cultural meaning imbued in the image of a disease, as her memoir attempts incessantly to untangle the interdependent sources of meaning making.

By writing her memoir and representing herself as a member of the Huntington's community she makes herself a representative of the community, as one of the actors in the long line of HD dramas she lamented beforehand. In doing so she is careful not to obliterate her other intersectional identity markers as setting her apart from many HD experiences. She claims to be "aware of my position as a white, Jewish, upper-middle-class woman" (A. Wexler, *Mapping* xxi). Nonetheless, her fears and depression, and her self-scrutiny are exemplifying a common experience of precariousness. Her parents' failed marriage, her father's affair, her mother's suicide attempt, and her own bouts of depression show a common suffering, despite her privileged position with all support networks in place – psychological as well as monetary. Wexler does not hide that all this suffering as well as the shame associated with HD for whole families are exacerbated by class difference but she establishes commonalities that obliterate this class difference to

---

20   Alan Petersen suggests that "more and more, in the health care arena, the concept of the active consumer, has come to replace the notion of the passive patient" ("Governmentality" 193). This represents a difference to Talcott Parsons's "sick role" which is usually associated with passivity.

a certain extend. She therefore writes a "community of (in)security" (Völz, "A Nation" n.p.) that is in need of protection by formulating their "narrative of injury" (Ahmed, *Cultural Politics* 32–33). Wexler's proclaimed intent, however, was not just the representation of a group for the outsider. In an article on life writing and responsibility she explains that she "tried above all to speak in ways accessible to those most affected by this story – people in the Huntington's community" (A. Wexler, "Mapping Lives"). This implicit audience of her memoir also determined her choice, which for her was an ethical one, regarding what to include in the memoir. And especially her decision not to reveal if she or her sister are going to be tested is explained with her "responsibility to this community of vulnerable subjects" (A. Wexler, "Mapping Lives" 169).

In making herself an example, she thus introduces an alternate security narrative to the overarching narrative of medical salvation. By narrating her life and assuming an HD identity she depicts her suffering to give the community a voice in the public sphere and therefore establish security by raising awareness. At the same time, she also negotiates and demonstrates her own way of coping with the disease. The life narrative as a process of understanding and knowing the self through the search for her mother's true identity, is thus not only an active negotiation of her risk and a process of finding the self but an act of establishing her own security narrative; one that subverts the normative security narrative of biomedical salvation. The life narrative is therefore a necessary act of making security

Wexler's search for her mother's true self, which I discussed above, and ultimately for herself as a form of knowing and understanding represents Wexler's individual process of "coming to terms with" the threat of Huntington's, which is comparable to her sister's and father's activism. Her narrative is not just a witness account and testimony of suffering but rather an act of "making security:" "If I could catch a glimpse of her whole, perhaps I could look into the mirror each day without the everlasting search for symptoms. Maybe if I could write her story, she would no longer push herself into my dreams, scratching my arms to drag me down with her" (A. Wexler, *Mapping* 5). The haunting presence of HD, embodied by the nightmarish mother "coming back" is connected to not "understanding her whole." This understanding replaces the certainty of a test with the reconstruction of her own identity at risk. Though with the image of the "glimpse" Wexler uses the same trope as biomedical narratives – the seeing of a truth inside as a form of self-empowerment – she does not limit "recognition" to a question of understanding based on observing as knowing. Rather it is the process of writing itself that carries the promise of security in terms of manageability. And though Wexler's life writing and her search for herself are deeply connected to and structured by biotechnology, foregrounding the biosecurity narrative of medical salvation this is not what offers assurance or security to Wexler herself. Rather the practice of writing, as the way of finding the self, becomes her most important practice of security itself. Writing provides the means to narrativize and thereby understand the self in terms of biological security.

At the same time, writing represents the most important proof that the disease hasn't set in, and might even be absent altogether. Writing thus becomes test and cure at the same time, replacing the biosecurity practices prescribed by the dominant security narrative of medical salvation. The book presents security of and for the author because it represents the proof that Wexler is not showing any symptoms of HD, *yet*. This is not only implicitly so but an explicit statement Wexler makes when commenting on beginning to write after her mother's death: "There were practical considerations too. I felt increasingly that my own time might be limited. If I were to go the way my mother, I had better start writing now" (A. Wexler, *Mapping* 166). Though the book and her ability to compose this narration are proof of the presence of security, the plot generator of the memoir is the absence of security. It is the perpetual and constant "might be" and "not yet" of the healthy present that dominates and directs action and narration. The text becomes witness to this "not yet" and turns into Wexler's own mark worn with pride, an "elaborate embroidery and fantastic flourishes of gold thread" (Hawthorne, *Scarlet* 50) that marks Wexler's belonging.

Wexler thus represents a dominant security narrative of science as salvation to subvert it both, discursively and narratively. What she proposes instead is the acceptance of ambiguity as the creation of a 3rd space, which she deliberately borrows from cultural critique, so a space in between as described by scholars such as Gloria Anzaldúa, that offers the possibility for a positive re-interpretation and space of creativity. In criticizing the propagation of the test she asks: "isn't it possible that those who opt not to know are more able to live with uncertainty and ambiguity?" (A. Wexler, *Mapping* 235). The community in Maracaibo embodies this possibility of ambiguity for her. While she acknowledges the dire situation describing it as paradise and hell at the same time, she nonetheless elevates them to an image of security in a decisively different form than offered in her sister's quest for cure. She reports "the way in which people with Huntington's seemed to be better integrated into their communities than those in the United States, who were often overmedicated and hidden away in hospitals or at home" (A. Wexler, *Mapping* 186). Despite obliterating the fact that this "integrative living" might not be as voluntary as it seems for the "outside observer," she projects her longing for happiness into this other. "Being at risk means feeling different from both those who are not at risk and from those with Huntington's. It's an emotional state all its own. The Venezuelans seem to understand this – better, perhaps, than North Americans, who do not tolerate ambiguity well" (A. Wexler, *Mapping* 199). The possibility of happiness materializes as another space and another culture. And though her quest of finding self ends with the union of mother and daughter when Wexler can "remember, I speak this language too, there are no more secrets and you and I are no longer strangers," the possibility of enduring ambiguity remains projected onto the other:

> My mother embraces me at the bottom of Lake Maracaibo. . . . Gently I let go of her arms and she releases me from her hold. As she falls away toward the floor of the lake, she turns into a beautiful golden fish with silky scales and emerald eyes. With a flick of her tail, she vanishes into the depths, while I swim up toward the surface of the water and emerge into the sunlight of the Venezuelan tropics. (A. Wexler, *Mapping* 239)

Repeating the symbolism of the fish, which represented the fearful discovery of the precarious normality, Wexler indicates her changed perspective. Here the mother as the stronghold of Huntington's risk releases Wexler. No longer seen as a carp the mother turns into a beautiful exotic fish. With a clearly colonial gaze of this exotic space of the tropics, Wexler expresses her chosen path of security.

The ambiguity that is the hallmark of the identity at risk is echoed on the discursive level of the narration. The general flow of the narrative in the life narrative sections is often interrupted by paragraphs in italics, which represent most frequently emotional or associative scenes, sketches, or dream sequences. Though all represent interruptions of the storyline, some of these are taken up and commented on in the following narration, others complement the narration in an almost Freudian subconscious mirror of the very reflected and thought-out narratives of the past. She thereby structurally creates a hybrid text with a formal subdivision of dream and "reality." However, over the course of the narrative Wexler starts breaking up the formal structure of the text that has been introduced to the reader as indicators of reality and "dream"; especially after the diagnosis of the mother and the subsequent identity change she is experiencing. She therefore narratively and structurally denies the reader the experience of certainty or security of a clearly structured story in these sections. Though these interjections merely represent short in-between sections in the otherwise clear-cut memoir, they re-embody the ambiguity she decides to represents her own biosecurity identity as.

The example Wexler sets with her memoir is thus a subversion of the dominant security narrative of scientific salvation, which would require a categorization. In opposition to the norms "perhaps I even enjoy the ambiguity, resisting sharp categories and binary definitions, the border guards insisting that we place ourselves in one camp or another" (A. Wexler, *Mapping* 238). Her didactic approach of educating is "in the hope that this story may encourage others to tell their stories as well" (A. Wexler, *Mapping* xxi). She thus aims to encourage others to take "her" path of making security by storytelling. She participates in the circulation of affect attached to an alternate object and participates in forming the Huntington's community that is the key to representation and research as much as for a support group of "shared sufferers." Her representation of HD and the HD community produces a visibility that is crucial for an improvement of the social and cultural construction of Huntington's. The visibility of HD produced by such expressions triggers more understanding in society potentially counteracting some of the social alienation and stigma associated with the disease. The book itself turns into a material object of the security narrative it depicts.

Though Wexler finds and represents her own way of dealing with being at risk by embracing ambiguity, she does not challenge the notion of undesirability of the HD body. The notion of "always already" that characterizes the precarious normality her family lives in reiterates a geneticized understanding of identity, or "genetics as fate," and thereby forecloses a dissolution or challenge of the categories "good" and "bad" life. The positive 3rd space that Wexler claims as her "happiness in ambiguity" is made impossible by this biologized understanding of security. "José has nine children. One son died of juvenile Huntington's at the age of nine. . . . José tells me firmly, 'All my children are normal'" (A. Wexler, *Mapping* 198). José understanding of "normal" remains projected onto the other as a potential but it represents a fundamentally different approach to the "always already" Wexler offers as her guiding logic of security. Furthermore, José remains marked as the voice of the uneducated Venezuelan from the poverty stricken village far away from the U.S.. In contrast, the individual at risk in the U.S. remains the other to the healthy norm under the "regime of total health" (Earle et al. 96). The ambiguity that Wexler represents as her positioning to, or rather between security and risk may describe her "category of identity," but it is a further promise rather than a fulfillment of the happiness she was seeking. Rather than a tangible alternative Wexler creates another hope that stands to contest the unquestionable urge for testing. It is a promise that "is 'ahead' of itself" (Ahmed, *Promise* 181) even after Wexler has seen her mother whole and finding a way to live in-between.

6. Performing Futures: Breast Cancer, Pre-emption, and the Biosecurity Individual

> Each woman responds to the crisis that breast cancer brings to her life out of a whole pattern, which is the design of who she is and how her life has been lived.
> *Audre Lorde*

While Wexler's memoir takes its heft from exploring a seemingly mysterious disease that few people know about, breast cancer narratives have a different urgency because the disease is so commonplace. One in eight women in the U.S. "will develop breast cancer over the course of her lifetime;" "in 2020, 276,480 new cases are expected to be diagnosed" and "42,170 women are expected to die" from breast cancer in the U.S. alone (Breastcancer.org, "Statistics" n.p.). The opening lines of Audre Lorde's iconic *Cancer Journals* describe the individuality of the experience and the incision that a cancer diagnosis represents as an injury not only of the body, but of the person. Her narrative stands out as her analysis reaches beyond the individual illness experience toward broader questions of gender, class, and racial injustice. Biomedical and biotechnological progress, as well as cultural representation such as Lorde's breast cancer narratives have changed the meaning of the disease and have created new forms of breast cancer experiences. Especially the focus on breast cancer risk and genetics has shifted the moment of crisis that Lorde described in the lines above. The possibilities of biomedical diagnostics in the field of breast cancer and the focus on diagnosing and treating risks have made preventive and pre-emptive security practices the dominant way of understanding and confronting breast cancer.

In this chapter I will examine the impact of biosecurity practices and the messianic narrative of scientific salvation in the context of breast cancer risk. I will turn to the "regime of surveillance medicine" (Armstrong 403) and the material effects produced by the security narratives of breast cancer prevention and pre-emption. Breast cancer is considered a national as well as global emergency and "a modern epidemic" (Schneider et al. 244). The war on breast cancer, however, is not only a national and global security concern but represents individual struggles. Nonetheless, the biosecurity practices in the context of breast cancer reiterate the omnipresent national security logic. I will therefore highlight how the individualized biosecurity practices follow the same pre-emptive logics and describe the place where national and individual biomedical security intersect. The existential uncertainty produced by the logics of national security narratives are reiterated in individual(ized) biosecurity performances pervading the public sphere and private lives in the U.S.. And these biosecurity performances give rise to a new form of biosecurity individuals: the breast cancer previvor.

Early detection and prevention of breast cancer has been a central element of the biomedical security narrative and its promise to "cure" for a very long time. The gospel of prevention proliferated throughout the 20th century focusing more and more on establishing and defining risk groups, and increasingly on defining risk individuals and practices of pre-emption. In place of a cure, the urge for testing has forwarded the detection of cancer, pushing the diagnosis to *before* a cancer develops and manifests. Improved screening technologies have facilitated the diagnosis of precancerous cells such as lobular carcinoma or ductal carcinoma in situ (DCIS), which are often medically and discursively treated as if they were breast cancer.[1] Driven by the promise to cure the body and eradicate breast cancer, pre-emptive logics of biosecurity are particularly salient in the post-millennial understanding and confrontation of breast cancer. Especially the possibilities of diagnosing genetic markers for breast cancer risk – facilitated by the discovery of BRCA1 in 1994 and BRCA2 in 1995 – have made interventions in the (still) healthy body to foreclose a potentially diseased future an accepted biosecurity practice in the U.S. (Fosket 339).

The diagnosis of a genetic marker such as the faulty BRCA1 or BRCA2 increases the "normal" risk of a woman to develop breast cancer to 65% on average. This is a frightening numerical reality that has garnered considerable public attention. These mutations only represent 0.1 to 0.6 percent of the population, however, they are on the forefront of most recent breast cancer representations.[2] The diagnosis of genetic markers for breast cancer risk is not a result such as the pre-symptomatic diagnosis of Huntington's disease. The genetic markers indicate an increased risk and a potential for a future cancer affliction. Nonetheless, "high risk" individuals are defined and treated as if pre-symptomatically ill in the biomedical security complex, and invasive strategies are used to treat the potential future cancer. Individuals diagnosed with hereditary breast and ovarian cancer have two choices. They can begin an increased and individual medical surveillance regimen with medical tests every three months and one additional annual Magnetic Resonance Imaging (MRI) to detect cancer in its earliest stages, or they have the choice to undergo chemoprevention (pre-emptive chemotherapy) or pre-emptive surgery. In this chapter I

---

1   Lobular cancer as well as ductal carcinoma in situ (DCIS) represent tissues that could develop into cancer, but do not represent a diagnosable cancer. Laura Esserman from the Carol Franc Buck Breast Cancer Center highlights that this name is misleading as it really is a marker for a risk factor rather than for an actual carcinoma (qtd. in Orenstein, "Feel Good" n.p.). Nonetheless, individuals with DCIS often opt for mastectomies (ibid.).

2   Other more common risk factors are "age, genetic factors (or heredity), poverty, diet and nutrition, and lifestyle" (Frisby 491).

will focus on the security narratives that legitimize such seemingly drastic material effects. I will therefore not focus on the extensive body of breast cancer narratives, narrative accounts of individuals afflicted with breast cancer, but rather narratives of individuals at risk of breast cancer, which "often take place at an uncanny locus of embodiment and disembodiment" (DeShazer and Helle 9).

While Barron H. Lerner, author of *Breast Cancer Wars*, still pondered the question of how such experiences of individuals treated for a breast cancer risk could be understood – in medical terminology they were called "unaffected carrier" – the term "previvor" is today an established label for these risk individuals. The neologism previvor is not a term created for the sake of academic analysis but a terminology that was first adopted by afflicted individuals. It was developed by Sue Friedman, founder of BRCA patient advocacy organization Facing our Risk for Cancer Empowered (FORCE), a previvor herself. The name describes the experience of individuals who live with an increased hereditary breast and ovarian cancer risk "surviving" a not (yet) existent cancer. I will turn to the security narratives produced by previvors, specifically the public representations of previvor "testimony," such as the celebrity accounts by Jessica Queller and Angelina Jolie published in *The New York Times*, as well as narratives published in forums and self-help groups. With these examples I will emphasize testimonies as public performances of biosecurity individuals which shape the public representation of breast cancer risk and of these new biosecurity identities.

Most analyses of previvor testimony place these texts in the context of health and disease and interpret them accordingly. They most prominently grapple with the simultaneous absence and presence of both of these categories (Herndl, "Virtual", Nye, DeShazer and Helle). I think this perspective neglects that these texts and experiences are articulated and constructed in terms of security. Though scholars assert that these narratives are expressions of radical uncertainty, I wish to show that the security narrative of medical salvation establishes a pervasive image of security which is at core performative. I will therefore read biosecurity practices as performances that help to shape the experience and understanding, and to a certain extent the reality of the affliction. I will show how the biomedical developments, specifically the growing possibility of genetic testing for breast cancer risk markers produce a new category of illness identity and thereby performatively produces an illness experience, which is premised on the understanding of security. By investigating the role and impact of cultural performances, I wish to demonstrate that current biosecurity is based on performance and theatrical methods to legitimize its pre-emptive logics. The representation of previvors and their security narratives heavily relies on the "history of meaning" (Bouwsma 285) established in the breast cancer movement. I will therefore first focus on the performances that have (in)formed the understanding and reaction to the "crisis" of breast cancer, establishing a narrative of survivability. I will then turn to individual accounts of previvors, to show how these acts of giving testimony represent a necessary acts in establishing biosecurity and the identity of the previvor.

Performativity, Biosecurity Culture, and the Breast Cancer Movement

> Previor or Survivor?
> If you have been diagnosed with cancer, you
> are a *survivor*. You're a *previor* if you have a
> family history of disease, an inherited
> mutation, or other factor that predisposes
> you to developing cancer and you've never
> been diagnosed.
> *Sue Friedman et al.*

Today's previor movement and the proliferation of security narratives of previors are – albeit decisively different in many ways – tightly connected to the narratives constructed in the cancer movement and its relation to the messianic narrative of scientific salvation. The material realities produced by the post-millennial security narratives can only be understood when analyzed in their relation to the "history of meaning" produced by a long line of female performances that have defined security in the context of breast cancer. The aim is here not to repeat medical history but rather to focus on the performances that have shaped both the research and the public image of the disease. The disease as well as its representations have a long history that has been well documented, and extensively researched.[3] Samantha King for instance asserts that the disease "has been transformed in public discourse from a stigmatized disease . . . to an enriching and affirming experience during which women with the disease are rarely 'patients' and mostly 'survivors.'" (S. King, "Pink Ribbons" 473). Accordingly, the security narratives concerning breast cancer represent a radical shift from passive patient to empowered subject, which is embodied by the biosecurity identity of the survivor as well as by the previor.

Though this change might seem radical the security narrative of controllability and hope, and the underlying messianic promise of scientific salvation have remained fairly constant. While the promise of finding a cure for cancer persistently remained ahead and out of reach, improved treatment options and diagnostics seem to have changed the prospect of a breast cancer affliction. In many ways it appears as if medical progress has simply changed the image of the feared disease from a definitive death-sentence to a manageable disease *if* it is detected early enough. Better treatment options and screening possibilities made "the survivor" a more tenable position, and therefore a more prominent symbol of security. However, besides scientific findings these changes have been closely related to and were facilitated by public performances – performances that have stressed the survivability and controllability of breast cancer when following the medical script.

Most historic accounts of cancer treatment emphasize the long line of mainly men and their heroic battles against the disease, such as the surgeon Professor William S. Halsted. The rise of breast cancer surgery is traced back to him and the turn of the 20th

---

3   Following the theoretic consent that disease is always both culturally and biologically determined (Sarasin, Davis and Morris), breast cancer has variously been argued to be a socially constructed disease (Kasper and Ferguson).

century. Halsted championed radical mastectomy – the removal of both breast and underlying muscle tissue – as the only way of preventing the spread of the cancer. Retrospectively judged as unnecessary and harmful in many cases, the practice "became the undisputed path that generations of surgeons trod with diligence" (Lakhtakia 167). The inability to provide security from breast cancer was not represented as an aptitude of the dominant security practice but as the failing of individuals and their ability to report possible symptoms. To provide the promised security it was crucial to establish a pervasive security narrative that would motivate individuals to consult a doctor as quickly as possible. The image of cancer as a definite death sentence as well as the ignorance of the warning signs of cancer had to be challenged by the dissemination of information marking "the beginning of an erosion of the public silence" (Carter 655).

This distribution of information and the normalization of biosecurity practices were decisively facilitated by female performances. In 1913 the first pamphlets informing about cancer and the security practices of cancer prevention started to circulate in the U.S.. The public health education, initiated by the American Society for the Control of Cancer (ASCC), was targeted at a female audience and published in women's journals (J. Patterson 74). Pamphlets circulated the narrative that cancer was survivable promoting a "'Message of Hope' – early detection – available to all Americans" (J. Patterson 76). In the 1930s the ASCC officially decided to "fight cancer with publicity" (qtd. in Lerner, *Wars* 43) by propagating the curability of cancer.[4] They relegated the task of cancer education to a newly established female subfield, headed by Marjorie Illig: the "Women's Field Army" (WFA). The information drives of the WFA represented public performances that staged biological security as a decisively female task on the home front against cancer. And the most crucial message circulated in these performances was that "delay kills" (qtd. in Lerner, *Wars* 47) while medical salvation stood ready at hand for those prepared. In 1940 the public representation of cancer was further increased by a public relations campaign that introduced the aspect of charity and fundraising to the struggle of the ASCC (J. Patterson 173). The campaign successfully raised more money than the ASCC's entire funding in its first year (Lerner, *Wars* 50). And it increased the stronghold of the messianic narrative of scientific salvation promising the coming of biosecurity as unquestionably ahead if scientific research was supported and funded.

The increased circulation of the security narratives of cancer prevention also established the proliferation of individual biosecurity practices that translated individual responsibility into individual embodied acts. In the 1950s the urge for breast self-exams started to circulate, teaching women to read their own bodies for signs of the disease (Lerner, *Wars* 55). The breast self-exams converted the biosecurity practice of surveillance into individual biosecurity practices – performances that are omnipresent today. These performances not only mandate individual responsibility for one's biological security –

---

4   Medical professionals also had to circulate the new image of security within their own circles with events such as the conference "Cancer is Curable" in 1932. The general sentiment of security granted by the medical profession led to the foundation of institutions with names such as "Cured Cancer Clinic" in Pondville (Lerner, *Wars* 42–43). Lerner calls this process for the post war years "inventing a curable disease" ("Inventing").

the self-reliant biosecurity individual – but make individual female performances a crucial constituent of biosecurity. As embodied and ritualized experiences, biosecurity thus
became a crucial part of female identity in the United States. Since 1963, when mammography was developed, the urge for earlier and more regular testing became louder
and more pressing, further emphasizing preventive security practices as the most crucial
element of improving mortality rates. At the same time, this growing "technoscientific
biomedicalization" (Clarke et al., "Charting" 88) made security increasingly unattainable
for the individual and a matter of expert reading.

In the 1970s, female performances of giving testimony further changed the understanding of breast cancer, which had remained a silenced and stigmatized experience
despite the public relations campaigns. Scholars assert that the personal stories of
women have decisively shaped the "history of the disease" (S. King, "Pink Ribbons" 476).[5]
Most famously, Betty Ford's breast cancer diagnosis in 1974 and her public testimony
is seen as paradigmatic in breaking the silence surrounding breast cancer. According
to Lerner, Ford's act of giving testimony led to an increased demand of the biosecurity
practices of early detection and boosted the publicity and desirability of projects such
as "The Breast Cancer Detection Demonstration Program" (*Wars* 175). In such public
performances women did thus not only share their struggle with breast cancer but
embodied the promised security if the assigned "sick role" (Parsons, "Sick Role" 257) was
performed properly: survival. Ford's post-surgery photo series (Kennerly), for instance,
represents an almost unchanged First Lady. The performative acts of giving testimony
thus represent both the imminent threat of cancer, and the promised security when
following a medical script, underlining the authority of the medical profession as arbiter
of security. But Ford also asserts in her speech to the ASCC in November 1975: "I just
cannot stress enough how necessary it is for women to take an active interest in their
own health and body" (Ford). Biomedical salvation, though relying on expert readings
was clearly also premised on the responsibilization of the individual.

At the same time as breast cancer became a much more publicly discussed and
recognized topic, female performances also began to renegotiate the security practices
prescribed by medicine and science, especially the Halstedean radical mastectomies.
Biopsy and radical mastectomy were at the time performed as a "one-step surgery" if
the probe tested positive, which left women disenfranchised. Influenced by the feminist
movement women began to challenge the medical authority which defined them as passive patients or cancer victims. As one of the pioneers of "medical feminism" (Mukherjee
199) Rose Kushner criticized the radical interventions into female bodies in *Breast Cancer*
published in 1974.[6] However, it wasn't simply the published critique but individual

---

5   In the 1950s Baba Zaharias publicly discussed her experience with the illness, followed by Shirley
     Temple Black, Betty Ford and Happy Rockefeller in the 1970s. Many scholars attribute the "des-
     tigmatization" (S. King, "Pink Ribbons" 476) of breast cancer to the act of giving testimony as well
     as the women's health movement (Kasper and Ferguson (Eds.), Klawiter, Ehrenreich, "Welcome").

6   Most crucially, her personal testimony emphasized that the practice of radical mastectomy had
     no scientific evidence to support it (Lerner, *Wars* 172). This fact was known but did not change the
     adherence to the practice and the belief in its promise of security of the mainly male practitioners.
     The medical surgeon George Crile had critiqued the generalized application of radical mastectomy
     in *What Women Should Know About the Breast Cancer Controversy* showing that radical mastectomy

performances that challenged the security narrative and ultimately changed the security practice. Especially Kushner was famous for her interventions in conferences and expert meetings, staging performative disruptions (Lerner, *Wars* 180). The performative acts of disobedience included not only activism but therapeutic choices. Kushner, as many women following her, refused to undergo the prescribed security practice of radical surgery (Mukherjee 200). Though the inevitability of the invasive practice was ultimately rejected by the biomedical institutional framework, the female performances of refusing radical mastectomies and the one-step surgical procedure, and campaigning against it were instrumental in advancing this change.

In the late 1970s and 1980s the medical authority over the security narratives was further challenged as the security practices garnered an extensive body of feminist critique in the rising genre of breast cancer narratives and art. Most of the works that emerged at that time "both inform and are informed by feminist activism and theory" (Hartman 155). Since the 1990s the long tradition of autobiographical accounts of breast cancer – beginning in the U.S. with Abigail Adams Smith's account in 1811 – has received academic attention. Many texts are today canonized examples of the literary negotiations of the "new" identities forged by the experience of breast cancer.[7]

In many breast cancer narratives, the question of identity and the injury to the identity and body are central themes (Herndl, "Virtual" 222). Becoming "wounded storytellers" (Frank) the individual narrators emphasize the need of re-establishing and re-affirming their subject position. These female performative acts of claiming an identity have changed the male and biomedically authored security narrative further redefining the responsibility allotted to breast cancer patients by the "sick role." According to Arthur Frank, these individuals have transformed the responsibility of becoming healthy again into the responsibility to define the meaning of the illness experience (13). As such, the writing of the individual breast cancer testimonials turns into a security practice of self-healing (Herndl "Our Breasts" 228).[8]

Audre Lorde's iconic *Cancer Journals*, for instance, emphasizes this need to recreate her identity after her mastectomy surgery and the loss of her breast. She highlights the emphasis on the use of prosthesis, which reveals the prescribed performative necessity to embody an image of security. The prosthesis in the case of breast cancer facilitates the appearance of an intact, normal and healthy body to the public audience – a performative act that infuriated Lorde in the 1980s and Eve Kosovsky Sedgwick still in the 1990s.[9]

---

did not alter mortality rates nor improve the outcome. Voices such as his did not, however, reduce the dominance of the practice.

7   These texts include Susan Sontag's *Illness and Metaphor*, Audre Lorde's *Cancer Journals*, Bobbie Ann Mason's "Spence & Lila," breast cancer poetry such as Katrina Middleton's "Mastectomy," or Adrienne Rich "A Women Dead in her Forties," Barbara Rosenblum's and Sandra Butler's *Cancer in Two Voices*, Margaret Edson's play *Wit*, Eve Kosofsky Sedgwick's "White Glasses," and Barbara Ehrenreich's "Welcome to Cancerland" to name but a few.

8   Today, the therapeutic importance of narrative and storytelling in the process of healing is commonly asserted and termed "narrative therapy." Yoe Gu even asserts that "[n]arrative therapy is regarded as one of the most influential trends in contemporary psychotherapy" (479).

9   In "White Glasses" Sedgwick delivers her breast cancer narrative in which she describes the anger she felt (and recognized in others) attending a support group meeting in which prosthetics were

Though offered as a therapeutic tool to establish a sense of security the unapologetic urge to use prosthetics came under scrutiny of feminist critics. This "prosthetic pretense" (56) as Lorde called it, did not only "perfect" the semblance of bodily security, it effectively made breast cancer survivors invisible, "passing" as normal in the public. It performatively erased them. For Lorde "[t]he emphasis upon wearing a prosthesis is a way of avoiding having women come to terms with their own pain and loss, and thereby with their own strength" (41). In contrast, Lorde renders the breast cancer survivor as warrior who wears her scar with pride. Finding her spiritual and corporeal heritage in the myth of the Amazons, she exclaims: "I am not a casualty, I am also a warrior" (Lorde 13).

Illness narratives are, thus, performative acts that provide alternative security narratives focused on the perspective of the individual, very much in the sense of Wibben. Today, the extensive body of illness narratives is seen as a crucial and ongoing challenge to the heteronormative male dominated knowledge production and the disempowered position of the female patient. In contrast to Ford's public performance, these testimonies were thus not intended to advance biosecurity practices. Nonetheless, they have at the same time further reinforced the symbolic position of the survivor. And while all these public performances have enabled a broad public discourse they have also created new normativities, such as facing cancer and becoming an empowered survivor.[10] Not surprisingly, in the late 1970s also the medical institutions revised their model of the cancer patient, making a conscious attempt to re-define the individual as survivor to further encourage the proselytization of the "gospel of early detection" (Lerner, *Wars* 248).

The symbolic position of the survivor as a stand-in for breast cancer security was further enforced by the institutionalization of the National Breast Cancer Awareness Month in 1985. The associated events procured a national stage for the struggle against cancer staging security as a question of early detection and cure. And also the growing number of non-profit breast cancer institutions such as Susan G. Komen Breast Cancer Foundation and the National Alliance of Breast Cancer Organization further increased the visibility of the survivor as a stand-in for security. Survivors quickly turned into the most important driving force of the breast cancer awareness movement. Though the movement was initially critical of medical authority and its heterosexist discourse, preventive measures have remained a central focus in their activism.[11] This emphasis on the survivor produced according to Susan Ferraro the expectation that "if you do your breast

---

promoted reducing the female body to the heterosexual male gaze that must be spared the corporeal reminder of mortality (203).

10   S. King asserts that these survivors "emerge as a symbol of hope" ("Pink Ribbons" 473) and six years later she even calls the figure of the survivor the "archetypal hero" ("Pink Diplomacy" 286).

11   A study set up to produce official guidelines on the age when testing should be necessary was inconclusive in its published suggestions. The evaluation had not been able to find statistical evidence for the necessity of early mammography screening. But breast cancer interest group and female legislators, most of them survivors, campaigned for the necessity and benefits of these early screening regimens. Still today, the generalized urge for testing in those under the age of 50 with normal risk is highly controversial. Breastcancer.org, as well as most other breast cancer institutions assert that the decrease in mortality after the 1990s in the United States cannot be correlated to early increased screening regimens.

self-exam and you get your mammogram, your cancer will be found early and you will be cured and life will be groovy" (n.p.).

The breast cancer movement quickly developed into one of the strongest and most widely recognized patient movements, represented and widely recognized by its pink ribbon. Furthermore, corporate and pharmaceutical interest have started to influence the breast cancer movement more heavily. Today, Breast Cancer Awareness Month turns whole cities pink and the emblem of breast cancer awareness, the pink ribbon is "little more than a fashion accessory and a marketing logo" (Hughes and Wyatt 281). The wide array of biosecurity performances that constitute Breast Cancer Awareness Month are sponsored by Astra Zeneca (Ehrenreich, "Welcome" 50), the leading pharmaceutical company in preventive breast cancer treatment. Not surprisingly, most events and performances further amplify the urge for preventive security practices. In 1996 *New York Times Magazine* described breast cancer as "This Year's Hot Charity" (Belkin) and it is often cited as a "favorite charitable cause" (S. King, "Pink Diplomacy" 476) for cause-related marketing.[12] These breast cancer awareness events dominate the public representation of breast cancer and its security narrative, forming an allegiance with corporate and pharmaceutical interests of the "Cancer Industrial Complex" (Ehrenreich, "Welcome" 52).

The magnitude of today's breast cancer performances become apparent when looking at the numbers of participant in such public events. According to the Komen Race for the Cure website the 3.1 km run took first place in 1983 with 800 people. Today it takes place "in 9 countries with nearly 140 Races globally" and 8.5 million participants (Komen.org). In every event, the importance of testing, and the unavoidability of medical intervention is reiterated and enforced. Survivor performances represent the center of these events as for instance the survivor ceremony, which is part of every awareness run. The performances reiterate the individual responsibility of every woman to take the right choice for security. Todd M. Tuttle et al. argue that these representations produce a "breast-cancer over-awareness" which is leading to a higher number of choices for more radical interventions.

This so-called pink movement has drifted far from its initial groundedness in second wave feminist critique. The performances that initially served to give voice to a "different" story of security have become more mainstream norm-conform expressions of able-bodied femininity. Breast Cancer performances are not only focused on inspirational sporting events but on the ultra-feminine healthy looking survivors, who dominate the movement's representations today and are the main vehicle to raise awareness for breast cancer prevention (Hughes and Wyatt 281). Carter asserts that since the late 1990s the movement performed a representational shift that stresses a "back to normal" (Carter 661) appearance. Breast cancer representation returned to the performance of bodily integrity as a visible sign of security. Indeed, even Matuschka, the icon of the breast cancer scar, had her breast reconstructed bowing to socio-cultural pressure, as she confesses

---

12   The variety of fundraising programs expand activism to everyday acts completely unrelated to breast cancer. Though benevolent, from a cultural critical perspective, programs such as the branding of regular products in pink risks to reduce activism and care into an easily consumable good which converts breast cancer into a commodified signifier, as scholars such as Samantha King point out ("Pink Ribbons" 480).

herself (Good Morning America). Emily Waples stresses that the "culturally emplotted cancer narrative" of survival (50) has been extended by the "subjects re-incorporation into a healthy body politics" (ibid.). The calls for representation and voice have been answered – but instead of the initially envisioned form of empowerment it has led to the "homogenization of the breast cancer patient" (Carter 657).

But the 1990s not only brought an unabashed coalition with corporate interests and consumerism and a return to a heteronormative representation of female able-bodied security. The revolution of communication and digitization revolutionized the distribution and authorship of biosecurity narratives. The internet and increasing digitization opened another performative space for the representation of security narratives, their exchange, and negotiation. Forums and digital support groups became a crucial part of breast cancer activism and a crucial resource for many afflicted individuals. Most of these forums were dedicated to cancer survivors. The technological revolution, especially the genetic revolution, however, had facilitated a new group that needed public representation, recognition, and support: the previvor.

Modeled on the survivor the experience of genetically inherited breast cancer risk was constructed as a form of "anticipatory survival" (Nye 107). The individuals, however, often sat uncomfortably between two chairs, that of the breast cancer survivor and that of the (still) healthy. In the late 1990s Betty Friedman founded the internet platform FORCE, which is dedicated to the rising number of individuals who live with a "high risk" for hereditary breast and ovarian cancer (HBOC). The platform has created another performative space for the new breast cancer experience and its security narratives to be performed, defined and negotiated. The experience of previvors and the activism giving voice to their experience was recognized in the Breast Cancer Education and Awareness Requires Learning Young Act (EARLY Act) of 2009, which supports the education and awareness raising of "high risk" individuals at an early stage. FORCE has successfully campaigned for national recognition and support which was officially instituted in 2010 with the National Previvor Day as part of the Hereditary Cancer Awareness Week.

Since 1995 the subgenre of "BRCA or 'previvor' narratives" (DeShazer, *Mammographies* 2) has emerged, which has further proliferated both, in number and in form since 2000.[13] Previvor testimonies do not predominantly exist in the literary form of a published book; they represent a mosaic of representations and performances, which is why I will focus

---

13   "Traditionally" published illness narratives of previvors such as Janet Reibstein's *Staying Alive: A Family Memoir* (2002), Elizabeth Bryan's *Singing the Life: A Family in the Shadow of Cancer* (2007), and Jessica Queller's *Pretty is What Changes: Impossible Choices, the Breast Cancer Gene, and How I Defied my Destiny* (2008), Masha Gessen *Blood Matters: From Inherited Illness to Designer Babies* (2008), and Amy Boesky's *What We Have: A Memoir* (2010) discuss the ambiguous position of the biosecurity individual defined as "high risk." And self-help books such as Dina Roth Port's *Previvors: Facing the Breast Cancer Gene and Making Life Changing Decisions: a Groundbreaking Guide with the Stories of Five Courageous Women* (2010) or Sue Friedman's, Rebecca Sutphen's, and Kathy Steligo's *Confronting Hereditary Breast and Ovarian Cancer: Identify Your Risk, Understand Your Options, Change Your Destiny* (2012) indicate more clearly how the exemplary life narratives should be read: as authentic exemplary narratives that help the individual understand their own biosecurity identity and position between health and disease to intervene successfully in the genetic prophecy facilitated by the biosecurity practice of testing.

on different forms of testimony. Platforms such as FORCE, Bright Pink, Young Survival Coalition, or Breastcancer.org all facilitate and actively encourage the exchange of testimony. Under forum pseudonyms previvors offer stories which are often fragmented and focused on specific parts of their biosecurity identity. They not only represent the post-modern life and individual with its diverse surfaces of representing and forming an identity but the increasingly fragmented sense of biological security which is defined by biomedical risk assessment and based on the construction of pervasive security narratives.

The previvor narratives represent paradigmatic examples of pre-emptive action taken in the present to foreclose the possibility of the future threat. Boesky asserts that the previvor testimonies express "a need to testify" ("Witnessing" 90) but I would go one step further. This need to testify is a necessary act to establish individual security narratives that negotiate the ambivalent situation between security and insecurity revealing the performativity of the new biosecurity identity.

Test and Testimony: Becoming a Previvor and a Biosecurity Individual

In 2005 Jessica Queller wrote the *New York Times* Op-Ed piece "Cancer and the Maiden", followed by an appearance on national TV, and the publication of her memoir *Pretty Is What Changes* in 2008. In 2013, Angelina Jolie's public testimony of her decision to have a pre-emptive double mastectomy was published in a similar Op-Ed piece titled "My Medical Choice." The same day Kristi Funk, Jolie's surgeon, published "A Patient's Journey: Angelina Jolie" as a complementary narrative on the Pink Lotus Breast Cancer Web site. Two years later, *The New York Times* published the sequel to Jolie's first previvor testimony "Diary of a Surgery" which describes the decision for the laparoscopic bilateral salpingo-oophorectomy, the surgical removal of fallopian tubes and ovaries. These texts mark two different historic moments in the popularization of the genetic test representing the "beginning" of genetic testing for breast cancer and its later more established phase. Furthermore, they represent different perspectives during the experience of the previvor. Queller's texts represent different moments in her process of becoming a previvor. Her first narrative was written after her diagnosis with a BRCA1 mutation but before deciding for and undergoing treatment. Her memoir is written after having undergone the double mastectomy and reconstructive surgery. Similarly, Angelina Jolie's testimonies mark two different moments. The first one was written after the mastectomy while the second was written while undergoing the process of oophorectomy, an even more invasive intervention since it changes the actual constitution of the body instigating premature onset of menopause. Both celebrity accounts represent their choice for radically invasive treatment – the pre-emptive surgical removal of healthy body parts – as an empowered act of overcoming disease.

Previvors are predominantly young and healthy. In the case of Queller and Jolie both were diagnosed in their early to mid 30s, ten to twenty years before the dominant security narrative of breast cancer frames women as at risk and in need of preventive breast cancer screening. The previvor narratives of Angelina Jolie and Jessica Queller are acts of bearing witness to an incision and change in identity triggered by the precarious experiential situation of being at risk exposed by the genetic test. The testimonies are often read as extensions of the genre of breast cancer narratives since they are closely related thematically as well as in form and function. As their early predecessors in the 1970s, previvor testimonies largely aim to expound the benefits of preventive security practices, in their case genetic testing and pre-emptive surgical intervention. They further share many aspects of more "traditional" breast cancer narratives with their emphasis on war metaphors, the fighting of a "disease" and overcoming it. The narrators represent themselves as self-reliant biosecurity subjects empowered by the diagnostic possibility to determine genetic predispositions for certain breast cancer variants and the medical choices they have made. They represent paradigmatic examples of individualized biosecurity practices that highlight the responsibilization of the individual for the possibility of biomedical salvation. However, there is a decisive difference between breast cancer (survivor) narratives and previvor narratives in how security and the body are understood and confronted.

Arthur Frank asserts that illness narratives are not only told by an afflicted individual but "by bodies that are themselves the living testimony" (140). In contrast to the "wounded storyteller," the narrators of previvor narratives cannot be easily subsumed under this category. The injury to the body caused by the "disease" which is being fought is in most cases not materially present as such. Neither Angelina Jolie nor Jessica Queller has been diagnosed with a pre-symptomatic disease, as in the case of Huntington's disease, but with an increased susceptibility to cancer. The positive test result shifts the body in its positionality to security – not its position in terms of health. Though not afflicted with a diagnosable cancer, previvor testimonies represent a renegotiation of identity caused by a biomedical emergency. In doing so, these life writing texts do not just testify and describe a "new" biomedical identity and the experience of this emergency but are performative acts claiming and producing the biosecurity identity of the previvor.

"Five months ago, I took a test for something called BRCA genetic mutation" (Queller, "Cancer" n.p.). Jessica Queller opens her testimony in The New York Times with the moment her identity shifts from that of a healthy young woman to a biosecurity individual defined by a genetic predisposition. The biotechnologically facilitated diagnosis plays an integral part in the testimonies of previvor experiences and their individual claims to a risk identity. In Queller's memoir the position and diagnosis is clarified already in the title and repeated in the preface. And Angelina Jolie, too, explains early on in her narrative: "I carry a 'faulty' gene, BRCA1, which sharply increases my risk of developing breast cancer and ovarian cancer" (Jolie, "Medical" n.p). Through these narrative acts of claiming the identity of the previvor the women foreground their biological make-up as a crucial element that defines their embodied selves. The individuals thus re-position themselves to a presupposed normal biological security. They thereby become primarily defined as risk individuals understood as a deviation from a biosecurity "normal." These claims introduce the testimonies as confessional statements, which reveal the "truth" about the self. They represent acts of exposing the self, making visible what would usually remain unseen. Previvors remain invisible, not only because corporeal problems are still considered one of the most private areas of one's life, but because there are no outside signs or symptoms that mark a previvor. The testimonies thus need this ascription to express their experiences and to make known the precarious normality they live with.

The two Op-Ed pieces, as texts published in newspapers and targeted at a broader audience, necessitate such a claim to the biosecurity identity as an introduction of the reader to the basic facts of these genetic risk markers. They provide an initial explanation for the meaning of the biomedical ascription. Especially Queller's first testimony from 2005, when the genetic marker and pre-emptive treatment of cancer were comparatively unknown to the general public, needed a translation of biomedical knowledge to establish bioliteracy of the reader (which follows this introductory confession). But also in "in-group" performances, such as forums or workshops, this act of identifying oneself as a previvor with the exact biomedical diagnosis holds a central position. In a forum hosted by Breastcancer.org, Lilypond identifies herself as "positive for BRCA2" (Lilypond) and Robin31 asserts that she "was negative for BRCA1 but positive for BRCA2" (Robin31). Though most prominent, the BRCA 1 and 2 mutations are only the best known genetic markers as the multiplicity of previvor testimony in forums reveal. Bc31 for instance "turned out to be BRCA1/2 negative, but positive for a CHEK2 mutation" (Bc31).[14] The self identification represents almost a ritualized and formulaic part of previvor testimony. The centrality of these confessional statements, which are comparable to the importance of the diagnosis in traditional illness narratives, indicates how crucial the biomedical description is for establishing the biosecurity identity of a previvor. The biomedical diagnosis represents the only way of describing and knowing the body. Since the body lacks a material or perceivable change, the act of naming the self depends almost exclusively on biomedical terminology and knowledge production. The narratives therefore represent the security practice and produced diagnosis as performative turning points. The genetic test result is represented not only as descriptive but as deeply performative, producing a changed understanding of the body.

This changed understanding is initially defined by the official risk assessment. Jolie explains that her "doctors estimated that I had an 87 percent risk of breast cancer and 50 percent risk of ovarian cancer" ("Medical" n.p.). The shift is not described as an intimate encounter of an individual with her body,[15] but with a numerical and statistical definition. The doctors, the border guards of the porous line between health and sickness inform the individual of her security status. Security is thus represented as lying beyond the realm of individual experience while biomedicine represents an unquestionable authority in deciphering the bodily signs and establishing a sense of security. The genetic test as a professional reading of bodily signs and their assessment in terms of security and risk is therefore of utmost importance to know "my reality," ("Medical" n.p.) as Jolie puts it. The biomedical knowledge repositions the individual in their relation to security – not health. In these representations, however, it appears *as if* the test provided a definite diagnosis that shifts the reality of corporeality.

---

14   Each marker represents a specific risk potential for a different set of cancers, not only occurring in different body parts but different in their biochemical characteristics. These "names" define the diverse experiences subsumed under terms such as previvor or "risk individual."

15   Though I will be writing about a female experience and the demands of biosecurity made on the female body in this chapter, it is pertinent to stress that the breast cancer previvor can be male as well.

The biomedical diagnosis of an increased hereditary cancer risk thus stands in for a material and perceivable breach. As a cancer diagnosis, the knowledge of one's risk represents a rupture that separates life in before and after. Queller asserts in her first testimony that "[i]t's akin to Eve taking a bite of the apple. Once you have the knowledge, there's no turning back" (Queller, "Cancer" n.p.). The testimony of the previvor and the positioning in the narrative act thus appear as a twice told tale in which the test itself is represented as testimony, a witnessing of the body – the truth inside which defines the identity of the previvor. And also the diagnosis and the chosen medical treatment are put into a seemingly causal relation to the diagnosis as if the statistical potential was expressive of a definable and definite truth, providing certainty. Jolie for instance asserts: "Once I knew this was my reality, I decided to be proactive and minimize my risk as much as I could. I made a decision to have a preventive double mastectomy" (Jolie, "Medical" n.p.).[16] The knowledge of the genetic mutation facilitates the confrontation of the risk offering the hope to control the future and initiating the script of previval. Not surprisingly then, most previvor narratives emphasize testing as the initiating performance, the most crucial act of becoming a previvor.

However, the biomedical ascriptions represent only a seemingly objective anchor of the narratives that are otherwise dominated by ambiguity and speculation. The use of medical terms and the emphasis on the exact statistical risks to identify the self disguises that the diagnostic test result is not descriptive of an empirically present threat but describes a potential future, a possibility which might or might not take place. The test does not diagnose a *certain* future as is the case in Huntington's disease but a *potential* future. Queller most clearly ponders this conundrum in her first testimony. She asserts that "modern science acts like a crystal ball," which promises to divine one's future and provide security.[17] The medical narrative of risk, however, "doesn't provide solace so much as open a Pandora's box" (Queller, "Cancer" n.p.). Describing the test as "Pandora's box" defines the knowledge of possible future cancer as a curse. But using this proverbial symbol of unexpected (and self-inflicted) calamity and misfortune also gestures toward storytelling. Pandora's box is not so much an object but first and foremost a myth, a narrative that has generated a plethora of stories imagining the curses that opening the box would unleash.[18] As the object in Greek mythology, the test does not represent an object that just uncovers the "curse" of the BRCA mutation. Rather, the test produces narratives of potential futures. The genetic test does not merely represent a testimony of

---

16   The temporality produced by genetic testing has been labeled "Genetic Time" (Nye) or "genomic time" (Conrad). In this genetic time people diagnosed with a genetic pre-disposition are regarded and represented as if pre-symptomatically ill, entering into an "anticipatory mode of patienthood" (Nye) determined by following the script of previving. The practices of previving thus effectively make the "high risk individual" a cancer patient without having cancer.

17   She further indicates the ambiguity of the knowledge provided by the test in the title of her testimony. "Cancer and the Maiden" refers to "Death and the Maiden" by Roman Polanski, a cinematic rendering of having to make a decision without knowing for sure, or ever being able to know for sure if one's decision is the right one. Both titles are derived from the Medieval Dance of the Dead.

18   Derived from Hesiod's "Works and Days" which originally described the act as a revenge. Interestingly, hope is supposed to be the last "item" left in the box. Throughout the centuries the arts have continuously used, rendered and adapted the myth.

a genetic mutation recognized in the body. It functions as a plot instigator producing future scenarios. These future scenarios, as in biosecurity exercises, are fictional narratives of security and threat. On the one hand, the test result opens the slim chance of remaining cancer free, on the other hand it gives shape to the more likely narrative of early and aggressive cancer affliction. The biomedically facilitated narratives do not describe the ambiguous position of the previvor as a third space between security and threat, however, but provide different narratives of competing futures. These narratives render the body as a speculative future which is formed on the basis of statistical risk assessment, a deeply collective security narrative. But it is not simply the biomedically produced narratives of the two competing futures that define the reality of the previvor.

The testimonies are necessary narrative acts to transform this abstract and collective narrative of biosecurity into individual narratives. The statistical probability of the projected futures defines the experience of the previvor and represents the changed perspective on individual security. The narratives represent "statistical panic" and lives "haunted, if not stalked by statistics of disease" (Woodward, "Statistical" 13). The testimonies foreground the different risk potentials and probabilities for different cancers and reiterate them almost like a mantra. "[S]tatistics show that having the mutation means it's almost certain that I will develop breast cancer at some point in my life" (Queller, "Cancer n.p.). Queller turns the statistical narrative into a description of her individual future. By representing the body as a speculative future the statistical narrative of biosecurity is, thus, individualized.

Scholars such as Coleman Nye assert in this context that the diagnostic practice represents "the enacting of immaterial disease" (108) which "charges these women's symptomless bodies with a pathology that is not diagnostically there in a strict clinical sense" (107). But the test result does not simply charge the body with a disease nor does it produce a definite security narrative defining the body as sick. First and foremost, the biosecurity practice and its diagnostic prediction turn "bodies into places of narratable disease" in the absence of the disease (Belling, "Narrating" 233). Rather than merely providing the narrative that charges the individual body, the diagnosis "invites" the individual to think through the future scenarios emphasizing the high likelihood of a future cancer affliction. The test as a "divinatory technology" (M. Locke 17) thus asks the individual to rethink and retell their life story within a different teleological structure: that of the "not yet" sick. The change indicated by the testimonies is thus primarily a cognitive, or rather narrative one.

Since becoming a previvor is initially first and foremost an experiential shift that is prompted by a change in understanding, the testimony of the test relies on the individual as audience or witness who acknowledges the implications of the security performance of the test. The retrospective narratives of this conversion often represent this transition as an instant event triggered by the performance of the diagnostic result, such as Angelina Jolie's quoted above. Queller, however, emphasizes that this becoming a previvor is a process. She dwells on this "moment" which keeps repeating until the biomedical term is appropriated and made her own. She describes how she receives the letter with her positive test results for the BRCA mutation, then hides it, coming back to it: "I read the report once, tucked it back into the envelope, put it in a drawer. / Then I blocked it out for three months" (Queller, *Pretty* 85). The next chapter starts with the description of her new biosecurity identity: "[w]hen I next opened the drawer, it was almost Christmas" (Queller, *Pretty* 86). "By December, a nagging internal voice pushed through my carefree veneer and urged me to set up an appointment at a reputable clinic for preventing women's cancer" (Queller, *Pretty* 87). Queller's coming to terms with the newly gained information shows that the identity of the previvor is not solely defined by biotechnologically facilitated reading of the body. Rather, it represents an acknowledging and reacting. The self identification thus echoes on a personal level what Burgess describes for security in general where the notion of security and what is understood as a threat is constructed by "permitting it to be shifted from the order of the ordinary politics to one kind or another of exceptional politics" (Burgess 2). Assuming and appropriating medical ascription in the case of the previvor represent therefore necessary speech acts. Rather than merely the test result, the identification of the self with the biomedical ascription represents the plot instigator of the new security narrative which negotiates the meaning of potential cancer affliction and "premature" mortality.

Becoming a risk individual and previvor thus relies on individual acts of giving testimony and rearranging the individual life narratives. In her memoir Queller reflects on the writing process of her earlier *New York Times* testimony, describing it as her personal turning point.[19] She represents her process of becoming a previvor as an act of reading and writing. Her research for the Op-ed piece for the *New York Times* – her first previvor testimony – describes the process of coming to know her own positionality as a biosecurity individual and understanding the meaning of her new identity. "For two months I came home directly after work . . . sat at my desk, and scoured the internet for articles on the BRCA mutation" (Queller, *Pretty* 100). Renegotiating her identity is not based on a different way the body is, or can be experienced but primarily on a process of learning abstract and largely scientific knowledge. Queller chronicles her way of learning starting with Wikipedia and "ninth-grade biology" on genes (Queller, *Pretty* 100) tracing her path of becoming a bioliterate biosecurity individual. She represents herself as an informed and self-reliant subject who forms her own opinions by actively seeking out knowledge and information.

This information, however, comes not only from biomedical institutions such as the genetic counseling in the Cancer Center but is marked by "new forms of knowledge production . . . distribution and consumption" (Clarke et al. "Biomedicalization" 163), which are described by scholars as a decentering of the biomedical authority over security narratives. Most important to Queller's process is the reading of the FORCE website "obsessively for months" (Queller, *Pretty* 170). She asserts that "[t]he FORCE website opened a whole new world to me" (Queller, *Pretty* 105) because it is providing a well curated database for the newest medical research on hereditary breast and ovarian cancer and also because it provides hundreds of the testimonies by other previvors. The process of reading and becoming a bioliterate subject chronicles the progression from abstract knowledge to individual identification, which the testimonies on FORCE also exemplify. Rewriting her life interwoven with the biomedical knowledge she acquires represents the narrative act which allows her to find and express her identity as previvor.

---

19   While Queller represents this process of conversion as following the knowledge of the genetic test, more often this experience precedes the test and is accompanied by genetic counseling.

The practices of reading *and* writing are thus crucial constituents in the process of becoming a previvor. In fact, the act of giving testimony represents a necessary speech act and a performative and narrative turn that does not only describe but facilitates and produces the "new" biosecurity identity.

The act of rewriting one's life with the new perspective of biosecurity appropriates traditional markers of difference, redefining them as crucial elements of the security narrative. Additionally to the biomedical ascription, family history, ethnic belonging, age, maternal status, and relationship status play a crucial role in the experiences of hereditary breast and ovarian cancer risk. And all of these characteristics are described as additional risk markers that sharply distinguish the meaning of biosecurity identities. The genetic test emphasizes the disparate likelihood of different ethnic groups to test positive for a particular genetic predisposition. Ashkenazi Jews and people of Caucasian and Eastern European descent are much more likely to test positive for the recognized risk markers.[20] Similarly, age and maternal status are defined as further risk factors that contribute to an increased risk of breast and ovarian cancer.[21] Most importantly though, the family history is used as a main indicator to predict the individual risk. To fully understand the risk, the individual is literally required to reestablish their family history in terms of a disease genealogy. On Bright Pink for instance, previvors are actively urged to "collect your family history" and guided in the pursuit as a practice of managing risk ("Personal Stories"). The previvor testimony is therefore further a necessary act to define the meaning of the diagnosed genetic risk and the individual disease potential. The testimonies are thus not just descriptive of a biomedical experience but necessary narrative acts that significantly determine the new identity of the previvor and their experience.

The testimonies represent curative practices of life writing as self-healing but are at the same time necessary narrative acts that produce material effects. Rather than just describing a coming to terms with the new risk identity, the testimonies require the individual to make choices. Jessica Queller describes this experience as "[a]lthough I am currently cancer-free, the knowledge of my genetic predisposition requires me to squarely face excruciating life choices" ("Cancer"). In the case of an increased hereditary cancer risk medicine does not establish a defined framework with clear suggestions of which treatment to choose. In medical discourse and genetic counselling an enhanced screening-program or the pre-emptive surgical intervention are represented as different choices of security. "[D]octors don't really know what to tell women with BRCA mutations except to be vigilant about increased surveillance. . . . The surest way to prevent breast cancer and ovarian cancer is to have your breast and ovaries removed. Recent studies show that undergoing these radical surgeries will reduce the risk of inherited breast and ovarian cancers by 90 percent" (Queller, "Cancer" n.p.). Medical literature, however, does

---

20   African Americans are less likely to test positive for mutations of BRCA 1 or 2. This assertion does not imply that African Americans are not prone to a different genetic mutation, and therefore more secure. Though less likely to be afflicted with a known genetic mutation and represented by lower numbers in cancer afflictions in comparison to Caucasian Americans, African Americans have a higher mortality rate than the average breast cancer patient (Frisby 489).

21   Early childbirth and full breastfeeding are crucial in reducing risk according to Breastcancer.org and represent therefore biosecurity performances.

not indicate a difference in mortality between increased surveillance and pre-emptive double mastectomy and oophorectomy, which means "the test is unaccompanied by any clear recommendations" (Queller, "Cancer" n.p.). Previvors therefore not only rewrite the self but need to establish individual security narratives that legitimize their choices. The testimonies do not represent a coming to terms with a diagnosis but a necessary act of determining the implications of the diagnosis by establishing a convincing security narrative. The construction of the personal security narrative is therefore necessary for the individual to represent the surgical removal of healthy body parts which seemed "crazy" and "outrageous" to Queller initially, as an act of taking "informed decisions" from a biomedically self-empowered subject position.

The testimony of the previvor is thus not just a representational act but a necessary narrative construction of a security narrative that produces the threat of the disease as an experienceable reality as well as the necessity to intervene in the body to foreclose the potential cancer affliction. To represent the previvor as an empowered biosecurity individual the testimonies rely on the two narrative elements of breast cancer doom and hope in biomedical salvation. The messianic promise of medical salvation as well as the threat and doom associated with a breast cancer affliction form dystopian and utopian narrative elements, as Völz puts it, that compete with each other. Both narrative strands are crucial to legitimize the biosecurity practices.

The Affective Fact: The Doom of the Breast Cancer Apocalypse as a Question of Time

Breast cancer strikes down on individuals, creeping up on "normal" life, interrupting it. The danger and threat is immanent and its effects physically and materially present. It is often described as an apocalyptic event that will remain a life-long presence for the afflicted individual: "not 'Apocalypse Now' but 'Apocalypse From Now On'" as Sontag phrases it in a different context (176). The previvor does not share the experience of such an apocalyptic strike but needs to establish the meaning of the threat posed by a possible cancer affliction narratively. They thereby create a radically different temporal relation to security. While the apocalypse of a cancer diagnosis has never really materialized for the previvors analyzed here, it is made present by collapsing past and future into the present narratively and performatively. The narratives convert the uncertain and temporally distant breast cancer prophecy into an apocalyptic event that is merely a question of time affectively producing the urgency to confront the absent disease in the present. They do so by turning to the past.

"My mother fought cancer for almost a decade and died at 56" (Jolie, "Medical" n.p.). "My Medical Choice," Jolie's first public statement, opens with the description of her mother's experience of cancer, and her second testimony "Diary of a Surgery," further includes her maternal grandmother's and aunt's cancer affliction. Though the intimate experience of breast and ovarian cancer is mostly physically absent from a previvor's life, the suffering and dying from these conditions hold a central place in the narratives. Much more than survivor narratives, previvors acknowledge the death and the corporeal suffering due to cancer (DeShazer and Helle 9). As Jolie's, Queller's testimonies both emphasize her mother's struggle with breast cancer and dying from ovarian cancer. In fact, in her memoir Queller dedicates ten chapters to her mother's breast cancer narrative. As a form of disease genealogy the early deaths of family members frame many previvor narratives. Mary K. DeShazer therefore asserts in this context that previvor narratives have a particular memorializing element that pays tribute to these relatives who have died from cancer (1). But as much as these family histories of cancer are memorializing their struggle and death, they also serve a crucial role within the security narratives provided by previvor testimonies.

Most obviously the accounts help to define personal risk, as shown previously. The disease genealogies are a mandatory part of rewriting one's life narrative when becoming a previvor. In shorter testimonies in online forums these narrative elements represent quick death counts such as the reports on the Voices of FORCE page, a database of previvor testimony: "BRCA 1 positive Father was a carrier of the gene. Lost 3 paternal Aunts to Breast, Uterine and Ovarian cancer" (Lisa J). Here the list of deceased clearly functions as a form of tagline defining the narrative, reflecting on the self and the inherited risk rather than being represented in their own right. The genealogy of family cancer gives the uncertain future of cancer affliction a material history. "My mother passed away from breast cancer 20+ years ago, at the age of 53. Her only sister (my aunt) also passed away at the same age from breast cancer, a few years before my mother. . . It was not until my cousin was diagnosed at the age of 48 that we got in touch with the genetics department" (Calgary 002). Rather than just functioning as a memorializing narrative reflecting on the past, these accounts serve as a narrative of fate that projects the future. It represents a legitimization for the biosecurity choices of the individual in which fear is the main motivation to "be proactive" (Jolie, "Medical" n.p.).

The testimonies of past family cancer afflictions make clear that for the previvor the crisis of breast cancer risk comes rarely unannounced. Rather, in most testimonies breast cancer is represented as a long determined prophecy that is looming ahead. "My mom died when I was almost 15. She battled cancer for about 6 years. Ever since, I've known in my heart I was at high risk of developing bc" (Ana). Many previvors such as Ana on FORCE articulate that they knew about their high risk. The threat of a breast cancer apocalypse has thus been part of the previvor's life all along and is not initiated only by the security practice of testing. Breast cancer apocalypse for the previvor is "a long-running serial" (Sontag 176), which is not an individual but a "transgenerational" cancer experience (DeShazer and Helle 9). The beginning of cancer is in these narratives thus not located in the body of the individual but in the bodies of their mothers, fathers, uncles or aunts, and grandparents.

The struggles of family members turn into the first narratable beginning of the disease though absent in the narrator's body. The family history – the perspective on the past – establishes the risk making it narratively present. The representation of this past turns the narrative of inherited genetic risk into a narrative of cancer, and therefore a narrative of illness. It depicts the genetic mutation not as an abstract numerical reality but as a "tangible" material experience. The testimonies, thus, render the inherited risk as an apocalyptic genetic legacy in which cancer affliction, not risk is understood as inherited fate. Queller's and Jolie's renderings of their mother's cancer afflictions represent the looming threat and foreboding of the apocalypse to strike. Rather than simply honoring the memory of their mother's, their testimonies represent the prophecy of cancer doom fixed as a genetic legacy. They thus do not merely reflect on the past but on the individuals prophesied future, conflating the two temporalities.

Nye foregrounds in this context the transition from an eventuality (*if* the disease will strike) to a certainty (*when* the disease will strike). The testimonies show how central the narrative act of rewriting one's life is for this temporal fusion. The probability of such a coming apocalyptic event is narratively turned into a question of temporality. While in the beginning Queller as well as Jolie emphasize the likelihood of their future cancer affliction, the following narrative portrays it as "almost certain" (Queller, "Cancer" n.p.) by representing a possible future as a narration of the past. Representing the "speculative future" framed by familial cancer past creates the sensation "that in all likelihood, cancer is coming for me" (Queller, "Cancer" n.p.). Future uncertainty is narratively domesticated and converted into an event that is merely a question of time. The narratives not only depict the future fate as a way "to look forward as though looking back" (Wald, "Future Perfect" 699) but by literally turning back. The past thus stands in for a possible future producing the threat of cancer as a concrete experience. In the security narratives provided by previvor testimony, future and past become a haunting present performatively establishing the potential future as an experienceable present threat.

But the previvor narratives do not simply describe a certain future of cancer affliction as the reason for pre-emptive and invasive treatment. An early cancer diagnosis could be confronted in time when detected since in "sixty-two percent of cases" the 5-year survival rate is 99 percent (American Cancer Society 10). Rather, the emphasis of past suffering emphasizes and defines cancer as a deadly foe that has been witnessed first hand, contrary to this statistical evidence. The portrayal of genetically increased risk is not only a biomedically facilitated narrative but is informed by the memories of what a cancer diagnosis might imply. In these narratives the threat of cancer is represented as a death sentence, confronting and reversing a century of contrary narrative efforts. The narrative elements of past suffering, thus, represents a chorus of doom that decisively contrasts the biosecurity narrative of survivability cultivated in breast cancer culture. "My mother had fought off breast cancer and she waged a ferocious battle against a second cancer, ovarian, when it ambushed her body seven years later. The cancer won" (Queller, "Cancer" n.p.). The previvor narratives dismantle the "fiction of security" embodied by the celebration of the figure of the survivor. Though Queller's mother had lived as a breast cancer survivor for seven years, her ovarian cancer left her with less than two years to live after the diagnosis (*Pretty* 20). The narratives stress that cancer cannot be understood as one specific cancer that can be fought and beaten but as a cluster of cancers that have to be understood in their relation both synchronically and diachronically. The testimonies pay tribute to the fact that in many cases the potential that a cancer reoccurrence signified for survivors has to be retrospectively judged as a fatal fact in most cases.[22] Affliction with cancer and the struggle with it are here therefore not characterized with pink

---

22   Today, the iconic breast cancer narratives are all published with postmortem prefaces, for many of the authors such as Kushner, Sontag, and Lorde, have died since the first publication, the majority of cancer.

teddy bears and uplifting quotes. Rather, it epitomizes Ehrenreich's controversial assertion in "Welcome to Cancerland" that being affected with cancer "IS NOT OKAY" (53). The thanatographic narrative elements serve as examples of what happens if cancer is not detected early enough and not confronted quickly and aggressively. They exemplify that reacting once cancer can be diagnosed is possibly too late and suggest that surviving is not enough anymore.

Opening with a thanatography, however short, makes the testimony of the previvor not (only) a witness account of the body of the previvor but a witness account of the cancer-ridden body of an other. The knowledge and understanding of the threat of cancer are defined as the watching and witnessing of a cancer apocalypse. The previvor do not render the suffering of the body in terms of a "restitution narrative" (Frank),[23] but as a long and painful process of dying. Over ten chapters Queller narrates the rather rapid demise of her mother once the ovarian cancer was diagnosed, as well as the fears and hopes that dominated the process. She describes her mother's fear of death which kept her literally moving, afraid of the bed as symbolic space of dying. Queller chronicles the progressive debilitation of her mother's body, describing how the cancer and related infections were dissolving it from the inside (Queller, *Pretty* 65). The mother is at that point on morphine and not aware of her own decomposing body. The scene appears rather as a gruesome spectacle for Queller and her sister, who are attending their mother's bedside around the clock.

The mother's body in dying is central to Queller's description and understanding of cancer. "As August wore on, her physical appearance grew startling. Each week she seemed to age a decade. It was impossible to reconcile my young, beautiful mother with the sick old woman she had become" (Queller, *Pretty* 71). The process of dying is narrated from the perspective of a spectator deciphering the bodily performance of dying. Watching the body slipping from a "paragon of health" ("Cancer" n.p.) to a body aged and debilitated beyond its age describes the body as a readable sign represented solely in the voice of the spectator. "Every breath she took was like drowning. The thick, heavy, gurgling sound of her gasping breath will forever haunt me. My mother's eyes were filled with terror, her mouth frozen in a permanent o" (Queller, *Pretty* 78). The description of the corporeality of her mother's deathbed leaves the most lasting imprint in Queller's memoir. And the suffering condensed in this dying scene indeed "haunts" Queller as well as her previvor testimony. The descriptions of dying as a witnessing and reading of the pain of an other remain caught in the unrepresentability and impossibility to understand it as scholars such as Sontag and Elaine Scarry have both pointed out. The Levinasean "face" of the other that will remain "refractory to all light" (Levinas, *Time* 75) does not decenter the individual, as he suggests, but is represented as a contemplation on the self.[24] In this

---

23   In 1995 Arthur Frank asserted in *The Wounded Storyteller* that most illness narratives follow the formulaic structure of a "restitution narrative" (77) of "[y]esterday I was healthy, today I am sick, tomorrow I will be healthy again" (ibid.).

24   Levinas asserts that the other's mortality takes ethical priority over the mortality of the self as the self recognizes the other as other in the moment of dying: "In that relation with the face, in a direct relation with the death of the other, you probably discover that the death of the other has priority over yours, and over your life" (Levinas, *Alterity* 164).

description the body of the dying mother is not just refractory but reflecting. It serves as a mirror into the individual potential future of the spectator-narrator. It is therefore not the cancer affliction but the cancer death which is depicted as inherited fate.

What is represented as at stake in these narratives is thus not a possible cancer affliction but a "bad death." "[H]aving watched my mother die a brutal, horrific death – to me, cancer is the worst thing in the world, I don't want to gamble with it. I don't want to gamble that maybe we'll catch it early enough. After going through a long, long process I came to the decision that I would do anything I needed to do to prevent it in the first place" (Queller, *Pretty* 165). The thanatographies forming the family history give shape to exactly this "worst thing in the world." These narratives give fear a tangible object. The mother's fate epitomizes that the possible future can only be foreclosed if eradicated before it materializes.

The narrative of death and dying represents the apocalyptic narrative strand that produces the urgency to confront and manage the future. The urge to act in the present to avert this apocalyptic future thus describes an "affective fact" (Massumi, "Future Birth") rather than a rational decision based on scientific facts. The narratives reproduce cancer death as inherited fate and as the event that has to be foreclosed by the biosecurity practices, which is a significant difference to a potential future cancer affliction indicated by the diagnosis of the genetic mutation.[25] The reasoning for pre-emptive surgery is based on the fear of the coming apocalyptic event made tangible and present by the narrative of the past. This fear replaces the fact that the disease is not there, and is not certainly coming.

The apocalyptic narrative element provided by the previvor testimonies depicts a hopeless situation at the same time as it offers hope. Though the previvor narratives exemplify stories of apocalyptic breast cancer doom, they also describe a katechontic turn and the possibility of self-empowerment and control. The narratives express the hope for a new beginning if the status quo is changed and challenged by radical intervention now. Framed by the impending apocalypse, pre-emptive logics and the practices of previving are illustrated as the only possibility to avert the coming apocalypse.

Hope and Fear: The Choice for Security and the Script of Previval

The genealogy marked by suffering and early death represents fate, which the security narrative of the previvor and the act of previving contrast and compete against. The perspective on the mother's cancer affliction is represented as an inability to do anything, or as Queller's psychologist phrased it: "Your mother is going to die from cancer, Jessica. There is nothing you can do but bear witness" (*Pretty* 49). In contrast, Queller as well as Jolie and many others, decide not to bear witness to their own bodies but intervene in them. "I now have something my mother did not: the warning that in all likelihood, cancer will be coming for me" (Queller, "Cancer" n.p.). Queller emphasizes as their distinguishing element the missing knowledge of the cancer affliction which she foregrounds

---

25   Nye asserts that to make this leap, or to bridge that gap between absence and presence of the disease it requires "affective labor" (Nye 114).

as fatal rather than the cancer itself. The feminist trope of "not becoming one's mother" with which Queller describes her mother-daughter relation pre-cancer becomes a life-sustaining narrative and performative act for Queller which pervades her entire previvor testimony. She asserts that "I see my life as a negative image of my mother's" (Queller n.p.).

While the narrative of cancer apocalypse is dominated by the testimony of the body of the other in dying, the previvor testimonies explain radical biomedical interventions within a narrative framework of messianic salvation. Previvors articulate a narrative of hope and give shape to the promise of future security, controllable and manageable with biomedical interventions. Instead of a "writing back" at the biomedical security apparatus, the previvor testimonies represent the radical biomedical interventions as empowerment. Framed by the breast cancer apocalypse described in the last section, the "burdensome knowledge" of the test is converted into the perspective of empowerment – "knowledge is power" (Jolie, "Diary" n.p.). The test thus becomes a salvational practice – a choice for security.

Queller's life narratives represent the test as a desirable and responsible decision, albeit a painful one. She highlights the different approaches she and her sister took – the latter decided against the test at the time of the narrative. Queller clearly hierarchizes the different decisions framing them in a teleological structure: "knowing that cancer is often a genetic legacy, I sought out knowledge that would allow me to make informed choices. Knowing that there is a 50 percent chance she did not inherit the gene, my sister is not yet willing to give up the luxury . . . to live her life freely, unaffected by the shadow of illness" ("Cancer" n.p.). Becoming a previvor is represented as a loss of innocence, a choice and decision to give up freedom in exchange for security. According to Queller's representation the sister is "not yet" ready to assume her position as a biosecurity individual. A position, she argues, that her sibling should and in time will (have to) assume. Because the biotechnologically facilitated testimony of the body is represented as necessary knowledge of one's fate and the possibility of being able to "defy destiny" as Queller puts it in the title of her book, and to manage one's own bodily security.

Queller describes the choice for genetic testing as an ethical necessity that seems unquestionable against the horizon of breast cancer death: "I can say without question that my mother would have traded those 51 years of innocence for the dark knowledge that could have potentially saved her life. My mother would have done anything to live" (Queller, "Cancer" n.p.). Diagnostic testing symbolizes the first act in the battle against cancer. And her choice of testing epitomizes here the choice for life, while choosing "not to know" means passively awaiting the fate of a breast cancer affliction. The test, thus, represents an "object of desire" which promises to provide the possibility of controlling the fate of cancer death with the knowledge necessary to take informed decisions. It describes the choice of an empowered individual who will face her trial and tribulations willingly and prepared. Previvor narratives thus represent paradigmatic examples of individualized biosecurity practices that emphasize the responsibilization of the individual for the possibility of the biomedical salvation.

Not surprisingly then, the positive choice for testing as an empowering act is highlighted in most previvor narratives. In fact, in many forum testimonies on Breastcancer.org the choice for testing is the main objective of the narrative. Especially in

Jolie's testimony the choice for the test exemplifies a foregone conclusion on the road to security. Her description reads almost like a line from an advertisement: "Cancer is still a word that strikes fear into people's heart, producing a deep sense of powerlessness. But today it is possible to find out through a blood test whether you are highly susceptible to breast and ovarian cancer, and then take action" (Jolie, "Medical" n.p.).[26] The test provides a form of relief that promises the possibility to control and change fate. Jolie asserts in her first testimony that "[l]ife comes with many challenges. The ones that should not scare us are the ones we can take control of" (Jolie, "Medical" n.p.). And also in her sequel she writes that, "it is possible to take control and tackle head-on any health issue." (Jolie, "Diary" n.p.).

Becoming a previvor is, thus, not just a shift of understanding and a narrative act, as described before, but a shift of doing and following a pre-established script of pre-vival. The genetic test is only the first step in the ensuing security regimen. The security narratives thus demand "to make choices that are right for you" (Jolie, "Diary" n.p.). More central than the ambiguous experiential situation of "radical uncertainty" (DeShazer and Helle 15) is the negotiation of choices implied in the act of genetic testing and assuming the identity of a previvor. Rather than the representation of despair in the face of these dawning numerical realities, choices of the different security practices to manage this precarious state of health are highlighted. The security narrative demands the individual to act and to confront the diagnosed risk by following a rigorous regimen of biosecurity practices that facilitate the act of previving. The testimonies are thus not just narrative acts but a deeply performative act which facilitates material effects.

As the test and the knowledge of risk produced by it, any further biomedical practice is thus represented as a form of controlling fate and preventing this apocalyptic threat. In the ascribed role of biosecurity individuals, previvors become "card carrying members" (Queller, *Pretty* 88) literally equipped with a cancer center ID, as Queller explains.

> I entered through the automatic doors and asked an official looking person where the clinic was. "Do you have a cancer center ID card?" she asked. "No – I'm just here for the clinic. . . ." She pointed to a desk to my left. "You need to get an ID card first. They'll tell you what to do next." I got in line behind the bald woman in the scarf. (Queller, *Pretty* 88)

Previvors are cancer free, nonetheless they enter the ranks of cancer patients because they are being treated in the same institutions and undergoing similar treatments. Pre-vivor narratives show that the narrators literally move into the *same space* and *role* of cancer patients initiating the possibility of "fighting and overcoming" the threat of potential future cancer apocalypse. As the competing narrative, the representation of practices of previving offer an alternative narrative strand which emulates the form of a "restitution narrative," which Frank defined.

---

26   In fact, critics have accused Jolie of having produced a promotional piece for the *Pink Lotus Breast Cancer Center* as well as for the test. This critique was deemed as preposterous by many members of the previvor community (FORCE "Angelina").

Entering the "anticipatory mode of patienthood" (Nye 105) is the initiating prerequisite for "restitution", clearly aimed at controlling and changing the genetic fate by following the script of previval. This script is most clearly chronicled in "A Patient's Journey" on the Pink Lotus Breast Cancer site. Dr. Kristi Funk reports on five stages a previvor will undergo when deciding for a pre-emptive mastectomy: "before diagnosis, after diagnosis, deciding for surgery, preparing for surgery, recovery from operation" (n.p.). Each stage represents different biosecurity practices as steps toward achieving future security. Starting with the family history of breast cancer and a BRCA1 or 2 diagnosis, stage one is described as accumulating information and becoming an informed and bioliterate individual.[27] After identifying as a person at risk and becoming a previvor that enables one to take the right choices, stage two describes the performative practices that define the new relation of the individual to her body. Funk calls "Stage 2: After diagnosis: Travelling the Road of Surveillance." As Funk's metaphor of a journey indicates, this "stage" is not a single act but a reiterative practice. This online supplementary material to Jolie's *New York Times* testimony asserts that in the individualized surveillance regimen the biomedically produced testimony of the body becomes a routine performance; one that defines and confines the life of the previvor. As for "normal" female risk individuals – so every menstruating woman – monthly breast self-exams are strongly advised security performances. Represented by a video link to a "how to"-video clip, breast self-exams are defined as necessary acts which allow the individual to read their own bodies for irregularities and risk signs: a lump, dimpling around the nipple, discharge, or pain. Though representing performances of security, these embodied practices also make the threat of cancer affectively present.

Additionally to the regular self-exams, previvors should undergo an increased screening regimen. Since the knowledge of corporeal security is ultimately unattainable for the hboc individual the body is turned into an unreadable cypher for the self, who needs ritualized biomedical readings to attain a sense of security. The surveillance regimen described on the *Pink Lotus* website, as well as on other self-help sites, consists of four annual medical screens (ultrasound, mammogram, and two clinical breast exams) and an additional yearly MRI screen. Each test represents a performance of security, a necessary ritual to know the present and protect the future security. This regimen begins – if the necessary biosecurity knowledge is given – "at the age of 18, or 10 years younger than the youngest relative with breast cancer" (Funk n.p.).[28] These security performances in medical settings, repeated every three months, offer a sense of security, which is temporarily fixed by the diagnostic result. They represent a certainty obtained *in* the present and *for* the present moment. A certainty which is complicated, however, by the temporality of a looming future threat foregrounded by the genetic security narrative.

---

27 Remarkably in the context of genetic testing, counseling is not mentioned in this guide to the hboc galaxy.

28 Mammograms are suggested only after the age of 25 because of the risks and side effects – both biologically and mentally – associated with increased screening regimens. In contrast to breast cancer surveillance, ovarian surveillance begins after the age of 35, according to Funk.

Despite the hope and promise attached to these biosecurity performances, they are at the same time characterized by fear which is only relieved temporarily after the embodied act. The threat of cancer in its perpetual mode of becoming is reiterated in the practices, made present affectively as a form of fear and relief. The screening appointments are anticipated anxiously and the anxiety is further increased if the readings show any indication of cancer. Especially Jolie's second testimony reveals how overwhelming her fears become after her yearly blood-test results showed inflammatory markers. "I passed those five days in a haze, attending my children's soccer game and working to stay calm" (Jolie, "Diary" n.p.). The threat of a(n early stage) cancer diagnosis clouds all other experiences, gripping the individual with anxiety. When the tests come back negative Jolie is relieved. However, this respite does not lead to a sense of security so much as to a sense of the precariousness of her corporeality. A sense of security cannot be found in the absence of cancer markers but only by the possibility of pre-emptively foreclosing the possibility of cancer with radical surgical intervention. "To my relief, I still had the option of removing my ovaries and fallopian tubes and I chose to do it" (Jolie, "Diary" n.p.). While the security practice of surveillance and prevention is represented by the interplay of hope and anxiety, only the pre-emptive practice seems to promise the desired security.

The step and decision for a surgery which removes a healthy body part does not solely hinge on performatively making present a non-existent, or "virtual cancer" as Diana Price Herndl describes the genetic cancer risk. Rather than establishing the "virtual cancer" as a co-presence of health and disease, the embodied acts reiterate the fear of the apocalyptic past which the biosecurity individual constructs as a proleptic narrative and identifies her fate with. "My mother's ovarian cancer was diagnosed when she was 49. I'm 39" (Jolie, "Diary" n.p.). Nye attempts to describe and analyze this "temporal dissonance" (108) with the comparison to "theatrical time" (108). She stresses the simultaneousness of health and disease that is paramount to the previvor experience. However, the focus on the individual security narratives and the biosecurity performances they are legitimizing rather suggests that the "healthy body" is overwritten temporally by the immanence of the threat that is afforded by the narrative construction of past as a proleptic narrative. Rather than health and disease existing alongside each other as in Nye's "theatrical time," the narratives of cancer apocalypse represent future cancer death which can only be averted by catching it before it materializes. The narratives thereby render the body a site of the pre-emptive strike.

In the temporality of the precarious normality and the perpetual becoming of threat the biomedically facilitated reading of bodily security is depicted as *not safe enough*, as with the breast self-exams. The fear of cancer death, epitomized in the apocalyptic past, showed that the beginning of cancer cannot be recognized in the detection of an MRI, ultrasound, or mammogram necessarily. "Having witnessed the death-grip of cancer, I am not inclined to wait around for it to strike, especially since exact surveillance machines do not always catch it at an early stage" (Queller, "Cancer" n.p.). The narratives emphasize the perceived unreliability of the surveillance regimen since cancer begins developing long before it is diagnosed. With the emphasis on the possibilities of missing the material beginnings or even the warning signs of precancerous cells, the narratives reveal that the surveillance regimen does not prevent the occurrence of cancer, nor does it control it. Previvor narratives therefore emphasize the "therapeutic lag" (Sunder Rajan, *Biocapital*

152) which ultimately betrays the promise of control attached to diagnostics as practices of security. Queller, for instance, questions if "there [was] a point in doing surveillance, waiting for cancer to strike, and then getting a mastectomy anyway?" (*Pretty* 148) when her doctor tells her that in the case of a breast cancer diagnosis mastectomy would be the recommended intervention. Similarly to not knowing, Queller represents surveillance as "waiting for cancer". The mastectomy, however, offers the means of control that diagnostics promise but cannot provide.

Similarly, Jolie's testimonies as well as Funk's complementary explanations to the narrative from a medical perspective represent pre-emptive surgery as the only possible way to effectively confront the risk of hboc. In "A Patient's Journey" for instance, surveillance is clearly described as a preliminary step toward more radical bodily interventions and security. Framed as a journey, the road of surveillance has a clear destiny: pre-emptive surgical intervention. Stage two is thus represented as an interim to "Stage 3. Committing to an operation" (Funk). Funk asserts that "in the course of these discussions, it becomes clear whether the patient will proceed to a mastectomy." She describes the mastectomy as an individual decision, however, to "proceed" expresses the teleological logic underlying these representations. The individual is in that regard progressing through predetermined steps approaching or approximating an imagined security. Such an image is similarly reflected in many previvor testimonies on FORCE. Though all previvor narratives indicate the individual choice that determines what the right decision to achieve security is, surgery is dominating the public presentation of the act of previving.[29]

This final act of security as a katechontic turn can only be represented in anticipation or retrospection. "A nurse led me into the OR and I climbed up onto the operating table. The room was too bright. I felt like I was in a play. The anesthesiologist asked me questions about writing for television while putting the IV in my arm. . ... I asked if they watched the show, but before I heard the answer, I blacked out" (Queller, *Pretty* 202). The act of security remains arrested in the in-betweeness of losing and gaining consciousness, which renders the individual passive in the hands of experts. "The operation can take eight hours. You wake up with drain tubes and expanders in your breasts. It does feel like a scene out of a science-fiction film. But days after surgery you can be back to a normal life" (Jolie, "Medical" n.p.) Both the surgery as well as recovery are represented as neglectably short. The acute phase and experience of physical impairment takes on a subordinate role in comparison to the decisions of exact procedures and their performative outcome. The surgery, as the concrete act of security seems to disappear behind the triumphant return to normality, the new beginning.

Most previvors emphasize the quick recovery as well as the new statistical reality gained by the surgical intervention ("Stage 5. Recovery from the operation"). "My chances of developing breast cancer have dropped from 87 percent to under 5 percent. I can tell my children that they don't need to fear they will lose me to breast cancer" (Jolie, "Medical" n.p.). Despite the fact that Jolie's statement is factually wrong, she expresses the promise and fiction of security attached to the katechontic turn of the pre-emptive strike. The

---

29   "A positive BRCA test does not mean a leap to surgery. . ... The most important thing is to learn about options and choose what is right for you personally" (Jolie, "Diary" n.p.).

pre-emptive logic of the narrative dissolves the ambiguity of security and threat in its future tense, presenting it as if it was stable, by temporarily fixing it. In the pre-emptive logic of the individual security narratives risk is domesticated. The testimonies represent empowerment and victory over the vulnerability and uncertainties contained in the body.

However, the mastectomy narratives are not closed narratives but in most cases part of a series, as I have indicated previously. Read as serials the narratives expose that the project of bodily security is always unfinished. The mastectomy is followed by increased screening for ovarian and uterine cancer, as Jolie describes in her sequel "Diary of a Surgery." These narratives challenge the initial celebration of having overcome one's genetic fate by the surgical biosecurity act. The sequels offer a relativism to the messianic narrative of medical salvation and the promised security: "I chose to keep my uterus because cancer in that location is not part of my family history. It is not possible to remove all risk, and the fact is I remain prone to cancer. I will look for natural ways to strengthen my immune system. . . . I know my children will never have to say, 'Mom died of ovarian cancer'" (Jolie, "Diary" n.p.). Despite this admission of "radical uncertainty" (DeShazer and Helle 15), the pre-emptive surgery is nonetheless represented as a katechontic turn and a necessary security practice the individual has to take. The swift return to "normality" emphasizes not only the performativity of security but its inherent relationality.

Performing Security: Able-Bodied Femininity and the Other

Though the understanding and representation of biosecurity in previvor testimonies is one of medical salvation, the narratives reveal at the same time that the imaginary of security encompasses a lot more than merely the pre-emptive reduction of risk. The decision for surgery represented in the testimonies is not only a consideration and negotiation of biological risk and the promise of biological security in terms of health, but a consideration of corporeality. It is decisively influenced by contemplations of whether one is able to maintain a "healthy" body image. Jessica Queller makes her deliberations explicit: "Aside from drastically interrupting my life, how might a double mastectomy adversely affect issues of sexuality? My romantic future?" (Queller, "Cancer" n.p.) The questions do not primarily revolve around the question of survival but her corporeality and its impact on her life and identity. Instead of just striving for absolute security her worries indicate that corporeal security is much more than just health and the foreclosure of a cancer death. In her anticipation the treatment and its possible repercussions take the representative place of illness, and project a fearful vision of the material effects of biosecurity. The risks of the surgeries themselves as risky procedures with negative side-effects such as wound infection, bleeding, phantom breast pain to name but a few, remain absent and disappear behind the questions of the speculative future life. Queller reflects on the security practice which promises control of future security as a threat to future life within the parameters of heterosexual normativity. The treatment is described as potentially impairing the normative life course based on the ability to perform able-bodied femininity. The security practice is thus not represented as only minimizing risk but as a threat to the ability to perform an intact bodily femininity. What is at stake when considering individual biosecurity is thus represented as the promise of happiness contained in the access to a normative life hinging on bodily performance.

The security narratives therefore emphasize the quick return to a "healthy body politic" (50), as Waples terms the urge for reconstruction, along side the quick recovery and reduction of risk. Jolie foregrounds this performative aspect of security as a central and reassuring aspect of "recovery:" "Nine weeks later, the final surgery is completed with the reconstruction of the breast with an implant. There have been many advances in this procedure in the last few years, and the results can be beautiful" (Jolie, "Medical" n.p.). Equally important as the return and salvation from breast cancer is the cosmetic result.[30] The greatest success of salvation and the return to the community of the healthy seems to be the seamless return to a normative body image which is necessary to merge back into normalcy. The "back to normal" thus implies the outward performance of security as bodily integrity, representing the norm and the normal. Therefore the testimonies stress the performativity of the body as a sign of security, which reveals starkly "ableist and heteronormative constructs of adult womanhood" (Slater et al. 409).[31]

Not surprisingly then, all three mastectomy texts, as well as the majority of the online testimonies on FORCE, or the BrightPink websites represent reconstructive surgery as the normal choice of security. In fact, neither Funk's nor Jolie's text even considers that a woman might not choose reconstructive surgery. Queller mentions one friend who decided against reconstruction. In contrast to the seemingly natural decision for reconstruction, her decision is explained: "She decided she didn't want any surgeries other than what was medically necessary" (Pretty 242). Queller further clarifies that this decision was also an act of memorializing a mutual friend who died from cancer (242). And on the FORCE website only one out of seven menu items under the headline "Breast Reconstruction or Going Flat" is dedicated to advice about not undergoing reconstructive surgery (FORCE Website). This information is furthermore situated at the bottom of the scroll down menu. The performance of security in the previvor movement thus seems to reiterate the representational dominance of the pink movement.

The preparations for the surgery therefore represent a balance of risk reduction and cosmetic result (Funk). More so than the question whether to undergo pre-emptive surgery, the exact details of the surgery and their security implications in regard to body image are foregrounded. Both Jolie and Queller meticulously chronicle their medical treatment, which can serve as an exemplary step-by-step guide to maintain heteronormative standards of female able-bodied security despite the necessary intervention. Especially Jolie's mastectomy testimony explains in detail the treatment she chose. Matter-of-factly she describes the surgery. She explains the preparatory procedures for the surgery: first "nipple delay" "which rules out disease in the breast ducts behind

---

30   In fact, many mastectomy narratives such as Queller's and Jolie's expound that the recovery period, in which the breast tissue is expanded by slowly increasing the size of the expanders, offers the possibility of choosing one's perfect breast size and "improving" one's body look.

31   The concept of able-bodied normativity is not new nor a contemporary societal category. Martha H. Verbrugge wrote in 1988 about the normativity of "able-bodied womanhood" in the context of 19th century Boston.

the nipple and draws extra blood flow to the area. This causes some pain and a lot of bruising, but it increases the chance of saving the nipple" (Jolie, "Medical" n.p.). Her elaborations make clear that the beautiful result she praised before not only consists in surgically reconstructed breasts but in a breast with all of its "natural" features. Jolie does not elaborate on the increased risk the procedure of "saving the nipple" carries according to the logics of preempting breast cancer. The more breast tissue remains, the accomplished risk reduction is lower. This correlation between biological insecurity and reconstruction is omitted in Jolie's narrative accounts.

In contrast, Queller's memoir reflects on this connection emphasizing it as a decisive part of her process of finding the right treatment. Taking the proper choices in confronting her risk becomes the "shopping for a doctor and treatment" that Clarke et al. have described. It outlines a process of choosing a version of security. One doctor tells her that with his method "'your risk will be reduced by eighty or eighty-five percent instead of ninety. But your new breasts will look fantastic'" (*Pretty* 155). As this quote demonstrates the choice for security is not one for or against reconstruction but for a particular form of surgery based on the desired post-surgery result. In the end Queller decides to leave L.A. where she lived to return to New York and have surgery there as she feels the doctors are more serious about her risk reduction than perfecting her body image. Nonetheless, in Queller's narrative all these considerations are also clearly connected to corporeal security understood as the ability to perform able-bodied femininity as a cornerstone of her future security and ability to achieve happiness.[32]

As with the pink movement, the previvor representations thus stress an "individualizing and heteronormative logic" (S. King, "Pink Ribbons" 477), which also pervades official representations of breast cancer previvors and survivors produced by the American Cancer Society, for instance.[33] This insistence on a healthy and normal way of recovery highlights the relationality and performativity of security. The emphasis on the appearance of the intact body surface emphasizes the importance of staging bodily security and the gaze of the other, who become a witness to the performance. Though the male gaze and the insertion in a sexual economy are clearly central elements in the performance of security, the testimonies also highlight a further form of relationality determining the women's lives and identities, which is motherhood.

Also in this context, security becomes a bodily performance for others: "It is reassuring that they see nothing that makes them uncomfortable. They can see my small scars and that's it. Everything else is just Mommy, the same as she always was. And they know that I love them and will do anything to be with them as long as I can" (Jolie, "Medical" n.p.). The performance of able-bodied security is narrated as a reading of the body by

---

32   The urge and representational dominance of breast reconstruction after mastectomy is criticized and opposed by initiatives such as the National LGBT Cancer Network who argue against the unnecessary practice which especially for sexual minority women seems threatening rather than providing relief.

33   The program Reach for Recovery in particular has been the focus of a considerable amount of critique as S. King points out ("Pink Ribbons" 477). Nonetheless, newer official representations are also incredibly heteronormative as Carter shows with a more recent video produced by the American Cancer Society called *A Significant Journey: Breast Cancer Survivors and the Men Who Love Them* (664).

others. In this description, security is never just for the self but inherently connected to the other and performed for an other. While in Queller's texts and many other narratives the heterosexual gaze and its desirability is foregrounded, Jolie emphasizes the gaze of her children. Their scrutiny similarly arrests her in an objectified role defining her as mother instead of a sexual object. More importantly though, her description shows that her surgery not only provides material security protecting Jolie's life. Rather, it has to be understood as offering protection for her children, who will be spared the sight of the non-normative "injured" body. While initially the risk of breast cancer affliction has to be produced performatively to become tangible, it is then reduced to small traces that should not be visible to others. The mastectomy and surgical reconstruction, thus, represent the possibility of making invisible again the suffering that the diagnosis and treatment have caused.

But the ability to perform able-bodied femininity extends from the body surface and cosmetic surgery to the ability to procreate, as expressed by Jolie's emphasis on her role and responsibility as a mother. Equally important as the injury to the body inflicted by the mastectomy is the more invisible injury inflicted on reproductive organs by the pre-emptive oophorectomy. For women who have achieved the normative milestone of motherhood in normative heterosexual female life course the decision for this procedure is depicted as rather straightforward. Jolie asserts that "in my case, the Eastern and Western doctors I met agreed that surgery to remove my tubes and ovaries was the best option" (Jolie, "Diary" n.p.). For her surgery symbolizes empowerment and femininity despite the pre-emptive onset of menopause which this intervention causes. "I feel feminine, and grounded in the choices I am making for myself and my family" (Jolie, "Diary" n.p.). By connecting her choice to the well-being of her children and her role as a mother the pre-emptive intervention becomes a selfless act of a mother. The individualist drive to survive and fear of death is veiled by the emphasis of performing (acts of) security for her children.

For women lacking this normative milestone, however, the considerations seem more troublesome. Queller clearly relates her decision for, or rather against the security practice with her vision of a successful and happy life which is connected to her being able to achieve the role of motherhood. In her first testimony she asserts that "I am single, dating, and want to have a family. I won't consider having my ovaries removed until after I've had children" (Queller, "Cancer" n.p.). Stronger than the urge for security, which is foregrounded in the mastectomy narratives, seems the imperative of procreation and thus the ability to perform able-bodied femininity in form of bearing children. The narratives thus express the "privilege of futurity" (Nye 112) in terms of being able to take advantage of pre-emptive measures as well as a form of fulfilling one's vision of a perfect and happy life: the modern American Dream not only includes both the self-reliant individual economically able to purchase a house as well as bearing the nuclear family that "belongs to it." The first testimony and her initial interviews stress the search for a husband and father while running against her own biological clock. Her later interview in 2008 more clearly indicates the option of biomedically procuring pregnancy by IVF and sperm donation, which she also discusses in her memoir of that year (CBS 5:06; *Pretty* 240).

The emphasis on motherhood and reproduction further emphasizes another level of relationality, which is specific to genetic security. Though the pre-emptive security practices seem to have stopped genetically inherited breast and ovarian cancer risk passing down from generation to generation, the threat of cancer does not end with the individual. For the ability to perform able-bodied female security this implies the necessity and need for further biosecurity practices, such as prenatal testing and Preimplantation Genetic Diagnosis (Queller, *Pretty* 240). But also if the knowledge of one's high risk identity comes too late to biomedically protect one's offspring, the responsibility for the self is also represented as an act of making security for the other as one testimony among many on FORCE expresses: "The hardest part of my journey was dealing with the fact that I may have passed this mutation down to my 2 little girls. I struggle with this every day. . ... However, I know that knowledge is power, and they will have the knowledge to make choices in their own journey if necessary" (Lisa J.). Though representing highly individual practices and individual security narratives the previvor testimonies show that the individual and the collective are inherently connected in the context of hereditary breast and ovarian cancer risk.

Making Security – Making Community [34]

Besides representing a necessary narrative act that establishes the apocalyptic doom and the salvational hope which legitimize the individual security choices, these previvor testimonies hold another, more collective function. While choice and the empowered self-reliant biosecurity individual represent the center of previvor narratives, the testimonies are at the same time never just individual security narratives but collective ones. Though biosecurity practices of surveillance and pre-emptive surgical intervention are crucial individual performances of security, and individualized biosecurity practices, they are at the same time performances that produce community and a sense of collectivity.[35] The testimonies therefore do not just emphasize new ways of understanding the individual but represent a relationality between self and other, which lends the narratives their biopolitical force and establishes them as acts of making security.

As previously demonstrated, the narrative construction of security rethinks familial bonds and their meaning by establishing a disease heritage marked by (mainly) matrilineal breast cancer doom as fate. In this context the choice for the test is a deeply ethical one that implies individual security as well as genealogical security and the responsibility for an other. The responsibility of engaging in biosecurity practices is reinforced by the implications for generations to come. Similarly, the act of giving testimony represents a choice and responsibility that are deeply ethical and relational. The sharing of one's biosecurity identity is rendered as an ethical choice which is represented as a crucial security

---

34   This subtitle is a rephrased quote from Maxine Hong Kingston *Tripmaster Monkey*, "We make theatre, we make community."

35   Similarly, as in captivity narratives, the individual fate is not just establishing the conversion experience and deliverance of the individual but reflects on the fate of the entire community.

practice. The performative shift of identity staged and performed in the narratives implicates the self as much as one's biological family, establishing close connections between relatives that would not necessarily be part of the immediate family. The previvor narratives can therefore never be just about an individual but always implicate the other. As a responsible subject one should inform siblings and parents about their potential risk, but also uncles and aunts, cousins, nieces and nephews. The act of giving testimony of one's own risk identity is, thus, a crucial act of making future security possible for others. Within the family, the act of giving testimony and identifying oneself as at risk is therefore understood as handing down of the information that will convert its audience to become self-reliant biosecurity subjects empowered to take the right choices. The responsibility of giving testimony is thus similarly entrenched as an ethical imperative and the process of responsibilization that is also produced by the test. The act of giving testimony and making one's identity as a previvor public is, thus, a choice which is tied up in the responsibility for others.

Furthermore, the testimonies as acts of making security create a collectivity and a broader community. Originating in the writing of breast cancer activism, previvor narratives have a strong and explicit ethical aim and claim. Jolie's texts for instance reiterate in different forms that, "I hope that other women can benefit from my experience" (Jolie, "Medical" n.p.). As most narratives, Jolie legitimizes her testimony with an explicit didactic and activist gesture. Representing herself and her experience as an example for others she repeats this message as a direct address to the implied reader: "For any woman reading this, I hope it helps you to know you have options. I want to encourage every woman, especially if you have a family history of breast or ovarian cancer, to seek out the information and medical experts who can help you through this aspect of your life, and to make your own informed choices" (Jolie, "Medical" n.p.). The change from the first person narrative to a direct address places the reader in the position of a potential previvor prompted to take responsibility for their own biological security.

The public performance of the risk identity is not only depicted as an individual conversion, a coming to terms, a self-actualization by taking control bravely, and an act of self-healing. Rather, the narratives are directed at the community of the not yet diagnosed as well. The narrative aim is thus awareness raising to expand the community of previvors, which is reiterated in most texts. The testimonies are thus performative acts that claim an identity as well as circulate a particular logic of security, which by and large promotes their chosen path of pre-emptive surgical intervention. The claim to such a biosocial identity articulated in the testimonies is therefore both personal and political, as Peggy Orenstein asserts for breast cancer culture. While survivor narratives are examples of "the benefits of early detection" ("Feel Good War" n.p.), the previvor narratives stage and circulate the benefits of pre-emptive intervention. Biosecurity performances are thus not just restricted to the biomedical and individual performances. Instead, they have to be understood as public performances manifesting biosecurity and spreading the security narrative, its logics and its practices.

While a generalized assertion of "reader response" is difficult to ascertain, the material effect celebrity performances such as Queller's Op-Ed piece and her performances on national TV, or Angelina Jolie's is potentially measurable. For instance, Sabel et al. have analyzed the influence of the growing numbers of celebrity testimony of double mastectomies as a possible factor in patients' decisions, which is often made prior to the consultation with a surgeon (Sabel et al. 1). Angelina Jolie's public performance of her risk status was compared to the public awareness raised by Betty Ford's testimony. It was predicted to produce an "Angelina effect," as *Time* described it. While many anticipated a widespread effect on women's choice for pre-emptive mastectomies (Grady et al.) her testimony rather publicized the possibility of genetic testing and increased the number of genetic tests, as a study from 2016 shows (Igoe n.p.).

But the previvor testimonies go beyond promotional biosecurity performances. They are crucial expressions of "disease communities" (Wald, "Future Perfect" 685)[36] and as public performances represent visible "signs" of "fellow feeling" (Ahmed, *Politics* 130). Broadening the meaning of life writing in its more traditional sense to encompass these proliferate forms of testimonies highlights the performativity of these narratives which reaches beyond the mainstream media. Jolie's and Queller's testimonies were not only followed by an uproar of publicity on national TV and in newspapers, but were discussed at length on the FORCE Message board (FORCE, "Angelina Jolie"). They became part of a network of testimonies and previvor performances, which are crucial in the context of the hboc community. The interconnections and effect of these testimonies might be less influential in measurable numbers, but represent an important constituent of the support network serving as a source of identification. On platforms such as FORCE large numbers of women are free to narratively expose themselves, making the body center stage for the description of the self discussing extensively the most intimate details of deconstructing and reconstructing breasts. The engagement in the forums and the positioning of the self as a biosecurity subject symbolizes the entrance into a "new" family as Suscet, a member on FORCE, posted on its Forum. Queller experiences it as a sisterhood with its own language (*Pretty* 105). She describes her first public post on FORCE as the final rite of passage in assuming her identity as a previvor. In fact, this public identification with the group in front of the hboc (online) community constitutes the second most important narrative and performative act (*Pretty* 169).

While scholars such as Orenstein or S. King criticize these disease communities for their over-emphasis on spiritual uplift, the previvor testimonies on forums serve not only as help for others spiritually but as a form of soliciting advice on how to medically confront the diagnosed risk. The narratives that establish the security narrative legitimizing the chosen course of biosecurity practices do so both for the individual and the community forged by the genetic defect. These previvor narratives are crucial for other previvors in balancing their choices. The assurance on decisions and the necessary information is often sought within these networks of previvor testimonies and information sharing as Queller asserts in her memoir (*Pretty* 105). The Bright Pink website, as many other platforms, offers different threads which follow distinct categories for specific "high risk identities" based on both diagnosis and on the choices made by the different individuals. They provide a special search function called "Connect to Support" which offers "One

---

36   Wald defines such communities as "clusters of afflicted people and those closest to them who come together for support, information, and sometimes activism" (Wald, "Future Perfect" 685) similar to what Rose and Novas have termed "biomedical activism" (Rose and Novas 18) as well as "biosociality" (Rabinow, *Essays* inter alia 99).

on One" mentoring. In these contexts, the narratives appear as a series of testimonies that form a body of possible futures and different "what if" scenarios. They enter into a conversation with each other, often introduced by a "me too" perspective. These other previvor performances are foregrounded as formative in assuming and forming one's own previvor identity and making the choices appropriate for each individual (Queller, *Pretty* 106). While it might seem that official medical security narratives govern these spaces and decisions, female performances of giving testimony, thus, take an important position in the authorship of the security narratives and practices. And such performances take place in chatrooms and in workshops and private meetings as a mixture of narrative and embodied acts of exposing the self in front of others as Queller and many other report (*Pretty* 133).

The texts of individual resilience and the self-reliant biosecurity individual thus do always appear as relational. The disease community that comes together in activism and as a support network furthermore consistently refers back to the nation. Jolie for instance asserts:

> [B]reast cancer alone kills some 458,000 people each year, according to the World Health Organization, mainly in low- and middle-income countries. It has got to be a priority to ensure that more women can access gene testing and lifesaving preventive treatment, whatever their means and background, wherever they live. The cost of testing BRCA1 and BRCA2, at more than $3,000 in the United States, remains an obstacle for many women. I choose not to keep my story private because there are many women who do not know that they might be living under the shadow of cancer. It is my hope that they, too, will be able to get gene tested, and that if they have a high risk they, too, will know that they have strong options. (Jolie, "Medical" n.p.)

Breast cancer, and in particular genetic breast cancer risk as "the shadow of cancer," is acknowledged as an individual challenge as well as a global crisis that needs to be confronted. While affecting a global community Jolie expounds the national emergency of this security threat, which is exacerbated by the capitalist structure in which risk is distributed unevenly. When Queller and Jolie were diagnosed with genetic breast cancer risk, Myriad Genetics, Inc. still held the patent for the expensive test. The decision on this patent was overturned by the Supreme Court just weeks after Angelina Jolie's testimony and the costs for the test have decreased and are paid for by health insurance if available.[37] Nonetheless, genetic testing for breast cancer risk is still deeply entangled in class differences, not only revealing them but producing them as differences of security.

Furthermore, the testimonies represent performances of citizenship and national identity, exposing the fault lines and divisions that mark the nation. The success stories of individuals, such as Angelina Jolie, stand in the lime light of the movement. The dominance of such representations excludes all those who cannot or do not want to partake in the scripted reality of the movement. Though previvor narratives do not omit suffering and dying, it serves as a horizon against which the previvor stands as a symbol of

---

37   The patent was overturned in the Supreme Court case, *Association for Molecular Pathology v. Myriad Genetics, Inc.* in June 2013. Today the costs for different tests and genetic predispositions range between $300 and $ 5000 (Breast Cancer Organization, "Genetic Testing")

security. Instead of representing the "radical uncertainty" of cancer, previvor identity is a story of success: "[t]he only illness story Americans really want to hear" (O'Brien 772). The performances communicating and enforcing the biosecurity practices thus exclude other experiences. The exclusion of individuals dying of cancer or refusing to follow the prescribed script of biosecurity practices represents the downside of the "new" normativities established by the movement.

The nation performed in the series of previvor testimonies is predominantly a white, heterosexist, affluent, and self-reliant individual that appears physically intact, as shown above.[38] While Queller or Jolie chose their affiliation and identification as previvors, both the choice of the test and testifying have to be understood as a form of privilege. As most biomedical developments in what Clarke et al. have termed the "Biomedical TechnoService Complex Inc." ("Biomedicalization" 162), the biosecurity practices as objects of desire promising a good life mark the difference that security makes. Especially in the U.S. preemptive biosecurity practices and therefore the position of the previvor mark an elite, privileged position.

> The particular configuration of time that is operative within economies of the "pre" –prevention, preparedness, preemption – relies not only on a relation to potential threats, but on forms of current security and on a particular form of "responsible" subjecthood. Often, subjects oriented toward an ethics of the "pre" are not vulnerable to the historical conditions of economic exploitation, social marginalization, and political disenfranchisement; they are not generally subject to the wearing out of their bodies and their possibilities through subtle, insidious forms of everyday violence that rob them of a secure or articulable future (Nye 113).

As Nye points out, the privileges expressed and reiterated in the pre-emptive logic of security are subtler than medical expenses that cannot be paid. Those robbed of the ultimate security are those who live in perpetual insecurity in their day-to-day lives and do not have the ability to invest in their futures. This form of biomedical separation or the "peculiar privilege of futurity" (Nye 112) can be read as a new form of classism and also extends to a "new" form of segregation.

---

38   The clearly heterosexist discourse is often coupled with a representational racism that pervades the previvor and the breast cancer movement at large and can also be identified in medical practice and research. The focus on white middle class heterosexual previvors and survivors has created a considerable gap in representations that is believed to affect the differences in mortality rates regarding breast cancer in African American and Caucasian women (Frisby 502). "Although research shows that African American women have a slightly lower incidence of breast cancer as compared to White women, mortality rates are greater" (Frisby 489).

7. Escaping Biosecurity? The Question of Security in Dying and the Possibility of Doing it Otherwise

> In this world, nothing can be said to be
> certain, except death and taxes.
> *Benjamin Franklin*[1]

Certainty in the sense of knowing (one's risks) has been a crucial element in the biosecurity narratives discussed in the previous chapters. However, the certainty of death as expressed in Benjamin Franklin's words in the epigraph represents a qualitatively different kind of certainty. Though death epitomizes the one certainty in every life, it does not coincide with the understanding of biosecurity outlined before. Rather, it represents the antagonist in the dominant biosecurity narrative of controllability and survival. The previous chapters have shown how logics of biosecurity are applied to non-contagious disease contexts, permeating the understanding of health and heavily influencing individual identity constructs. The biosecurity narrative discussed up to now relies on the promise of survival and the prolongation of life, and more specifically and systematically the controllability of the body. The analyzed security narratives show that these security practices which promise control and manageability represent the main stakes in the gospel of biosecurity. But what happens when this promise ultimately fails? In this chapter I will turn to the moment when the biosecurity narrative of survival, good life and control fails, namely during the process of dying.

Though death and dying seem to represent the ultimate failure of the messianic narrative of medical salvation, security narratives play an important role in the understanding and experience of this last biological process of life. And while unquestionably a biological process death cannot be regarded as neutral, rather it is almost compulsively judged and evaluated as good or bad depending on the understanding of security. Today, a good death is largely perceived as a quick and painless death at the end of a long (and

---

1   This quote is often attributed to Benjamin Franklin. However, it exist many different versions attributed to different people, including in Christopher Bullock's *The Cobbler of Preston* from 1716: "Tis impossible to be sure of any thing but Death and Taxes."

ideally fulfilled) life.[2] But even more important than how long life lasted is the absence of prolonged physical and mental debilitation before death finally occurs. The evaluation of death is thus bound by the temporal period preceding it and is determined by the process of dying. It is rather a question of dying well or badly which defines security in death. Therefore it is imperative to analyze the *process of dying* rather than *death* as the mere end point.

In dying the original biosecurity promise of "survival" and "good life" is substituted and replace by the security of dying well – of dying with dignity as it is called today. What that means exactly, however, has changed throughout history. Today, competing narratives of dying well reveal the failure of the promise of biosecurity and their security practices.[3] The security narrative promising to die well with physician-assisted dying (PAD), which is the focus of this chapter, represents one of the counternarratives to biosecurity and an escape from its prescribed security practices. I will argue that the narrative provides a revision or reinterpretation of what security in dying, or "dying well" means and what threatens its success. By discussing PAD as security practice I wish to focus on the turning point of the security narrative: the moment when a new promise is replacing the old.

The documentary *How to Die in Oregon* provides one of these narrative efforts and will serve as an example for the construction of a security narrative in and of dying. With the documentary I will turn to a further discursive formation, one that is both visual and auditory. Similar to the life writing genre discussed in the previous chapters, documentary filmmaking has its own implications regarding authenticity. Life writing texts and their supposed adherence to mimesis still create the appearance of truth and "veracity" based on the "autobiographic pact" (Lejeune 3–30), though they are widely acknowledged for their inherently "fictional" characteristic: the creation of a "truth" and a life through the telling of the story. Likewise, images (both photography and documentary) are commonly bestowed with a similar authenticity perceived as a mimetic representation of a reality. The director Peter Richardson uses this claim to authenticity in his construction of a pervasive narrative representing self-administered death as a valid and necessary security practice. As a full length documentary dedicated to the right to end one's own life, *How to Die in Oregon* is rather unique and was crucial in the debate and circulation of the security narrative of dying well in the United States.[4] The construction of the secu-

---

2　Clive Seale asserts that "[i]n the Anglophone world, confessional deaths in which terminally ill people fight, face, and eventually accept their deaths, reconciling themselves with their loved ones, retelling and sometimes reconstructing personal biographies, presiding over their last days" ("Media Constructions" 967) is represented as a good death. For a more detailed exploration of dying well today see T. Walter *The Revival of Death* (1994), or Susan Orpett Long "Cultural Scripts for a Good Death in Japan and the United States: Similarities and Differences."

3　Lydia Dugdale demands in "The Art of Dying Well" that it is the responsibility of bioethics to rewrite a directive for dying well (a modern *Ars Moriendi*). Others argue for a more spiritual approach (Ayeh, Derek), Nursing Studies are often calling for life writing conduct to create heroic life narratives (Seale and van der Geest "Good and Bad Death").

4　It was such an important representative milestone that the documentary is featured in the short history of aid in dying on the *Compassion and Choice Homepage* alongside the history of legislative changes and groundbreaking cases such as Terry Schiavo's.

rity narrative supporting the practice of assisted dying in this documentary is therefore paradigmatic for the necessity of narrative in creating a pervasive understanding of what security in dying means. I will first interrogate the cultural history of dying well to then turn to the security narrative that juxtaposes the "beautiful death" with the loss of dignity in dying. I will question if this challenge to the normative biosecurity narrative of surviving can represent an escape from the normative power of biosecurity. I aim to argue that the narrative construction of security in dying relies on a normative understanding of the able body and "the human," and is established in relationality to the other.

Dying Well and in Time: A Shifting Narrative of Security

Security narratives almost never emerge out of nowhere, as the previous chapters have shown. They relate and refer to previous versions of security, representing alterations or re-interpretations of older narratives rather than entirely new ideas or concepts. Also, the understanding of attaining security in death and dying – so the security practices in dying – have repeatedly shifted throughout history, depending on the changing narratives constructed by different narrative perspectives and voices. According to the historian Philippe Ariès, who has published extensively on the history of Western attitudes toward death and dying, the practices surrounding these changed very little over long periods of time.[5] The 20th century, however, has been marked by faster and more radical changes than before: "In our day, in approximately a third of a century, we have witnessed a brutal revolution in traditional ideas and feelings. . . . Death, so omnipresent in the past that it was familiar, would be effaced, it would disappear. It would become shameful and forbidden" (Ariès, *Western Attitudes* 85). This "brutal revolution" was facilitated by changed living conditions and cultural changes, but most crucially it was driven by the increasing medicalization of life which went hand in hand with changed practices in death and dying. In fact, not only the attitudes and perceptions have changed, but the process of dying itself has been altered by the all-encompassing reach of biosecurity.

For the longest time – the seminal text on the attitudes toward death by Ariès spans over "the last one thousand years" (*Hour of Our Death*) – death and dying were religiously determined practices governed by the Church. In the Christian context the security practices were derived from the Catholic *Ars Moriendi*, a Middle Ages text elaborating rituals that were supposed to guide and console both the dying and the bereaved.[6] Ideally, dying was a time of preparation that took place in one's home surrounded by family and friends and with the guidance of a priest who administered the last rites. This tradition of the deathbed represented a security practice that made the process of dying a necessary conclusion of a life and gave meaning to the suffering in dying. This last act can

---

5   In this chapter I will exclusively refer to Western ideas and conventions of dying. Every culture has its own very complex understandings and rituals concerning death and dying. The processes in different cultural contexts can thus not be conflated to one biological process that every person experiences at the end of life.

6   Similarly to the Christian *Ars Moriendi*, in Tibetan culture the *Bardo Thodol* is another example of such a security narrative.

be structurally compared to a performance in which all participants enacted prescribed roles following a common script that described the process of dying (securely). The process of dying, thus, consisted of highly ritualized practices that were largely "organized by the dying person himself, who presided over it [the ritual of dying] and knew its protocol" (Ariès, *Western Attitudes* 11). This means that the dying individual had an active role in the deathbed rituals: resolving remaining affairs, distributing responsibilities as well as possessions and speaking the last farewells (Ariès, *Hour of Our Death* 448). The knowledge of one's nearing end – the awareness of death – was therefore crucial to facilitate the rituals of the deathbed, which represented security practices that prepared for a good death.

Furthermore, dying was a public event that stressed the importance of awareness and of acceptance as the prerequisite for a good death. Though not always necessarily welcomed initially, death was to be accepted as the divine act summarized in the Christian tradition with the biblical citation "the Lord gave, and the Lord hath taken away" (King James Bible, Job 1.21). Accordingly, the individual was expected to die in peace, humbly receiving their handed fate. Since the time of the deathbed was regarded as highly important the solitary and unexpected death was feared. It did not provide the opportunity to resolve earthly matters, confess sins, and receive the sacraments and therefore represented a great threat at the end of life. The acceptance of death at the time determined by God also meant that the intentional death – suicide – was condemned, as life was only to be taken by God. It was understood as a violation and an unforgiveable sin, which was sanctioned with the exclusion from security in the beyond and was symbolically often marked on earth by a burial place outside of the boundaries of the graveyard, as it represented a bad and shameful death (Kellehear, *Social History* 86).[7]

With the normative power over the process of dying shifting from religion and priests to medicine and doctors the cultural rituals, such as the gathering at the deathbed, were challenged and changed by new security narratives that rendered the former practices a threat. During the first half of the 20th century dying turned from a ritualized public practice into a hidden and denied part of existence. The new arbiter of security promised the controllability of the body, and highlighted the potential possibility of cure, which raised new expectations of security. The process of dying, however, made visible the deceptiveness of this security promise. Dying, therefore, became more and more closely associated with loss caused by a failure of medicine and the individual alike (Ariès, *Hour of Our Death* 586). Individuals were blamed for diseases supposedly caused by irresponsible behavior: drinking, smoking, unhealthy diet, not enough exercise, too few preventive medical exams, the list is inexhaustible.[8] The loss against "nature" was no longer regarded as a "natural" end but as a loss caused by the misconduct of the individual and the shortcomings of medicine.

---

7   This stigma attached to suicide still exists in a secularized form as moral judgment, ranging from pathologization to the judgment of simple cowardice.

8   The blame for disease is not a new phenomenon but prevails in the long history of the cultural construction of disease. For a detailed study see Ariane Schröder *Biological Inf(l)ections of the American Dream*.

Furthermore, the new arbiter of security and the new security practices converted the dying into the sick as "death has been replaced by illness" (Ariès, "Reversal" 140). Dying well now meant to deny it, or rather to refuse to die and to fight for life until the very end. In a way, it meant not dying at all, but rather transitioning directly from being sick to death.[9] Various studies and reports emphasize the dilemma for medical practice which is "adept at sustaining life" (Dugdale 22) but not at letting people die, let alone helping them to hasten the process.[10] Accepting death and "giving in" became therefore perceived as diametrically opposed to the normative security narrative established by biomedicine, which is based on fighting and survival, as discussed previously.

The representations of death and dying became increasingly dominated by fear, sorrow, and threat. With the growing influence of medicine and the waning power of the Church, suffering in dying became a meaningless experience within the scientific framework that defined the new security practices. With this shift, the experience of dying was altered from a familiar to an abject event, and death was increasingly perceived as a "nauseating spectacle" (Ariès, *Hour of Our Death* 569).[11] The changed attitude went hand in hand with the change of practices in dying and ultimately the displacement of the space of dying. The public practice of the deathbed became first a private gathering of the closest family and friends, who had the moral obligation to bear the sight of the suffering in dying and whose presence would not humiliate the dying individual. In a changed form the deathbed gathering was still practiced until the 1930s, while most other accompanying traditions were lost. The home as the setting for the deathbed – the iconic space of security – was in the following two decades increasingly replaced by the hospital. There, medical professionals were able to administer necessary treatment to maybe save the life (one more time) and avert death. The hospital represented the new security practices in dying, and the new symbolic space of security. However, since people were rushed off to hospital, death and dying seemed to have disappeared from the public sphere. The changed security narrative which stressed survival and the utopian idea of the controllability of the body had not, of course, eradicated dying but had made it "invisible."

The deathbed gathering was ultimately abandoned in the middle of the 20th century, because the presence at someone's dying was perceived as increasingly uncomfortable

---

9   Marelli and Moses point out in their analysis that modern obituaries often include the cause of death and explicitly state "after (long) illness" (129).

10   Lydia Dugdale, among many others reports in the Hastings Center Report 2010 about how individuals are kept alive, such as the "elderly woman with end-stage dementia readmitted to the hospital for the fourth time in three months for anorexia, now with a feeding tube" (22).

11   The increasingly widespread use of sedatives was also progressively better able to control and alleviate the pain in dying. At the same time, these medications also decreased the visible, or rather audible, suffering of the patients, which represented alleviation also for the "audience" of the deathbed scene. Similarly, post-mortem rituals reflect the important role of the survivor in determining the understanding of security in dying as Elizabeth Klaver asserts. Embalming has been an established practice in the U.S. since the Civil War. It primarily preserves the corpse but it also eradicates the traces of suffering as visible signs of dying. Jessica Mitford shows in *The American Way of Death Revisited* that the funeral industry in the U.S. has used this argument of "therapeutic" benefit for the bereaved to legitimize the excessive and expensive post-mortem procedures. The signs of incontrollable suffering are erased by the mask of security that fits more neatly the biosecurity fiction of controllability.

and intolerable for those witnessing it. Furthermore, the knowledge that one was dying was deemed unbearable for the afflicted individual. The biosecurity promise that life could be controlled and disease cured became so strong that the knowledge of a fatal condition was perceived as an insurmountable burden for the afflicted person. The dying were therefore often not informed about their fatal condition. Ariès explains that, "it was unquestionably clear that the primary duty of family and doctors is to conceal the seriousness of his [their] condition from the person who died" (Ariès, "Reversal" 138).[12] This "new" security practice represents the reversal of the understanding of security in dying that stressed anticipation, consciousness, and acceptance as core elements of a good death. Awareness in and of dying, which represents one of the cornerstones of the security narrative that promised a good death up to the beginning of the 20th century, was reinterpreted as a threat. "What today we call the good death, the beautiful death, corresponds exactly to what used to be the accursed death: the *mors repentina et improvisa*, the death that gives no warning" (Ariès, *Hour of Our Death* 587). Awareness of immanent death was perceived as obstructing the belief in and struggle for survival that was the ultimate goal of the new security practices.[13] By withholding the information of a person's nearing death the experience of dying was made impossible and the process of dying itself was in part eradicated. Though the rituals that once promised security in dying were lost, the process of dying remained "ritualized." However, today the rituals are often dominated by hospital routines, dictated by doctors and nurses and frequently aimed at life: the here not the beyond. So while the rituals and practices of dying have changed, the performances surrounding the process are still governed by protocols and scripts that are now controlled by (bio)medicine instead of religious dogma.

The "regime of silence," as the era dominated by the practice of withholding the knowledge of one's imminent death has been called, extended until the 1980s when more and more people perceived the security practices designed to cure and save life dictated by hospitals and medical staff as precarious.[14] Dying had become a fully medicalized phenomenon but instead of providing the promised security, the new practices lead to the incapacitation of the patients who in part started to feel threatened by the

---

12   Ariès asserts in a later publication that the arrival of the priest was delayed "until his appearance could no longer come as a surprise" (*Hour of Our Death* 562).

13   This awareness of death was not only important in religious considerations but represents the center piece of Heidegger's *Being and Time*. He defined the awareness of death, so the knowledge of one's end, as the core characteristic that distinguishes humans from animals. The denial of death that has dominated the second half of the 20th century would in that sense be the eradication of what makes us human. But Heidegger also stresses the importance of awareness in dying and approaching death in his existentialist philosophy by ascribing it the unique possibility of authenticity – the falling away of *Dasein* making *Sein* recognizable to the dying individual. He argues that dying is one's "ownmost" (Heidegger 294) and grants the individual the possibility of experiencing "an impassioned freedom towards death – a freedom which has been released from the Illusion [sic] of the 'they,' and which is factical, certain of itself, and anxious" (Heidegger 311). Today this notion of authenticity is echoed in bioethics stating that "[t]he approach to death offers the dying person a kind of understanding of himself that perhaps no other period in life can provide" (Curran 254).

14   Elisabeth Kübler-Ross was one of the first who broke the silence and denial of death and dying already in 1969 with *On Death and Dying*.

prescribed scripts of survival championed by the dominant biosecurity narrative. The hospice movement, amongst other reform movements for dying, called for a renewed awareness of dying to facilitate the possibility of dying well. And Psychological Studies have shown that the horror of death and dying today is the most intense it has ever been, which is often attributed to the lack of social ritual (Kübler-Ross, "Fear of Death" 211, Wouters).

The demand to reconsider and renegotiate the understanding of and attitudes toward dying represents a return to the older security narrative that centered around awareness and acceptance. Today, the time of dying is increasingly rendered as a time of preparation again, which includes arrangements that are in place to safeguard the dying as well as the bereaved. Though the practices today are thoroughly secularized, awareness represents again the prerequisite for the security practices in dying that promise the possibility of dying well. However, the importance of awareness is not directed (exclusively) toward the end point – so the security in the beyond – but the security during the process itself, as noted before. Acceptance as the proper and safe way to die, however, hinges on the awareness of dying to be able to follow "specific cultural scripts" (Seale, *Constructing Death* 40). The new security narratives not just problematize a lack of awareness, so the ignorance of one's impending death, but at the same time re-evaluate the life prolonging measures and the treatments that are focused on survival. The overall medicalization of life – the pillar of biosecurity – and the core practices of biosecurity are in the context of dying perceived as potential threats themselves. This becomes obvious when looking for example, at the changes in the "documents" preparing for one's death. While once the last will was the symbolic object preparing for death, the "living will" has become the modern addition to the testament. It was "instituted" in 1977 when California passed the "right-to-die" law, which allowed patients to be disconnected from life-prolonging technology and treatment, or to deny resuscitation. Though biosecurity practices are not a threat to life, they came to represent a threat to the person and their dignity.

The all-encompassing medicalization of society facilitated not only the prolongation of life and the changed attitudes toward dying, it further altered the process of dying by decisively lengthening it. Today "the average American male . . . is debilitated for five years before he dies, and the average female for eight years" (Hardwig 37). Hence the actual process of dying has changed fundamentally. The thanatologist Allan Kellehear points out that in some cases "the expectation of 'dying soon' comes and goes as a psychological and social experience and may do so – not over days or weeks – but perhaps years" ("On Dying" 389). The experience of dying is therefore oftentimes an experience of waiting for the end. Today, the rise of biomedicine as a normative power has been so radical that people are not only afraid of death, but of death not coming "quickly enough," or in other words of waiting for death for too long and of being overtreated.[15]

---

15   For the aged, Hardwig asserts that "the traditional fear of dying to soon" shifts to being "afraid that death will come too late" (Hardwig 37). And also in other cases, most famously Terri Schiavo's case, people are afraid of being kept alive – of becoming living corpses. In 2014 Compassion and Choice reported that 25 million people per year experience unwanted treatment.

Rather than the fear of dying too early, it becomes a question of dying in time, i.e. early enough so as not to lose dignity in suffering. Escaping the dominance of biosecurity with a living will, a do-not-resuscitate order, or the right to die represent the new practices of security in dying. They promise to ward off the loss of dignity and inhumanity that often seems to be encountered at the end of adhering to the gospel of biosecurity. Today, the positions within the medical community drift apart and are apparent in the distinction between "Hippocratic Medicine" and "New Medicine" (Colbert). While the former restricts its intervention to the alleviation and the withdrawal of life-prolonging measures, the latter supports PAD. The practice is legal in 11 states, based on the argument of unnecessary and inhumane suffering.[16]

The Hemlock Society is seen as a decisive factor in starting this development. Founded by Derek Humphrey in 1980 after the death of his wife the organization was renamed End of Life Choices in 2003 and merged in 2005 with the Compassion in Dying Federation to become Compassion and Choice.[17] Together with Death with Dignity they are the leading institutions advocating change to prevailing security narratives and practices of dying to legalize PAD as a crucial civil right. All of these shifts of understanding and practice are accompanied and facilitated by narrative efforts that render the (new) visions of security in dying. The documentary How to Die in Oregon is an example of such a narrative effort, which provides an exemplary narrative in which biosecurity practices of prolonging life become a threat to the security of the person.

Fearful Visions: The Threat of Dehumanization and the Relationality of (In)Security

> I would prefer not to
> Herman Melville

The HBO documentary How to Die in Oregon by Peter D. Richardson represents the security narrative of dying well facilitated by the practice of physician-assisted dying, or Death with Dignity as the practice is also called. The documentary was released in 2008 and won the Sundance Film Festival in 2011. It enters into a growing debate in the U.S. about the way to die well and the choices that should be available to dying individuals to guarantee security in dying. It is therefore part of a narrative effort advocating legal changes that allow for the widely prohibited practice in the first place. It does so by putting dying on screen, which a Sundance reviewer called "emotional, provocative stuff" (Chr. Campbell). The opening scene sets the tone for the documentary and represents without further introduction the deathbed scene of Roger Sagner in form of a handheld

---

16   In 1995 Oregon passed the Death with Dignity Act; in 2008 the Death with Dignity Act was approved in Washington and in Montana. Since then, eight more states have authorized the practice: Vermont, New Mexico, California, Colorado, Washington DC, Hawai'i, New Jersey, Maine, and New Mexico.

17   Compassion and Choice is an advocacy group that institutionally supports the practice in states that have enacted an act modeled on the Oregon Death with Dignity Act and organizes the struggle for legalizing the practices in states that have not.

home movie: him drinking the fatal medication, his last words, his last breath and finally his lifeless body. The narrative is roughly divided into two storylines. It tells the story of patients choosing to end their lives (and dying) by making use of the possibility granted by the Death with Dignity Act in Oregon. At the same time, it represents the activism of Compassion and Choice working to legalize PAD in Washington under Initiative I-1000. Each storyline follows primarily one personal testimony as representative for the group of the dying and the group of activists.

Cody Curtis is a 54-year-old woman diagnosed as terminally ill with recurring liver cancer and the main protagonist telling her story of dying well with Death with Dignity. She is supported in both, her dying and her storytelling, by her husband and two children (Jill and T.) as well as her doctor (Dr. Katherine Morris). Cody's narrative of dying safely is further contextualized with smaller episodes narrated by other dying individuals who also chose Death with Dignity. These short episodes of Roger Sagner, Gordon Green, Aideen Wakefield, Barbara Lucke, Peter Scott, Ray Carney, and Randy Stroop introduce the documentary and interlace the first half of it. They illustrate that PAD is not a rare occurrence but a well institutionalized practice in Oregon. The episodes are narratively connected by the Compassion and Choice volunteer Sue Dessayer Porter whom the documentary accompanies to home visits with most of these individuals. Her work also represents the bridge to the parallel main storyline represented by Nancy. She tells her story of becoming an activist and volunteer for the legalization of the practice in the state of Washington, which is successfully instituted at the end of the documentary. In doing so Nancy represents reiteratively the story of her husband's suffering in dying as a negative example of what happens if Death with Dignity is not available. The two narrative strands are woven together by the alternating exposition of Cody's dying and Nancy's activism. The combination of the two storylines represents both the personal as well as the political and institutional side of the security practice of physician-assisted dying.

In representing PAD as a benevolent and necessary practice (to protect security) the documentary constructs a narrative that needs to render a radically different understanding of security from the dominant narrative of biomedical salvation. To establish the legitimacy of the "new" security narrative, the threats to dying well have to be narrativized and made pervasive. Accordingly, the documentary represents what is at stake by establishing and re-defining the threat in dying not as death but as survival. Further prolongation of life threatens the loss of dignity caused by unnecessary suffering due to continued medical treatment and the uncontrollable corporeality in dying. The security promised formerly by life-prolonging measures is represented as standing in the way of security, so in the way of dying well and with dignity. The documentary therefore exemplifies the shift in the understanding of security where medical treatments turn from security practice to a fearful vision of humiliation and dehumanization.

The main storyline of Cody's dying starts after an introductory frame with a direct interview in which Cody reports how she was diagnosed with cancer (How to Die 16:54) and how her cancer returned. Cody's diagnosis of only "six months to live" based on the lack of effective treatment for her form of recurring liver cancer is, thus, foregrounded from the beginning on. This introductory information on Cody's medical history makes unmistakably clear that this woman will be dead soon and that the possibilities of biomedical security practices have been exhausted. While a cure and biomedical salvation are out of

reach, life prolonging measures are here represented as not only obsolete, but as potentially damaging. "95% she will only gain a couple of extra months, that will be a lot of extra
pain, and a lot of extra cost" (*How to Die* 26:45) as Cody's son explains in one of his many
interview fragments. The medical treatment and the inability of controlling the body in
dying are understood as producing "extra pain," contributing to the likelihood of losing
dignity in dying, thus representing insecurity.

Cody herself articulates it this way: "I would prefer not to die, thank you very much.
But given that I know I am gonna die, is an extra three months of...em... fluid leaking
through my pores sound that great? Well, no. I rather go when I am still feeling okay and
when I can still communicate with my family" (*How to Die* 21:58). This interview segment
is followed by Cody bending in pain, which embodies and manifests the severity of the
threat the audience has just heard about. Since Cody's appearance does not otherwise
indicate that she is sick and much less that she is dying, this *showing* of her pain – the
inclusion of this scene in the documentary –is crucial to make visible the suffering and
pain. But medical treatments are not only framed as prolonging suffering. The normative
biosecurity practices are also represented as increasing a loss of self-determination:

> It's very comforting to have them [the medications] here. And I don't have to go
> through any more bureaucracy, or take another trip to the pharmacy, ...em... they are
> here...It's whenever I decide. It's nothing that I have to do, it's not like in the hospital
> where I was told, "you have to have another CT scan," or "we are gonna take you down
> to do another procedure." It's my choice when to take them, and whether to take
> them. (*How to Die* 23:15)

The continuation of medical treatment is represented as merely facilitating more and
longer suffering enhanced by the loss of self-determination within the symbolic space of
security: the hospital. The biomedical practices geared toward saving life are thus clearly
detached from the promise of security. The endurance of pain and struggle for survival is
narrativized as unnecessary suffering since survival is unattainable and the prolongation
of life does not promise the continuation of a quality of life. In foregrounding this threat
the documentary shows that security relies on a normative understanding of the able
body and is established in relationality to the other.

Security cannot be found in survival for survival's sake but is oriented toward the
normative understanding of an able body. When Gordon reserves the right to die for the
time when "I am wrecked up and in this bed" (*How to Die* 12:43) he articulates at what
point his life would not be worth living anymore. The security narrative of dying well established in the documentary therefore makes clear that security is not just a promise
of life, but of "good life." The narrative thereby also makes more obvious the normative
understanding of corporeality that underlies this understanding of "good life." The documentary explains the reasons that lead to the decision of PAD as well as the necessary
legal preparation "from buying to dying" by following the volunteer Sue Dessayer Porter
of Compassion and Choice in her work with the prospective patients. Almost every in-
terviewee foregrounds the fear of disability and suffering as the leading motivation for
taking advantage of the Death with Dignity Act. Peter, one of the patients the documen-

tary introduces with the volunteer's home visits, explains: "I can still walk, but when that ends I will be making that decision" (*How to Die* 9:56).

In contrast to the loss of self-determination associated with continuing medical treatment, the interviews with the dying stress that the individuals seek a form of control, which is also indicated in sociological studies of the Death with Dignity practice.[18] The Compassion and Choice volunteer articulates the desire most explicitly: "These people have lost so much control. And they will tell us repeatedly that they want the medication for control" (*How to Die* 9:23). Throughout the different parts of the documentary the endurance of pain and suffering in dying is represented as unbearable and inhumane because of its uncontrollability. Likewise, in the scenes dedicated to the legalization of the practice represented by Nancy this question of controlling or managing suffering in dying is central. When Nancy's co-interviewee on a radio show cautions that she is troubled by the practice since there are so many things that can be done to alleviate suffering, Nancy responds: "There are diseases where you cannot control it, my husband had one of those, and that is why it should be an option" (*How to Die* 50:33). The documentary leaves this question with Nancy's explanation and her opinion as the last word. The threat in dying is mainly marked by the suffering of the individual and the declining materiality of the body that proves uncontrollable and therefore threatening the dignity of the individual.

The driving force in both main storylines – Cody's dying and Nancy's activism – is the impaired body, the loss of control over bodily functions, and the reliance on care. Loss of dignity is thus also described as the loss of agency due to the debilitated body which serve as the negative horizon of dying well taking advantage of the possibility of PAD. In Nancy's case it is the memory of her husband's agonizing suffering in dying, which motivates her to dedicate herself to the Death with Dignity movement. The narrative of her husband's process of dying is the counterpart to Cody's experiences leading up to her decision for Death with Dignity. Losing dignity is in both these stories based on the physicality of dying and the increasingly debilitating body. The threat of losing dignity is made present by the reiterative narration of the impaired body, however, it narratively only exist either retrospectively or in anticipation.

The dehumanization in dying is made tangible through Nancy's witness account of her husband's dying. She reports the excruciating pains her husband had to suffer without the availability of Death with Dignity. Introduced halfway through the documentary (*How to Die* 35:00) her story is characterized by slow piano music in a minor key, setting the mood for the portrayal of how her husband wanted to die but couldn't – or rather wasn't allowed to. She details his suffering in dying as torment that could have and should

---

18   A study on the leading reasons for seeking physician-assisted dying states that the "most fre-
      quently reported concern among patients include loss of autonomy (90%), loss of meaningful ac-
      tivities (88%), loss of dignity (84%), and loss of bodily function control (57%)" (Drum et al. 5). While
      most people die confined to their bed, "[s]eventy-nine percent of DWD patients did not wait until
      they were bedridden to ingest lethal medication" (ibid. 6). They even state that "physicians per-
      ceived their patient's desire for DWD as stemming from the patients' inability to adjust to disabil-
      ity" (ibid. 7). Courtney S. Campbell and Jessica C. Cox elaborate in their 2010 paper "Hospice and
      Physician-Assisted Death: Collaboration, Compliance and Complicity" that the large majority (88.2
      % to 95.1 %) of patients who decide for PAD already receive "high quality palliative care" (27).

have been prevented: "He was in a hospital bed, he couldn't control his arms, probably worst was that he became incontinent and he had to be in diapers. He hated that. He lost his vision and then his eyes started popping out from the tumors so he couldn't close his eyes" (*How to Die* 35:14). The threat of dying within the system of biosecurity is described by Nancy retrospectively as a dehumanizing process. Showing pictures of before and during his dying Nancy describes his visible outward bodily change as the transformation of a "50-year-old man into an 80-year-old man within just a year" (*How to Die* 36:00). The narrative thus relies on the reading of the body in dying to describe the loss of dignity and testify to the failure of available biosecurity practices. Nancy's reading of the body in dying shows that the body and bodily security is indeed performative most forcefully so in its disguise as natural as Butler puts it ("Performative Acts" 522). Neither Nancy nor the documentary in general explains why for instance incontinence should be regarded as inhumane. Without a further elaboration this meaning is represented as if it was inherent in the materiality. Since it follows a well-established discourse of the able and controllable body that "naturally" opposes the impaired body the missing explanation does not produce a break in the narrative but seems like a logical causal narration.

The understanding of a certain kind of impairment as dehumanizing and unnecessary, while others such as depression, are not, shows that the visibility on the body surface, a material deterioration is crucial for our understanding of security in dying. It further shows that this materiality should not be simply understood as a natural entity but rather as a performatively established meaning. Butler rethinks the relation of body and power in which "the fixity of the body, its contours, its movements, will be fully material, but materiality will be rethought as the effect of power, as power's most productive effect" (*Bodies* 2). The suffering in dying can therefore not be understood outside of pre-established categories of meaning that are recognized in the performance of the body. Though the body in dying does not enact the demands of an internalized power discourse, the understanding of what is dehumanizing very much does. What is frequently represented as the bodily expression that follows a natural order are instead "socially instituted and maintained norms of intelligibility" (Butler, *Gender Trouble* 23). The security read in the materiality of the dying body as something dehumanizing thus needs to be acknowledged as pre-established cultural categories that are applied to the body rather than an inherent meaning.

The understanding of what (in)security in dying is thus depends on the construction of a narrative that has an author, aim and perspective. It is therefore important to always keep in mind what Spivak calls the "place of 'interest'" (279)[19] when looking at security narratives of dying and at the claims of a normal in contrast to a dehumanizing body. In the documentary the dehumanized suffering body serves as a comparative horizon to legitimize the claims to what constitutes security. The problems and pitfalls of the security practice of Death with Dignity remain unquestioned in the documentary in the same

---

19   Spivak criticizes the position of intellectuals speaking for and representing so-called subaltern individuals problematizing invisibility of their speaking position: "intellectuals, who are neither of these S/subjects, become transparent in the relay race, for they merely report on the nonrepresented subject and analyze (without analyzing) the workings of (the unnamed Subject irreducibly presupposed by) power and desire. The produced 'transparency' marks the place of 'interest'" (279).

way that the underlying assumptions of good and bad death, or the sheer possibility of dehumanization in dying remain uncontested. The documentary does not confront what exactly is implied when Cody says she will opt for Death with Dignity when "her life isn't worth living anymore" (*How to Die* 23:23), which keeps the security narrative supporting the practice of physician-assisted dying straight forward and easier to understand.

The juxtaposition of Nancy's husband's dying and the narratives of those being able to choose Death with Dignity establishes dying without the security practice as unnecessary suffering for the patient as well as for the caregiving family. Though the documentary renders the process of dying as much more than "just" a material process of bodily decline, the physicality is represented as significant, if not determining the impact on the individual's life and willingness to live, as shown above. This understanding of physical decline is not a solitary process but very much a social one. The sociologist Clive Seale suggests understanding "the 'bodily' symptoms as the body's communicative interjection into social life" (*Constructing Death* 2). This emphasizes that the body and its projected trajectory in dying are not just "read" and evaluated by the dying individual but also by others, whose perspective is reflected in the opinions voiced by the dying. Cody, for instance, claims that, "I will not be humiliated with losing control of my bodily functions again" (*How to Die* 28:25). The humiliation feared and anticipated is based on the implied audience of the process of dying. It relies on shame which is an inherently relational affect and an important force in the understanding of security, as well as in the dying person's experience. Cody's assertion that "this will be tidy" is therefore not only referring to the security of the dying self but to the witnessing other.

The control and eradication of the uncertainty of dying is paired with its relationality to the other: "it is a weird limbo...except with Death with Dignity you know what's going to happen and you can give that to your family" (*How to Die* 24:15). Cody asserts again and again that "I don't wanna put my children through that;"[20] "I'll come to the point where I am not enjoying things and I am a burden" (*How to Die* 1:15:04). Cody's repeated mentioning of her responsibility toward her family is also mirrored in Gordon's position, who asserts that "I just wanna lie down and never wake up. And do the decent thing. Once in my life I will be decent" (*How to Die* 15:17) looking at his uncomfortably smiling wife. This fear of becoming a burden represents what Kellehear has termed in *The Social History of Dying* "Birth of the Shameful Death" (213), where "[t]iming [d]eath" (234) becomes an important and complex exercise. This timing of death is governed by the security narrative, which determines the appropriateness of practices and the exact moment when this appropriateness ends. The security of the self in dying is not just contingent on the experience of suffering but seems to be understood through the "gaze" of the other. Security, in other words, is defined in relationality. Cody's son puts this relationality into words when he explains: "She [Cody] is also very dignified. And when she looks sick that

---

20   This comes in response to Cody telling the volunteer in tears that "I am really afraid of being a coward at the end" (1:02:46), which is answered with "we call it death with dignity not death with cowardice. Do you think its coward to die instead of suffer? That is a message our society gives over and over again; that only, hm ... if you..., that only the truly courageous are the ones willing to suffer" (*How to Die* 1:03:02).

is very hard for her because she wants to present herself as being healthy" (*How to Die* 21:23). The insecurity caused and "revealed" by the body to others is thus crucial.

The humiliation associated with the failing body in the documentary thus shows that it is not just the reading of the self and an intimate feeling of suffering but also the reading of others – family, friends, caregivers – that influences the experience of dignity in dying. And it is this relationality between self and other that ultimately defines security/insecurity. The documentary thus exemplifies that the intangible fear of death is often eclipsed by more mundane fears. The fear of death and of suffering in dying are further increased by social expectations as sociologists such as Charles O. Jackson point out: "Individuals die through a whole cluster of societal definitions and value-laden categories. The worth of their particular type of death is assessed. . . . Social assignment is made also on the 'appropriateness' of death" (4f). The documentary thus shows that suffering in dying is exceedingly influenced by society. Dying thus materializes through the encounter during the process: between self and body as much as between dying and those present and witnessing. Though the regression in dying is pathologized and is not attributed to the responsibility of the sufferer in the documentary, it nonetheless seems inherently connected to the feeling of humiliation and shame.[21] The complexities of security in dying therefore indicate a change in materiality, medical technology, and the ever-growing presence and importance of bio-medicine in U.S. culture and society. They also indicate a changing relation to "what is human," what is dignified, what is the "we." And this "we" is reinforced in affective terms against the ostracized other.

The affects attached to the deteriorating body, such as shame and humiliation function similarly to affects in national discourse as Sara Ahmed has described it in "Politics of Bad Feeling."[22] Ahmed asserts that "[e]xposing the failure of the ideal is politically important" ("Politics" 79) because it reinforces the ideal, not in representing it but in defining what its opposite is. The representation of the feared dehumanizing bad death thus reinforces the border between good life and unlivable life, between proper and improper "decline." It is this exclusion from a "normal" and good life that defines the question of when a life is not worth living (anymore).

Since the other is so important in negotiating the meaning of dying and its evaluation, the act of witnessing plays a crucial role in establishing the security narrative in the documentary. The representation of loss of dignity in dying, so the representation of insecurity, relies largely on Nancy's witness account which she represents in the interviews. Her husband might have experienced his dying as excruciating and humiliating, but it is Nancy's witness account of reading and interpreting his body that defines

---

21   This shows that the affects determining the worth of a death are never only the feelings and experiences of the dying patient, but also those of the relatives or friends and of healthcare professionals. Emotions regarded as a "window to the truth" or "a different kind of intelligence about the world," as Nigel Thrift calls this perspective (60), are therefore problematic. Thus, I would rather suggest that the process mainly materializes in the affective encounter between self and other and dying materiality, an encounter of almost compulsory assessment.

22   Ahmed asserts in the context of the "National Sorry Day" in Australia that the expression of negative feelings such as shame toward the failures of the nation does not only reveal acknowledge the negative but at the same time reaffirms the positive qualities of the nation and therefore reestablishes an ideal rather than deconstructing it.

his loss of dignity. This reading and interpreting of the body shows that the drama of security in dying is played by the body as actor while the dying self and the attendees represent an audience that is reading the body for (in)security. The notion of theatrical performance is thus profoundly important for the understanding of security in dying inscribing a structure of witnessing and staging. The narrative construction of threat/insecurity in dying thus relies on the bodily process as a performative act. It can be regarded as a performative act because it is staged and closely observed by doctors, friends, and family – if present – and the self. Though the deteriorating body thwarts any intentionality of the subject, the corporeality is always and already in society, always on display, "impressed upon by others, impinging upon them as well" (Butler, *Precarious* 27). As such bodily decline relies on similar structures as staged theatrical performances of spectator and actor. As performativity is essentially based on communication to produce its effect it requires a second person that is similar to Austin's interlocutor.

Narratives of death and dying usually rely on the witness of dying to establish the "survivor's tale" retrospectively after the death of the individual, as represented by Nancy's story line. In the security narrative of physician-assisted dying represented in *How to Die in Oregon* this temporality is reversed, since the loss of dignity is a future threat. The retrospective narrative is turned into a proleptic narrative of what would or could happen without the access to the security practice of PAD. In the security narrative of dying well provided by the documentary the feared loss of dignity is not experienced and therefore not present. It represents a threat that can and has to be foreclosed by the security practice. The narrative construction of the threat therefore relies on anticipation, which is marked by fear. As previously argued, the modern way of dying is more frequently than not a process of waiting, an anticipation determined by expert knowledge, diagnosis, and prognosis. The perspective dominates the documentary which takes place in this temporal space of anticipation. It uses this temporality in its narrative perspective to establish the security narrative of dying well. Dying is represented, as in Thanatology, by emotions – mainly pain,[23] fear, and distress – which are caused by the prospect of the deteriorating body.[24]

This fear is in part based on past experiences of suffering, which foreshadow the potential menace of losing dignity. The threat of "losing dignity" in dying is exemplified by the retrospective narrative of Cody's diagnosis and her suffering after the first surgery. Within Cody's story the retrospective narrative of her illness narrative serves to foreshadow the expectations for her potential future. Images of Cody in a coma after her first surgery and her suffering during recovery are shown in a photo montage with her voice-over explaining her bad surgery results. The scene is summarized by her husband's recollection of her saying that "I don't want another night like that" (*How to Die* 18:26). The

---

23   In the 1964 Cicely Saunders published the article "The symptomatic treatment of incurable malignant disease" which challenged conceptions of what causes the suffering in dying with her concept of "total pain." This approach recognizes "not only physical symptoms but also mental distress and social or spiritual problems" as constituents when describing the pain of dying for the diseased individuals (C. Saunders 430).

24   In dying, affects, as expressions of inner feelings, are often the main source of "knowledge" about the process. Many studies, such as Kübler-Ross' interviews with the dying, define dying in affective stages such as anger or depression.

narrative of suffering is so forceful that the discovery of new signs of cancer literally represents the decision for the security practice of assisted dying in the documentary. Temporally, this mirrors the pre-emptive logic of the security narratives in previous chapters. The narrative of past suffering makes the potential future suffering of the final stages of dying present and to a certain extent experienceable. In more abstract terms this means that a projected future (threat) is narratively made present triggering an action in the present to foreclose this future.

The temporality that defines Cody's experience and her decision to take advantage of the Death with Dignity Act is also emblematic of all other stories of the dying. It is the potential future threat that is estimated according to a comparative horizon. What in Cody's case is represented by her illness experience is Gordon's experience of his father's dying: "I saw my dad twelve years with a stroke and one whole side was gone ... and he just kept saying 'I just want out'..." (*How to Die* 13:12). "But I'll handle it until something like that happens" (*How to Die* 13:27). The narrativization of this past suffering makes present the future threat which is then foreclosed by the security practice of physician-assisted dying. The practice eradicates the uncertainty of "nature taking its course," which is contrasted by the desire to control and author one's own death. This also shows that also the security narrative of dying well with physician-assisted dying follows a pre-emptive logic of security.

The narrative of suffering is represented interchangeably with scenes of happy family life as a competing narrative representing security. Cody's assertion that "we did not let animals suffer" (*How to Die* 21:24) is concluded with a cut to photos of her happy and healthy. The feared suffering represents the comparative horizon for the effective narrative of the new security promise of dying well.

The Promise of Security and the Proper Way to Die: Agency, Choice, and Acceptance

> he raised the cup to his lips and cheerfully and quietly drained it. I have heard it is best to die in silence. Keep quiet and be brave.
> *Plato*

Physician-assisted dying promises security in dying in form of dignity, controllability, and agency. The beginning of the documentary, which shows Roger Sagner's dying at home after drinking the prescribed medication represents this opposition clearly, as I previously argued. This prelude offers a shocking and highly emotional scene since the audience witnesses Roger's last moments of dying and his death, which is a rarely staged moment and an unfamiliar one for most people. However, the scene becomes an emotionally ambiguous one as Roger states that "it [the medication] will kill me and make me happy" (*How to Die* 2:08). This "last act" serves as introduction and frame for the main narrative. It establishes death as welcomed and the practice of taking one's own life as security. The first thing the viewer learns is that Death with Dignity is not an imposed practice but an individual choice, which is experienced as a blessing by the individual.

The practice represents the promise of security, showcasing the controllability of the body and agency of the individual which is established in opposition to the negative horizon of humiliating and uncontrollable bodily decline, discussed above. But the re-interpretation of death – the moment that otherwise represents and manifests insecurity – is more complex than showing one scene of a self-administered death. It relies on the narrative construction to establish agency and acceptance as core constituent of security in dying. This renegotiation of security in dying represents a return to core elements of dying well that preceded the rise of biomedicine as the arbiter of security and its all encompassing promise of controllability. The documentary foregrounds agency and choice as well as awareness and acceptance as the foundational pillars for security in this last passage of life.

In order to represent PAD as a way to die well it is fundamental to divorce the security practice from its negative connotations, especially suicide. Already the name of the security practice used in the documentary exemplifies this detachment. The interviewees consistently use the term physician-assisted dying instead of physician-assisted suicide.[25] This choice of nomenclature linguistically separates the association of suicide from the security practice and thereby detaches it also from the moral judgment of suicide as a cowardly and selfish act that is condemned by religious groups and society at large. Nancy puts the importance of this distinction into focus in an interview with a Canadian journalist: "No, it's very offensive to me to call it suicide. Suicide is something someone does who is otherwise physically healthy and has their life ahead of them, is clinically depressed and don't [sic] wanna live" (How to Die 50:58). In this representation the stigma attached to suicide remains unchallenged. Instead of denouncing the narratives condemning the act of ending one's own life altogether, suicide is pathologized and represented as mental illness while PAD is rigidly separated from this practice. This distinction between "sick" behavior, compulsively enacted by non-competent individuals and the rational choice for medical aid in dying is crucial. It creates a definitive dichotomy of good and bad forms of ending one's life, or rather of good dying in contrast to bad suicide. Suicide as such remains configured as a threat to the individual, a preventable tragedy and failure based on irrational or pathological problems – something to be averted. In contrast, in the security practice of PAD the act of killing oneself becomes exemplary for "good dying" and a salvation of the individual from the irredeemable body suffering from physical health problems.[26] In fact, Death with Dignity becomes the epitome of good death as the term euthanasia would literally indicate. However, the history of involuntary euthanasia makes this terminological link problematic as well.

Not surprisingly then, the practice is also disassociated from the dark past of euthanasia and the term euthanasia as such. Studies have shown higher public approval

---

25   The organization Death with Dignity dedicates an extra page on the website to the "Terminology of Assisted Dying" insisting on the importance of using value-neutral language, which is not hurtful to patients and their families.

26   The invisible suffering from mental illness in Nancy's explanations is not acceptable as a legitimate reason to choose death.

ratings for PAD when promotional texts do not use the term euthanasia.[27] The movements institutionally supporting the practice and its further dissemination are therefore meaningfully named Compassion and Choice and Death with Dignity. The practices
of euthanasia of the past are not explicitly mentioned but any connection to coercion,
persuasion, or intimidation is eradicated by an insistence on the agency of the individuals choosing Death with Dignity. The documentary stresses again and again that the
practice is not based on coercion but free will and that it is a choice that is not violating
rights but representing a right itself. The security narrative of the documentary therefore
stresses not only the inhumane and unnecessary "suffering" experienced without the security practice of PAD but the agency of the individuals using Death with Dignity.

Agency is primarily foregrounded by marking the practice as an empowering choice
of individuals. This choice for security in dying is emphasized and detailed in the depiction of the home visits of the Compassion and Choice volunteer Sue Dessayer Porter.
The short episodes reveal single steps in securing the right to die at a chosen moment
averting the otherwise seemingly inevitable humiliation and loss of dignity encountered
in dying. Dying is here not constructed as "the self coming to an end" but as an active
"ending of the self." Security is based on individual active decisions and therefore on the
responsibility of the self. The responsibilization for the self thus reaches beyond the obligation to stay healthy to the process of dying and how one dies. After the first scene at
Roger's deathbed, Gordon is accompanied on the way to the pharmacy to buy the prescribed drug and is then shown calling the volunteer to inform her that he has obtained
the medication; and Aideen is informed about which drink she should purchase as there
are two options – "Nembutal costs over a thousand dollars, Seconal is 130 dollars" (How to
Die 11:46). It is made clear that PAD is not a quick and easy act possible on an impulse by a
suffering individual, nor a "fast way out" that is imposed on a helpless individual by others. PAD is represented as a practice that requires extensive organizational and logistic
effort on part of the dying as self-reliant responsible subjects.

The detailed representation of the practice in the documentary shows that security
in dying does not rely on one but on multiple choices, each one representing a step of
an able individual on the way to security in a pre-emptive sense. After deciding to take
advantage of Death with Dignity the further necessary choices for security consist in obtaining a prescription for the medication and the decision if and when to take it. The
patient thus pre-emptively gets a drug in case suffering becomes unbearable for the individual and then pre-emptively takes the medication to foreclose the possibility of losing
one's dignity. Every step is marked by agency and self-reliance stressing the importance
of bioliterate subjects and the care of the self. To prepare and provide for one's end is thus
decisively the responsibility of the individual.

In addition to the insistence of choice and agency, the security practice of physician-
assisted dying needs to eradicate any suspicion of coercion, especially hidden and implicit forms such as social expectations, or purely financial considerations. Each episode
stresses the agency and choice of the practice, as the volunteer explains: "There is a fine

---

27   The Hasting's Center Report in 2010 asserts that "Field testing prior to passage of the Oregon law
in 1994 disclosed that when the process was described as "suicide" or as a form of "euthanasia,"
popular support declined by 10 to 12 percent" (Campbell and Cox 28f).

line of never ever wanting to think that we are selling a process here. We are not. We are offering a choice" (*How to Die* 11:02). By representing the practice as a rational and institutionalized choice it is further detached from its negative connotations which are judged as irrational or non-consensual acts. When Porter states that "we represent choice not death" (*How to Die* 13:39) she articulates the walk on a tightrope when it comes to defining assisted dying as a security practice. Her interview scenes highlight the importance of precluding any accusation of coercion in the very carefully formulated sentences informing the individuals about the different details of the practice. She uses almost formulaic phrases such as "If you were ever to make the choice to take this medication" (*How to Die* 13:47). Porter says this to Gordon, who already has the drugs at home and has clearly made the choice. She thereby highlights her consulting role which remains in all comments impartial, neutral and in the conditional when referring to the act of ending one's life. All these carefully selected scenes place the (mentally) able subject at the center of the practice.

To protect individuals from coercion the Death with Dignity Act prescribes that patients have to be of sound mind and be able to self-administer the drug. The documentary recreates this guarantee of the free will and choice in its narrative construction, especially its voice. The documentary is carefully narrated and constructed *as if* told by the people themselves and has no traditional voice-over narration. Subjectivity and free will are thus represented in the voice of the individuals providing their own narratives.[28] This is achieved by the exclusive use of direct testimonials combined with a "fly on the wall" perspective. Large parts of the documentary are structured by "behind-the-scene" elements. The audience accompanies Cody into the hospital, the volunteer to her home visits and witnesses Nancy's activism. As a "character-driven documentary" it "approach[es] broader issues through one or a few social actors; that is, they combine the typing, portrait, and testimonial functions that other documentaries might keep separate" (Cagle 56). In doing so the director mirrors the core method in the study of dying applied in the different fields of Thanatology. Many studies are conducted as interviews with the dying or their caretakers, such as Kübler-Ross's famous "Interviews with the Dying."[29] The narrative voice of the documentary echoes this structure of "learning from the dying" which represents the dying as "native informants" for the still healthy. The voices of these native informants are pivotal in contradicting the established security narrative of biomedical salvation, and embodying free will and choice.

The narrative voice emulates, or attempts to aesthetically increase, authenticity by representing the dying as experts, and their stories as undeniable truth. The narrative of the documentary aims to capture the "authentic" experience by "showing" and thereby

---

28   Bill Nichols provides a historically oriented classification for distinct documentary styles: the "direct-address style of the Griersonian tradition" ("The Voice" 17), the *"cinéma vérité films" (ibid.)*, the interview-based documentary as "direct-address," and the reflective documentary, which "mixes observational passages with interviews, the voice-over of the film-maker with intertitles" ("The Voice" 18).

29   Elizabeth Kübler-Ross is one of the pioneers of studying and reforming the modern practice of dying. Her psychological studies, such as *On Death and Dying*, established a five-stage model of dying comparable to the process of mourning, a crucial period at the end of life which needs professional attention.

revealing the "truth." The stories represent the lessons to be learned from the dying them-selves. The documentary genre in general is a narrative formation aiming "to represent 'things as they are'" (Nichols, "The Voice" 17). Or rather, as Patricia Aufderheide claims, "[a]ll documentary conventions . . . arise from the need to convince the viewer of the au-thenticity of what they are being told" (11). In *How to Die in Oregon* interviews with experts that are typically used to guarantee the veracity of what is shown are replaced by the dying themselves. Their comments on their own intimate experiences therefore substitute the expert talk *about* the experience. Thus, Richardson uses the aesthetics of the documen-tary genre to "provide" authenticity by testimonial narratives as an almost uncontestable "real."

The aesthetic strategy aims to reinforce the semblance of unaltered reality, and thus actively obscures its constructedness and the narrative agency of the director. Though the documentary style aesthetically enhances a "truth value," selection and edits are creating a version of the truth as much as a "traditional" narration would. The narrative develops its argument in an inductive structure, by showing evidence of the "beneficial" value of Death with Dignity. The audience follows the different personal stories, their perspec-tives, and their relation to Death with Dignity. The observational structure of the docu-mentary furthers this implicit exposition. The direct interviews that represent about half of the documentary hide the interview situation. The face and voice of the film-maker remain invisible and silent, though the testimonies clearly emerge out of interview sit-uations.[30] The testimonial narratives dominate the aesthetics while the editing controls the narrative by cuts, voice-over, and establishing the timeline. In other words, by assem-bling the selected material it determines the meaning of the story.

Nonetheless, by giving a voice to those who often remain unheard when dying and death are discussed, the dying are represented as subjects rather than objects of the se-curity narrative of dying well. In the narrative representation the dying individuals, and in particular Cody, therefore preside over their dying as a governing agent similarly to how it was practiced in the traditional deathbed scenes. This representation of the new security practice of Death with Dignity approximates, and appropriates the old security practice of the deathbed, adapting it to the modern way of dying. The passivity of the "sick role" (Parson) dominated by medical procedures is narratively substituted by activity and subjectivity represented by the individual's role in their dying. But the dying are not only narratively re-constructed as the agentic subjects of their dying, equally important for the rendering of security in dying is their attitude towards dying as acceptance.

The native informants vouch for free will and choice and serve as examples of what dying well looks like. To provide a narrative in which suicide becomes the convincing way to "die well" and with dignity the documentary relies once again on its expositional character: Cody's dying exemplifies what good, and thereby dignified dying is. Her pro-cess of dying represents the competing narrative to the suffering and fear attached to the images of hospital routines. Her process is visually accompanied by nature scenes that dominate the largest part of her dying. Cody is shown on strolls through woods, walks on the beach, and working in the garden. The information that she plans to take the Seconal on Memorial Day (25th of May) (*How to Die* 23:23) is visually accompanied by an

---

30   There are but a couple of instances where the voice of the director enters the narrative.

ocean scene. The security practice is thus visually described by nature. Though physician-assisted dying cannot be described as nature taking its course, it is nonetheless aesthetically represented as natural in contrast to the "artificial" interventions in a hospital setting. The documentary consistently reiterates the opposition of uncontrollable suffering with the planned and peaceful farewell facilitated by the security practice of Death with Dignity. Though not without grief and mourning – every member of the family is shown or interviewed in tears – the peacefulness of the wide nature scenes lends their grief a righteousness; it is represented as the "proper" or "appropriate" performance in response to inevitable death: the healthy way to act. Dying well with PAD is thus able to circumvent the threat foreshadowed by the past suffering that is marked by distress, panic, fear, and uncertainty.

This representation of Death with Dignity shares a crucial aspect with the older (religious) understanding of security in dying though the current form is characterized as a completely secularized practice – and in fact is opposed by most religions. The narrative stresses that dying is more than merely a biologically determined end, but rather a closure of a person's life, which relies on awareness and acceptance. Rather than the ending of a person, Cody's story reflects the active "bringing to an end of the person." She is introduced as she crosses off things from her Bucket List (How to Die 16:04), saying farewell, and giving away things. She is aware of her nearing end and is able to close her own life (narrative) by telling her own story. It is thus not only the materiality of dying – the suffering – that determines the understanding of (in)security, but also the prescribed attitude toward and behavior in dying. Her dying embodies and exemplifies this acceptance when Cody is still feeling well, but, more importantly, also closely before her last act of drinking Seconal. Her liver has begun to fail and Cody is shown in her physical suffering, while appearing mentally stable and in good spirits. She teaches her son the family Christmas cookie recipe and the camera team accompanies her to the hairdresser for a last haircut. She is shown in an over-the-shoulder shot in the mirror while her hair is being cut with a voice-over providing her reflections on dying (How to Die 1:25-35). Cody closes her own narrative by telling her story in the documentary and by deciding actively how she will be remembered. Her process of dying represents what she asserts already early in the documentary: "everything will be fine; I've written them letters" (How to Die 27:43). The ability to close one's own life narrative mirrors the prescribed "healthy" behavior in dying also foregrounded in thanatological studies supporting pastoral interventions such as "life review conduct."[31]

This positive nature of awareness and acceptance as a healthy and proper conduct in dying is further accentuated by the musical score that characterizes the different scenes of dying. In contrast to Nancy's and her husband's musical characterization, Death with Dignity is introduced with the comparatively "happy" folk song "In My Time of Dyin[sic]" performed by Tom Brosseau (How to Die 4:39-7:00). Creating the mood for the scenes representing self-administered death with a folk adaptation of a Psalm might seem counterintuitive as it expresses the most fervent opposition to physician-assisted dying. But it

---

31   Cody's dying exemplifies this acceptance that is also defined as the good way to die in Thanatological Studies. It represents the possibility to reconstruct biographies and can also be seen as a form of narrative healing, so a security practice itself.

directly associates the "easy" and good death found with Jesus's help and the good death represented in the documentary. The soundtrack further underlines that the claim to dignity that the documentary makes draws on centuries-old cultural narratives of dying well, meaning dying prepared and aware of one's death, which has been reiterated in newer thanatological versions of the same narrative. Security in dying is here understood as awareness and consciousness, as a conclusion to life that reflects (on) the person. It represents a reversal of the denial of death and dying that dominated up to the 1980s as described before. Every dying protagonist who decides to take advantage of PAD represents this awareness in dying. They know they are dying and have accepted their "fate."

The documentary further stresses the necessity of acceptance as the proper way to die well by juxtaposing it with two short episodes of dying without taking advantage of Death with Dignity. The documentary allows a short glimpse of the feared downside of the practice. It dedicates four minutes to the problematic eventuality that people would be expected to use the Death with Dignity law as a form of implicit coercion. In showing "The Other Side" the documentary cuts to a Trailer Park (*How to Die* 52:06) which marks a different socio-economic environment than that of the other characters. Randy Stroup has final stage prostate cancer and reads out a letter which informs him that his Medicaid only covers palliative care or physician-assisted dying but no further treatment. Randy is angry and desperate, offering a contrasting understanding of dignity: "dignity means to me that I can hold my head up high and I can't see how anyone can take [sic] through life and hold your head up high while doing this" (*How to Die* 55:00). What could have instigated an interesting discussion on the different visions of "dying well" is cut short in favor of a clear cut security narrative in which awareness as well as acceptance are crucial to dying well. Randy's story ends after a few minutes with a black panel explaining that after his strong objection to PAD he received another round of aggressive treatment, yet died shortly after nonetheless. His experience and behavior in dying is marked by denial, which is not untypical for the process of dying,[32] but it is here clearly depicted as "harmful." The story of his dying is not further represented. The meaning and affective charge of his dying is dictated by the intertitle following his story: "Despite receiving chemotherapy treatment for 4 weeks, Randy died from cancer" (*How to Die* 55:16). His dying while fighting the disease with aggressive and physically debilitating treatment is represented as pitiful and unnecessary, ever more so as the security of dying well would have been accessible had he taken the right choice for security. The omission of his story's exposition represents the general exclusion of "another truth."

In contrast, Ray Carney's dying, which also occurs without the use of the medication, is defined by "self-determination" (*How to Die* 55.20). He has fully accepted his diagnosis, has obtained the prescription drug to end his life and is planning his own funeral (58:00). In contrast to Randy, Ray was only diagnosed as terminally ill with an estimated

---

32   According to psychoanalysis, the fear of death is motivated by the inherent denial of one's own death because "in the unconscious every one of us is convinced of his own immortality" (Freud, 'Thoughts" 291). This notion is psychoanalytically attributed to the impossibility to think our own death, and indeed Kübler-Ross describes denial as the initial phase in her five-stage model of dying. She cites multiple interviews in which the patients, in rare cases until the very end, deny the possibility of their own passing with words such as: "no, not me, it cannot be true" (*On Death* 51).

six months to live because he refused the offered treatment to save or at least prolong his life – the removal of his voice box. His voice and voice box are central parts of his identity as Ray, a former TV host and singer, explains, and he cannot imagine a life without it. He declines treatment as it would mean a radical loss of an essential part of his identity. Ray is interviewed and accompanied to the studio where he records his own eulogy. His story also ends with a panel information: "Ray never had his voice box removed. / He died in hospital, physically unable to give himself the lethal doses of Seconal, a requirement of the Oregon law. / His eulogy was played" (*How to Die* 1:00:49). While tragic all the same, as he was not able to fulfill his wish and take the medication, his acceptance in dying nonetheless marks his process of dying as good and dignified; even triumphant as he defied the biosecurity narrative of survival which prescribed further treatment. He *chose* to die without having his voice box removed and closed his own life narrative. The juxtaposition of the two dying narratives of Ray and Randy reveal the normativity of the performance of dying in security. It is not the biological facts of dying that can be judged as inherently good or bad, but it is the behavior and attitude of the dying person.

The acceptance of death as the proper performance of security in dying is further accentuated in the conclusion of the documentary, which ends with Cody's deathbed scene. This scene is introduced by an intertitle that only reads "Saturday," two days before the set date for ending Cody's life. In the last days preparing for the final act Cody's suffering is shown close-up, highlighting the corporeality of the threat Cody is preempting (*How to Die* 1:32:42-1:34:36). Though her deathbed scene depicts grief, pain, and crying, it is explicitly marked as happy: "You must not think that only because I am crying it's not happy" (*How to Die* 1:38:45). The next intertitle reads "Monday" (*How to Die* 1:38:54) and introduces the final gathering: the house is shown from the outside, it is dark and only the windows are lit. The preparation of the drink is shown while the actual deathbed scene is represented by the audio from inside and the image of the window from the outside. It depicts a deathbed scene with singing, thanking, crying, the act of drinking the medication and heavy breathing. The scene culminates in Cody's last words: "This is so easy; I wish people knew how easy this was" (*How to Die* 1:44:10). The documentary ends with almost the same words that opened the documentary representing the iconic convention of last words.[33] The symbolic meaning that is according to Diana Fuss traditionally bestowed onto these words is here emphasizing the final truth of something that will remain forever out of reach for the living: the moment of truth associated with death.[34]

The last part of her long process of dying represents a return to the "beautiful death" of 19th century *sentimentalism*. The documentary represents an iconographic deathbed scene as the climax of the security narrative serving as *the* example of good and dignified dying, which is depicted as peaceful and natural, and strangely culturally familiar. Cody's deathbed scene echoes the iconic deathbed scene of the "beautiful death" (Ariès, *Hour of*

---

33   Despite the invisibility of the deathbed today "the convention of last words survives into the present, outliving the circumstances that produced it" (Fuss 894), which reveals the importance they have for our concept of dying.

34   This moment of truth is important in the concept of death and dying in religious and spiritual as much as in secularized understandings. As previously noted, also in Heidegger's existential philosophy death held the promise of truth.

Our Death 473) that for instance Harriet Beecher Stowe has enshrined in her depiction of Little Eva's dying. In this sentimentalist rendering death is not only beautiful, it is triumphant; instead of doubtful anxiety, Eva dies happily and in a manner that consoled her bystanders for whom the spectacle turns into a spiritually enlightening moment: "'O, Eva, tell us what you see! What is it?' said her father. A bright, a glorious smile passed over her face, and she said, brokenly,—'O! love,—joy,—peace!' gave one sigh and passed from death unto life!" (Beecher Stowe 257). The heavenly vision of the beyond that Little Eva grants her bystanders is in the deathbed scene of Cody secularized and thoroughly detached from any divine reference. Nonetheless, the last words as a message from beyond uttered by the "native informant" of death resemble the same idea. Both deathbed scenes framing the documentary – the opening and closing scenes – "console" the bystander corroborating the security found. However, the security found in the escape from the normative biosecurity practices of survival replaces the promise of controllability only seemingly. Awareness and acceptance emphasized in this new security practice do not indicate an acceptance of fate but re-enforce the primary role of medical practice and controllability.

Not without my Doctor

The practice of physician-assisted dying represents a counter-narrative to the dominant biosecurity narrative of survival and to the traditional understanding of medical practice. In fact, some people, such as a counter-protestor interviewed in the documentary claim that Death with Dignity "is not medical practice" (*How to Die* 1:10:10) and a violation of the Hippocratic Oath. But though assisted dying clearly represents a counter-narrative to the biosecurity narrative of medical salvation geared toward survival, the security narrative supporting the practice cannot be divorced from medical practice and the normative power of medicine. Rather, the documentary makes clear that PAD represents yet another facet of biosecurity. It functions as a replacement and a changed version of the original promise, but it is a biosecurity narrative nonetheless.

From obtaining the prescription to the taking of the medication and the final deathbed, every step of the process is accompanied by medicine as the arbiter of security. The security practice of PAD heavily relies on medical authority and represents a medically facilitated death rather than an escape from the normative power of medicine. It is the unchallenged biomedical power that decides the legal availability of this alternative security narrative – the safety net. Since the diagnosis of "six months to live" is the prerequisite for the security practice to be attainable the process of dying has to be literally "named into being" by a doctor. The authoritative voice of medicine is thus comparable to Austinean performative words, which create the reality in the moment the words are uttered. The process of dying can rarely be recognized and experienced without this performative shift. In the case of physician-assisted dying, however, it not only informs the individuals about their security status, and thereby making dying experienceable, this "naming into being" determines the availability of security. The diagnosis represents the prerequisite for accessing the security practice of "dying well" referring to both, the awareness and the medication that together promise the security in dying.

This reliance on medical diagnosis to instigate a performative turn defining the shift from "sick" to "dying" also becomes obvious in the representative problem of the documentary. Most of the dying individuals in the documentary do not embody the corporeality associated with dying, some do not even necessarily appear sick. Visually and narratively it is thus the representation of diagnosis, symptoms, and reading of CAT scans that define the individuals in the documentary as dying. Since individuals who decide for Death with Dignity have to be of sound mind and have to be capable to self-administer the prepared medication, the dying bodies fail for the larger part of the documentary to represent the corporeality that is culturally expected in dying. Cody, for example, is introduced initially while hiking with two friends laughing and joking about her preparations for dying – she invites her friends to "shop her closet" (0:15:22). Her body is marked by heavy breathing but her positioning as dying relies entirely on the intertwined medical history and final diagnosis of the recurring liver cancer: the authoritative voice of the medical narrative.

Shortly after introducing Cody the documentary starts skipping back to explain why this seemingly healthy woman has decided to take advantage of Death with Dignity. Cody explains how inexplicable pain prompted her to see her doctor, which represents the transition to the medical narrative. It is followed by an interview with her doctor explaining Cody's diagnosis and showing images of her first ultrasound exam. Her illness narrative is represented alternatingly by Cody's voice-over commenting on her bad surgery results, a short section of an interview with her husband quickly followed by more post-surgery images, and the voice-over of the daughter explaining further the long and difficult recovery. Without the knowledge that Cody is dying the narrative would represent the common and familiar structure of illness narratives of fighting an illness. However, Cody cannot leave her temporary "sick role" behind (Parsons) but becomes part of the "remission society" (Frank).[35] The next CAT scan cuts short this illness narrative of fighting disease and reclaiming life: The voice-over of the doctor explains the meaning of the visual image (the scan), which represents the onset of dying. This scene uses the medical and technically facilitated image of cancer to performatively represent dying, or at least its beginning. The image makes (affectively) present the reality of dying, producing it in the very sense of performativity. Since this diagnosis and performative turn obviously preceded the timing of the documentary the moment is recreated visually with the images and the doctor's voice-over emulating the shift of reality for the audience. The doctor's voice is needed to explain the technoscientific image as a representation of dying: she asserts that there are "no options" (How to Die 19:30). This performative turning point is crucial and shows how difficult it is to determine the onset of dying.

This central positioning of the doctor, the professionalized and sanctioned authority over life and death, shows that dying requires an authoritative voice to create the perceivable reality of dying. Though such a diagnosis is ambiguous and not always feasible,

---

35   Arthur Frank defines individuals who are part of the remission society as "effectively well but could never be considered cured" (Frank 163).

it is nonetheless crucial to instigate the change of reality from illness to dying. The documentary reinforces this perfomative turn from sick to dying with an intertitle: "Cody was diagnosed with 6 months or less to live on February 16th. / She plans to take the lethal dose of Seconal on May 25th, Memorial Day" (*How to Die* 23:28). The intertitle not only reiterates the diagnosis as a necessary performative shift but ties the onset of dying to a decision. This decision, however, is not whether to die but how to die and when to die. Thus, the promise of Death with Dignity rests not just on the promise of dignity but of total control. Though a liberating counter-narrative to the biomedical security narrative of survival, it nonetheless relies on the elements of the normative security narrative, namely controllability. The loss of control feared in the prospect of an un-administered death is contrasted by controlled temporality and physicality. Security in dying and dignity is represented as the foreclosure of uncertainty, which is offered by the physician.

The turn from illness to dying is important on a legal, but also on a personal level. Medical diagnoses are crucial for the experience of dying to "institute" the process as well as to define and explain the different phases. The documentary shows that today patients are often unable to "understand" the severity of their condition because the knowledge of the terminal illness does not always coincide with the physical signs of decline that are expected, as sociological studies point out (Kellehear, "On Dying" 389). The ambiguity of Cody's experience of dying shows how important professionalized readings of bodily performances are for the understanding and experience of dying. Accompanied by nature shots and contemplative flute music the audience is informed that Cody has outlived her prognosis. Though this shows that death and dying is not just "created" and defined without referencing a materiality, the representation at the same time indicates the normative experience of dying. At the doctor's office Cody states that, "I am lucky not to be feeling sick" (*How to Die* 47:13) but she is confused because her body does not conform to the imagery of a dying body. She feels as if she is not experiencing dying properly, nor acting like "a person with a terminal illness" (*How to Die* 1:01:32). That she understands her body as failing to represent the risk that it poses to her life emphasizes the importance of the performance of the body "surface" to understand and experience one's security status. Cody asks jokingly: "I am ready to start to decline, and I am not declining. What's the matter?" (*How to Die* 1:02:06). Cody is only able to understand the meaning of her bodily symptoms on the basis of the medical explanations. And she can only time her death on the basis of this medical narrative of decline. Medical estimations are thus not only necessary to be eligible to access PAD but are crucial to facilitating the awareness and acceptance that are core elements for the security practice of dying well.

The inability to fully understand her bodily processes and the absence of symptoms of decline without her doctor's explanation is structurally decisive for the security narrative of dying. Again, it is the other – this time in form of the medical professional– and not the dying self who relates and explains, and thereby determines the meaning of dying. Medical explanations both explain symptoms and provide "the language" to describe and understand the experience. Accordingly, Cody's suffering and increasing pain is described primarily by medical markers, namely pain medication. The doctor explains that "about three weeks ago Cody was on a very minimal amount of pain medication, within the last three weeks she has gone to needing the equivalent of 10 milligram of IV [intravenous] morphine an hour, which is a lot" (*How to Die* 1:26:51). Likewise, Cody details her suffering by the amount of morphine she needs an hour (by then 75 mg) (*How to Die* 1:35:37). Suffering and pain in dying are thus firmly positioned within a biomedical model.

The importance of biomedicine in the story of dying with PAD is further increased in the narrative construction exemplified by Cody's storyline. The testimony of Cody's dying – the "truth" told by the native informant – represents rather a shared story of patient and doctor than an intimate account by one narrator. Cody's failing body and the onset of the last part of the process of dying is introduced by an intertitle informing the audience about the physical problems and the needed procedures accompanied by slow piano music. The documentary cuts back to the doctor's treatment of the physical symptoms such as the changing of tubes and draining of liquid to alleviate the painful swelling of Cody's stomach due to fluid build-up (*How to Die* 1:15.52). In fact, the doctor takes over the narrative quickly after Cody's introduction (*How to Die* 17:17). Medical language dominates her narrative sequences which represent a guiding and equal element in the story of Cody's dying. Cody's story starts with her first symptoms of pain but it is the doctor's reaction that explains the gravity of the situation: "she [the doctor] called me into her office and then she burst into tears, and she said, 'You have a big mass in your liver'" (ibid.). These shifts in narrative voice between the doctor and Cody emphasize the necessity and predominance of the medical perspective in dying, especially for the practice of PAD. The dying depicted is a shared story told from different points of view, which make clear that the doctor is an important actor in determining and evaluating the process of dying and facilitating security beyond the initial diagnosis.

The representation by the interchanging narrative voices thus do not just dominate the onset of dying but the entire narrative of dying. Most poignantly, before the difficulties of the decision for Death with Dignity within Cody's family are mentioned the documentary shows the doctor's emotional reaction to the diagnosis and her moral dilemma. The doctor's decision to write the prescription stands at the beginning of Cody's storyline as she explains: "It kind of shocked me thinking about it in an intellectual realm … versus I am gonna write a prescription which will end someone's life" (*How to Die* 19:59). Cody's and everyone else's decision for physician-assisted dying is in contrast represented as a foregone conclusion – a decision already made. The conversations, quarrels and negotiations that presumably precede such a decision are only represented temporally following the doctor's explanation in the narrative.

Considering this central positioning of the medical narrative it is not surprising that it is the doctor's narrative perspective that reveals the important turning points of the narrative of dying. She tells Cody that the cancer has returned and she is the one that narrates Cody's decision for Death with Dignity: "She [Cody] said, if this comes back I know there are no good treatment options. I will want that in reserve, the death with dignity law" (*How to Die* 19:50). She announces that "this is the change" once Cody starts to visibly decline (*How to Die* 1:22:00), affirming the onset of "acute" dying, and it is the doctor who announces the moment when Cody decides it is time to end her life (*How to Die* 1:26:55). And finally, it is the doctor's schedule that determines the actual time of taking the medication. Cody's process of dying, and the security narrative for that process, are thus narratively represented as a shared story between Cody and her doctor.

The professionalized reading of the body in dying also marks the decision of the "timing of death" that is so crucial in the modern way of good dying as discussed previously. Cody asserts at the doctor's office: "Actually, the main thing we wanted, is to get a decision tree from here" (*How to Die* 1:23:08). When the doctor explains how life-prolonging measures could get her to Christmas, Cody declines, deciding that she could not do it. The last preparations at the hairdresser are really just the visual and narrative anchor for the doctor's voice-over that dominates the scene. She elaborates on Cody's pain, what her dying without Death with Dignity would look like and finally how she had been asked to attend the deathbed and "made a date for her life to end" (*How to Die* 1:31:04). It is the doctor's voice that introduces the deathbed scene proper starting with the intertitle "Saturday" (*How to Die* 1:31:40). The story is thus not just told by interchanging narrative voices of Cody and her doctor, but it is the doctor's voice that ultimately dominates the narrative determining the timing of death and introducing the deathbed scene – the climax of the achieved security in death. Though the self-reliant autonomous subject is foregrounded in the security narrative promoting physician-assisted dying, the narrative construction and therefore security itself is highly dependent on the other. Furthermore, rather than contradicting the dominant idea of biosecurity in terms of controllability, the narrative emphasizes this foundation of understanding security. The security practice of self-administered death is not just a decision to (let) die but the decision when to die. This controlled and chosen time forestalls the possibility of losing dignity in suffering.

The security narrative of physician-assisted dying, thus, does not simply contradict and resolve the failed biosecurity narrative of survival and life. The promised security recedes and slightly changes, but the core elements of controllability and the understanding of what good life is, remain stable. Furthermore, the source of security remains the same. Security cannot be found "alone" but has to be professionally prescribed and guided. The documentary represents the simultaneous failure and success of biomedical security: "We had the one chance of surgically removing it all and hoping that would be enough for her" (*How to Die* 17:46). The importance of medical knowledge and practice which is highlighted in the documentary, shows that physician-assisted dying cannot be seen simply as "escaping biosecurity" but rather as representing a further facet of the pervasive biomedicalization of life. It shows that the "new" security narrative of dying well represents a displacement of the "original" promise of survival which is substituted with the promise of dignity guaranteed by ultimate controllability.

Making Security: Disease Activism and Affective Legislation

> My dream is that every terminally ill
> American has access to the choice to die on
> their own terms with dignity. Please take an
> active role to make this a reality.
> *Brittany Maynard*

Though *How to Die in Oregon* is rather unique as a documentary and as a representation of PAD, the filmic documentation of dying has become a more common phenomenon, which is also used by Brittany Maynard quoted in the epigraph. For a brief moment at the end of 2014 she became internationally famous and a heroine for many people around the globe who followed her video posts. She was diagnosed with a terminal form of brain cancer and chose to die on November 1st using her right to die under the Oregon Death with Dignity Act. But that is not what singled her out from all people who opt for the security practice,[36] nor was it the fact that she was a comparatively young woman who died "before her time" as the cultural script would categorize it. What was most important was that Brittany made her process of dying public on the Compassion and Choice website in an attempt to raise awareness for the importance and legitimacy of Death with Dignity. The videos about her decision and process of dying "went viral," producing a publicity for this understanding of security in dying that forced public debate internationally.[37] The circulation of her videos and the encouragement and compassion for the woman's suffering that these generated were so pervasive, that the Vatican felt compelled to intervene and condemn Brittany's decision to end her life before her disease could. Brittany's videos are perceived to have directly influenced the Californian legislation, which was passed as the End of Life Option Act a year after Brittany's death. The president of Compassion and Choice Barbara Coombs Lee even commented in the anniversary video "Brittany Maynard's Legacy": "[The] wind of Brittany's message filled our sails...I don't think anything can stop us now" (Compassion and Choice 5:58). Since Compassion and Choice aired Brittany's videos 15 new bills have been introduced to hearing proceedings (Compassion and Choice News March 10, 2015).

The documentary as well as the video posts epitomize a predominant method of "disease activism" based on testimonials. They are a key element in providing narratives legitimizing the practice as a necessary right. As in the context of breast cancer discussed in the previous chapter, the production of such testimonies is crucial to the Compassion and Choice movement, which calls on individuals – both dying and bereaved – to become storytellers. The documentary echoes this reliance on personal narrative by making the dying the storytellers and authors of their own dying. For Compassion and Choice, the personal stories provide the main vehicles of promoting PAD, which the documentary reflects with Nancy's storyline. The prospect of changing the law to legalize the practice forms her motivation for sharing her husband's story of dying which represents the central practice of her activism. Nancy's and her husband's story are thus not just told to and for the audience of the documentary to represent the threatening horizon of dying without the possibility of PAD, they also emphasize her main role in the movement to legalize Death with Dignity: giving testimony.

The documentary reflects that dying well symbolizes a return to both awareness and acceptance of death as well as to the public nature of dying. And also today the public characteristic of the process of dying can be described as an act of making security,

---

36   According to the annual report of Death with Dignity by the Oregon Public Health Division 105 individuals have ended their lives taking advantage of physician-assisted dying in 2014. Altogether 859 patients have died using the law since it was enacted in 1995 (1–2).

37   Her first video "A Video for All My Friends" was released in October 2014 by Compassion and Choice has now had over 12 million views.

though for disparate reasons than its 19th century predecessor. Today, the public character of dying does not refer to the deathbed but rather to the documentation and circulation of a way of dying. While the documentary as well as the storytellers of Compassion
and Choice are more clearly aimed at activism, video testimonials of dying are remarkably more commonplace. The rise of blogging and social media, and especially v-logging
have changed and challenged the narratives of dying by allowing "everyone" to share their
own stories. In these representations the act of storytelling often also functions as a form
of healing similar to traditional illness narratives.[38] Storytelling is thus one important
element of making security on two different levels: On the one hand it is seen as a form
of healing, a "pastoral intervention" also reflected in "life review conduct" (Howarth 181,
Kellehear, "On Dying" 392). On the other hand, in the documentary, the testimonials are
more importantly a form of activism explicitly connected to the legalization of the security practice.

As shown above, the juxtaposition between a "good" and "bad" death establishes dying
without Death with Dignity as dehumanizing and unnecessary suffering for the patient
as well as for the caregiving family. The only solution offered in Richardson's documentary is the quest for legalizing Death with Dignity in states where it is still banned. In both
storylines the narrative forms a climactic development toward the completion of two success stories: Cody's peaceful death thanks to Death with Dignity and Nancy's triumphant
delivery of all the necessary signatures to the Washington State Capitol in Olympia. The
euphoric "happy end" of the story of activism is further highlighted by the closing scenes
of this storyline. A dramatic emphasis in the close up of the women counting the signatures leads up to Nancy's final speech where she elaborates that "My husband ... didn't
feel that any government or any religious leader had the right to tell him how long he
had to suffer" (How to Die 49:51). It represents the end of a struggle that places Death with
Dignity clearly within the discourse of Civil Rights and the promise of security expressed
in the Declaration of Independence. This relation between nation and individual is also
summarized by Roger's last words which introduce the documentary: "I thank the wisdom of the voters of the State of Oregon for allowing me the honor of doing myself in of
my own volition, to solve my own problems, thank you all" (How to Die 3:00).

The narrative connection of dying well and legislative change to make this "right to
die" possible represents two crucial elements for the security practice of dying well. It
further establishes the documentary itself as a crucial object for the struggle to make security possible. Rather than a controversial discussion of the competing security narratives of dying well, the documentary represents a clear-cut didactic narrative supporting
the practice of physician-assisted dying. Though the documentary carefully represents
the right to die as a necessary choice that every American should have the right to, other
choices and possible practices remain largely absent from the narrative. The representation of palliative care, hospice care and pain management, or end of life directives would
complicate the unambiguous security narrative Richardson offers with the dichotomy of

---

38   Dying V-loggers are usually younger individuals such as Charlotte Eades (16–19) who chronicled
her dying from a brain tumor between 2014–16 (Brain Cancer: Dying to Live, Living to Die), the
blogger Eva Markvoort (65_RedRoses) in 2010, Miles Levin (18) in 2007, Michelle Lyn Mayer (39) in
2008, to name but a few.

choosing to die well versus a continued struggle for survival. Rather, the documentary represents a call to legalize the practice, representing it as an essential right of American citizens and becomes therefore itself part of the effort of making security. The documentary offers a sympathetic portrayal of the practice of Death with Dignity with an underlying educational agenda of "giving a voice" to what supporters call the quest for the ultimate civil right. It is not a balanced representation of a controversial practice but a carefully composed exposition of the Death with Dignity Act as a necessary and important legislative act. The testimonies of the dying and their claim to authenticity are thus a decisive tool for the ulterior motive of the documentary. Storytelling becomes in the documentary not only a last act of closure, but a last act of activism and of making security.

As the epigraph at the beginning of this section shows, this patient activism is firmly situated in an American rhetoric tradition. In her appeal for support of the Death with Dignity cause Brittany Maynard's call for the right to die well references one of the most famous and widely quoted civil rights speeches, namely Martin Luther King Jr.'s "I have a Dream." She thus puts herself and the support group championing Death with Dignity in a long line of civil rights activists who demand the protection of their rights as American citizens. This protection is not meant as a form of government intervention, however, but rather the opposite. Derek Humphrey, the founder of the Hemlock Society, proclaims in his manifesto "Liberty and Death" that "In a spirit of compassion for all, . . . every competent adult has the incontestable right to humankind's ultimate civil and personal liberty – the right to die in a manner and at a time of their own choosing" (n.p.). The reference to the foundational text of the American nation, the paraphrasing of the Declaration of Independence, is crucial. The claim to civil rights remains a stable – if not staple – element of the security narrative provided. Throughout the documentary Death with Dignity is represented as a right of a person in need of protection, while the prohibition of the practice symbolizes a breach of authority into the privacy of the individual. To establish the meaning of dying the documentary therefore follows the dominant argumentative elements of autonomy and choice, that define the practice, as I have discussed above. The narrative remains in the realm of privacy presenting physician-assisted dying as an individual and personal choice (for security), therefore establishing a link to core American values and identity narratives. It strongly rests on the opposition to government control or intervention in dying as a private individual practice. Furthermore, the narrative references the myths of U.S. American self-reliance – the ability and right to choose and take care of oneself.

This right to die, however, rests on affects, which were already central in the construction of the security narratives in the preceding chapters. The established meaning of dignity or rather its potential loss in the process of dying is based on fear attached to suffering in dying while death "in time" represents hope. It is thus affective attachments that determine the evaluation and understanding of suffering and fear (of losing autonomy and control). As shown in the analysis of How to Die it is not a logic argument that proves the inevitable "goodness" of Death with Dignity, or inversely the inevitable inhumanity of pursuing treatment up to the last moment. Rather the right to die is based on a call for compassion with the decision of a person in such a situation. The argument for the possibility and legality of this security practice is therefore based on "affective facts"

(Massumi, "Future Birth"). As such, affects do not only determine the understanding of dying but are productive on a social scale leading to changes in medical practice in a cultural as well as in a legal sense.

Affects therefore determine both the way security in dying is understood, and how the experience itself is perceived, as well as influencing to a large extent the process itself. Medical practices, which govern most deaths in the U.S. today are thus based on both facts and affects. Affects therefore determine the attitude and understanding of dying as well as legislative measures such as the Oregon Death with Dignity Act in 1997. Since the understanding of dying well with PAD is not just a personal attitude but ultimately aiming towards legislative change, the documentary represents an instance of "affective legislation."

8. Failed Futures: Biomedical Security and the Biosecurity Individual in Fiction

> Failure is simply the opportunity to begin again.
> *Henry Ford*

The most prominent representations of the biosecurity individual come from the field of fiction. The countless renderings of the conjunction of science and the human represent a big body of texts that go far beyond the contemporary biosecurity individual and their stories, which I have discussed in the previous chapters. It is therefore hardly possible to examine these identities and the narratives that forge them without including a reading of the biosecurity individual in fiction. With this chapter I will turn to the limits and limitations of science and security, or rather the end of the legitimacy of the scientific security promise and how it is tested in fictional narratives. As in the last chapter I will turn to the failure of the messianic narrative of scientific salvation, the failed futures. I will focus on fictional narratives that represent the failure of established security narratives promising controllability. While the last chapter stressed the continuation and renegotiation of the security promise here I will turn to the bleak endings represented in dystopian speculative bio-fiction. By reading fictive texts I wish to focus on how a security practice and an understanding of biosecurity is made to appeal and how it is integrated into individual identity.

In contrast to the fairly contemporary biosecurity narratives discussed in the preceding chapters I will turn to dystopian fiction in two very different historic periods, the mid 19th century and the 21st century: Nathaniel Hawthorne's "The Birth-Mark" (1843) and Gary Shteyngart's *Super Sad True Love Story* (2010). I will consider both texts as dystopian, although "The Birth-Mark" precedes the emergence of dystopia as genre of science fiction.[1] However, the interconnections between biology and fiction are complex and man-

---

1   Jameson asserts in "Progress Versus Utopia" that "it is a commonplace of the history of SF that it emerged, virtually full-blown, with Jules Verne and H.G. Wells, during the second half of the 19th century" (149). For a more thorough definition of dystopia and utopia see Pfaelzer and R.M.P "Parody and Satire in American Dystopian Fiction of the Nineteenth Century," or Ruth Levitas *Utopia as Method*.

ifold and cannot be restricted to the temporal limitations of narrow genre definitions.[2] Many of these texts circulate "what if"-scenarios that frequently depict utopian ideas gone wrong and often serve as a testing ground for social and scientific developments.

The wider genre of science-fiction is complex and has proliferated in the last 50 years with various subgenres and many questions of terminology arising; most important in the context of this book would be bio-fiction, bio-punk[3], cyborg writers, or medical futurists, to name but a few. Jay Clayton in "Convergence of Two Cultures: A Geek's Guide to Contemporary Literature" even introduces "a new genre of contemporary literature that focuses on science and technology. . . . Indeed, the increase in fictional explorations of scientific issues is one of the most striking developments in American literature at the turn of the century" (808). Though I will focus on texts belonging to this group, a genre definition is not attempted nor intended here as they are notoriously slippery and not essential for the purpose of my discussion.[4] Like many others, I will use the term speculative fiction (Bieber Lake), or rather speculative biofiction, which indicates the increasingly important role of biotechnological developments in contemporary U.S. American culture. With Hawthorne I will therefore read an early expression of dystopian speculative fiction at a point in time when medical science did not represent a consolidated field of study and had not it assumed its position as the arbiter of security. With Shteyngart, in contrast, I will turn to the contemporary when biomedicine and biotechnology have turned into the unquestionable authority over body and life.

Dystopian speculative bio-fiction serves as an important element in articulating the fears of society regarding the increasing possibilities of biotechnological developments. Science fiction scholars such as Sheryl N. Hamilton assert that "Sf texts in a variety of popular media have been active in exploring and constructing the boundaries of the biotechnological imagination" (269). Eugene Thacker points toward the bifurcate relation of science fiction and biomedical technoscience. "[S]cience fiction is necessary in order for biotech and biomedicine to continue constructing their narratives of technological advancement and increasing sophistication of a biotechnology of the population" ("Science Fiction" 157).[5] I wouldn't dismiss this interrelation of fiction and science as a "common-sense position on the anticipatory nature of SF" (Jameson "Progress" 150).

---

2   Some of its most iconic texts include Nathaniel Hawthorne's "The Birth-Mark," and "Rappaccini's Daughter," Mary Shelley's *Frankenstein*, H.G. Well's *The Island of Dr. Moreau*, Aldous Huxley's *Brave New World*, Robert Louis Stevenson's *The Strange Case of Dr. Jekyll and Mr. Hyde*, Philip K. Dick's *Do Androids Dream of Electric Sheep*, Margaret Atwood's *The Handmaid's Tale*, George Saunders' *Tenth of December*, Kazuo Ishiguro's *Never Let me Go*, Jodi Lynn Picoult's *My Sister's Keeper*, Gary Shteyngart's *Super Sad True Love Story*.

3   Jeff Prucher defines this subgenre as "science fiction which explores the societal effects of biotechnology and genetic engineering" (16) such as Interzone (1997) or Frankenstein's Daughters (1999).

4   For a discussion of genre definition of science fiction see John Rieder "On Defining SF, or not: Genre Theory, SF, and History."

5   And also speculative fiction changes and reacts to developments in biomedicine. The rise of the gene and the discovery of the structure of the DNA as a Double Helix changed the imagination represented in Science Fiction from evolutionary species change to genetic modification (Clayton, "Ridicule of Time" 327). While Theodore Sturgeon still imagined a new human based on "genetic mutation" in the sense of species development in *More than Human*, in Margaret Atwood's *Oryx and Crake* genetic engineering is the explanation for the existence of its protagonists.

But I would like to stress a different facet of this anticipatory mode. I will argue that these texts circulate affective attachments, which dominate the representation and understanding of scientific research and its security promise. And today these narratives are virtually everywhere. They appear as references in negative media reports, and gain an even wider audience and increasing proliferation in movies.[6] Despite its status as popular fiction, science fiction has been widely recognized as a genre dedicated to cultural critique, most explicitly in theories of posthumanisms.[7] Speculative bio-fiction challenges the representation of the imaginable, the confines of what is human(e). In doing so many texts form connections between science and cultural theory that make them objects of biocultural investigations *par excellence*. More so than in the limits of the imaginable, however, I am interested in the construction of pervasive security promises and their failure.

In this chapter I will therefore focus on the question of desirability and ask how biosecurity practices that are doomed to fail are represented as desirable? How are they produced as a legitimate and convincible force in these fictional tales of biosecurity? While the texts analyzed in the previous chapters establish the security narratives legitimized by their claims to authenticity, the fictive texts establish the security narrative despite the failure of the promise, or rather to then let them fail. They therefore more clearly reveal their narrative constructedness of the understanding of security and show that, though not everything is security, the understanding of what represents security depends on narrative construction and affective attachment.

In the first part of this chapter I will focus on Nathaniel Hawthorne's "The Birth-Mark" and then turn to Gary Shteyngart's *Super Sad True Love Story*. The texts question or reconceptualize the boundaries of what is human. However, they also emphasize the process by which science constructs, or is complicit in constructing security and the security narrative that determines the "affective attachment to what we call 'the good life'" (Berlant "Cruel" 97). As literary examples the texts grant an insight into the logics and dynamics of biosecurity, offering a complex representation of how an understanding of biosecurity is produced as an essential part of identities. In the analyses I will therefore focus on how security is constructed in terms of belief, hope, threat, and fear.

The two texts deal with different structures: in Hawthorne's "The Birth-Mark" it is a markedly individual structure in the 19th century, while Shteyngart's *Super Sad True Love Story* is more obviously describing security in a broader, collective structure. However, both are based on the erasure of bodily marks as readable signs of threat. And both represent science utopias and their failures, emphasizing in different ways how the security narratives supporting these utopias are based on faith. In reading the two texts together

---

6   The following is a selective list of examples, which seems inexhaustible: *Blade Runner* (1982), *Gattaca* (1997), *The Fifth Element* (1997), *A.I.* (2001), *Eternal Sunshine of the Spotless Mind* (2004), *The Island* (2005), *Inception* (2010), *Never Let Me Go* (2010), *In Time* (2011), *Prometheus* (2012), *Cloud Atlas* (2012), *Elysium* (2013), *Blade Runner 2049* (2017). The theme also increasingly appears in TV series such as *Black Mirror* (2011, 2013, 2017, 2018), *Orphan Black* (2013–2017), or *Westworld* (2016, 2018).

7   There are distinct branches of posthumanism, hence the plural s at the end. Hayles represents a disembodied form of posthumanism while Wolfe represents the posthumanist. Both concepts are vastly different from conceptions of transhumanism (Nick Bostrom, Young), which are sometimes also subsumed under the umbrella term of posthumanisms.

I want to point out the continuities and changes in the representation of the biosecurity promise and its threats.

Failed Future in Nathaniel Hawthorne's "The Birth-Mark"

> Knowledge, absolute sure of its infallibility,
> is faith.
> *Yevgeny Zamayatin*

The quest for perfection and immortality did not just emerge with the rise of biosecurity as a normative power, nor did the warnings against new scientific developments only surface with the birth of biotechnology. Rather scientific developments have always been eyed with suspicion. The proverbial scientist playing God has a long tradition reaching back to Daedalus and beyond. Nathaniel Hawthorne wrote about science and scientific experiments in many of his texts. "One of the plainest attitudes in Hawthorne's writing is a contemptuous distrust of science, which he personified in villain after villain of Rappaccini's stamp: Cacaphodol, Aylmer, Brand, Chillingworth" (Rosenberry 42). It is a recurring theme in Hawthorne's fiction. Undoubtedly one of the great figures of American Literature and known as a fervent critic of Puritanism and its haunting presence, Hawthorne both epitomizes the Romantic period and slightly transgresses its associated distance to any "real" society or politics.

"The Birth-Mark" was published in 1843 in *The Pioneer* and then later in 1846 as the first short story in *Mosses from an Old Manse*. It tells the story of the scientist Aylmer and his newly wedded wife Georgiana. It is set in the late 18th century "in those days when the comparatively recent discovery of electricity and other kindred mysteries of Nature seemed to open paths into the region of miracle" (Hawthorne, "Birth-Mark" 628). A little hand-shaped mark on Georgiana's cheek is identified by Aylmer as a "fatal mark" that he cannot tolerate, and which turns his and consequently her life into misery. He sets out to erase this imperfection of his otherwise ideal wife, experimenting on the consenting Georgiana together with his laboratory assistant Aminadab. Although he succeeds in removing the birthmark, Georgiana dies in the process.

The short story is usually read as a cautionary tale about the dangers of the uninhibited pursuit of science.[8] The narrator himself describes it as a story with a "deeply impressive moral" (Hawthorne, "Birth-Mark" 628). Critical analyses, however, have provided a more complex picture. For some the story is a representation of how Hawthorne understood humanity (Wentersdorf),[9] others see it as a rendering of the conflict of science and art (Rucker), or the practice of editing (Howe). More recent research often reads it as "a study of misogyny or racism" (Person 57), aspects which had been neglected in the earlier studies of the story that focus on perfection and idealization. Feminist readings

---

8   The short story is set before the advent of science and Aylmer as well as his experiments are marked as part of Alchemy. Nonetheless, the story is most commonly read as a comment on modern science.

9   Karl P. Wentersdorf describes how Aylmer "overlooks the claim of humanity and so destroys the very being whom he hoped to perfect" (174).

have pointed out how Georgiana is sacrificed on the altar of male pleasure: sexually objectified and reduced to her outward appearance, her story aligns well with today's plastic surgery craze. Judith Fetterley has famously highlighted the violence that is the source of Aylmer's supposed veneration: "'The Birthmark' demonstrates the fact that the idealization of women has its source in a profound hostility toward women and that it is at once a disguise for this hostility and the fuller expression of it" (24). Cindy Weinstein, on the other hand, stresses the representation of Georgiana as a reflection of the gendered market economy and labor. Relating the story to its contemporary political and social history Goreman Beauchamp sees Aylmer as a reformer, while Leland S. Person highlights that "'The Birth-Mark' illustrates the consequences of eugenic efforts to perfect and purify race and gender characteristics" (Person 57–8).[10] In the field of bioethics "The Birth-Mark" has become the standard example emphasizing the errant strive for perfection –both aesthetically and metaphysically. It was famously used by Leon K. Kass in his "Welcome and Opening Remarks" in the 2002 session of the President's Council on Bioethics on human cloning which led to the Report of the Bioethics Committee that proposes a moratorium on cloning for medical purposes and a ban for reproductive purposes.[11] The text is, despite its age, used in bioethics classes to explain "what can happen a when scientists becomes so preoccupied with his science that he disregards the dignity and worth of people" (Singleton et al. 284). While all these aspects are crucial I wish rather to focus on the construction of security, its promise, and its failure. I will focus on how the utopian hope is betrayed by the dystopian ending and how the scientific promise of security and its failure are narratively constructed. Hawthorne's short story not only represents the experiment of removing the birthmark as a failed security practice but emphasizes the importance and necessity of constructing a pervasive security narrative in the first place.

With the focus on how security is constructed I will turn to earlier readings focused on "idealization" and religion, such as Heilman's and in part Fetterley's feminist reading though they are not the cutting edge of more recent readings of Hawthorne. I will first turn to the relation of science and faith, and how the removal of the birthmark does not just represent a transgression of divine rule but becomes a religious practice itself (Heilman). Science does not replace religion, which remains absent from the text as such, but is represented as faith. I will then turn to the construction of threat that allows for the belief in the promise of Aylmer's powers in the first place, which Hawthorne renders in affective terms. Rather than a practice of revelation and truth, as a religious as well as scientific framework would suggest, Hawthorne emphasizes the use of fiction in order to maintain the dynamics of faith and fear that represent the gendered reality of security in "The Birth-Mark."

---

10   "Written in the early 1840s, shortly after the Trail of Tears culminated years of white efforts to displace and even exterminate Native Americans, shortly before the women's movement would gather momentum" (57–8), Person points out that the mark is red, not black referring to the ethnic cleansing that was being executed in the United States at that time.

11   For a discussion of this reading and its problems see Newman *Promethean Ambitions and the Quest to Perfect Nature* (1–6).

Hope, Belief, and Science

The mark as an evident flaw in Aylmer's otherwise perfect wife destroys the gendered security embodied by matrimonial happiness, putting at risk their relationship but also their well-being. Hawthorne makes clear from the beginning that Aylmer's quest to rid Georgiana of her birthmark is a Promethean pursuit bound to fail.[12] The protagonist, however, is "convinced of the perfect practicability of its removal'" (Hawthorne, "Birth-Mark" 631). The attempts to remove the mark and save Georgiana from the threat embodied by her imperfection are therefore represented in terms of hope and belief rather than by the empiric foundation and rational practicability. Science and its promise are personified by Aylmer, who is a "philosopher" of the highest calling. He "had made discoveries in the elemental powers of Nature that had roused the admiration of all the learned societies in Europe" (Hawthorne, "Birth-Mark" 632). Aylmer is often read to represent the purity of science and intellectual pursuit since he epitomizes the rational role in the Cartesian split of body and mind. He is "a type of the spiritual element" (Hawthorne, "Birth-Mark" 633) who is paired with his laboratory worker Aminadab who "represent[s] man's physical nature" (ibid.).[13] In his laboratory library Aylmer aligns with "Albertus Magnus, Cornelius Agrippa, Paracelsus, and the famous friar who created the prophetic Brazen Head" (Hawthorne, "Birth-Mark" 636). What all of them have in common is not their incredible achievements but that they "were believed, and perhaps imagined themselves to have acquired from the investigation of Nature a power above Nature, and from physics a sway over the spiritual world" (ibid.). Hawthorne emphasizes that Aylmer's, as well as his predecessors' achievements do not generate the claimed power but the alchemists *imagine* it, believing in their own powers. This hubris leads Aylmer to believe in the feasibility of an "elixir vitae" (634) and to regard it arrogantly as a manageable task for him. According to this conviction he claims powers higher than nature and also convinces others, or so it seems. Georgiana and Aminadab at least do not question him.

This faith and recognition is the central axis around which Aylmer's ambitions revolve. His research is not without reflection – he refrains from creating eternal life as "it would produce a discord in Nature which all the world, and chiefly the quaffer of the immortal nostrum, would find course to curse" (Hawthorne, "Birth-Mark" 634). It is not a potential moral transgression – Heilman calls it the understanding of evil (36) – that restrains Aylmer from this goal. Rather, the material ramifications that the creation of eternal life would cause deter him from this pursuit. Moral boundaries seem to be absent here as much as in the description of the attempt to eliminate the mark on Georgiana's cheek. In contrast, what Aylmer is seeking is recognition and fame. He exclaims that it "will be my triumph when I shall have corrected what Nature left imperfect in her fairest work!" (Hawthorne, "Birth-Mark" 632). He understands his actions not as a transgression or the cruel imposition of male power, but rather as a heroic quest to reach the perfection that

---

12   According to Greek mythology Prometheus stole the fire from the Gods and gave it to humans. For this act he was punished for eternity. He iconically stands for the human quest of knowledge and the unintended consequence due to the transgression of boundaries.

13   Wentersdorf emphasizes this dichotomy which he compares to the construction of Prospero and Caliban in Shakespeare's *The Tempest* (186).

seems so tangibly close, and so deserved by Georgiana. Hawthorne renders Aylmer's urge to establish security in perfection as a utopian endeavor and as an utter failure. Aylmer could not "find the perfect future in the present" (Hawthorne, "Birth-Mark" 641) and destroys "the mystery of life, . . . the bond by which an angelic spirit kept itself in union with a mortal frame" (ibid.). The attempt to tinker with nature is punished in Hawthorne's tale in the same way as in most Promethean quests – with the death of the loved one.[14] He thus depicts a tragic end that is foreshadowed again and again throughout the narrative. Aylmer had dreamed of the failure of his attempt, every trick he performs somehow fails revealing the unpredictability of the quest, and all previous experiments in his career have been failures in comparison to their high aims. However, "poor Aylmer" does not perceive the warnings due to his eccentric belief in his science. The faith in his own powers is so strong at first that he does not even understand his own failure. It is Georgiana who recognizes when she exclaims "I am dying" (Hawthorne, "Birth-Mark" 641).

The scientific genius and uninhibited pursuit of science is based on such a delusion of grandeur that Aylmer forgets his previous "unwilling recognition of the truth" (Hawthorne, "Birth-Mark" 632). In studying the "human frame" he had accepted that "our great creative Mother Nature . . . is yet severely careful to keep her own secrets, and, in spite of her pretended openness, shows us nothing but results. She permits us, indeed, to mar, but seldom to mend, and, like a jealous patentee, on no account to make. Now, however, Aylmer resumed these half-forgotten investigations" (ibid.). Hawthorne emphasizes that Aylmer forgets the "mortifying failures" (Hawthorne, "Birth-Mark" 634) of his past because he is preoccupied with the belief and hope in his science. Instead, he sees himself closing in on the "triumph" of science: to creation itself. With "thought[s] which might almost have enlightened me to create a being less perfect than yourself. Georgiana, you have led me deeper than ever into the heart of science" (Hawthorne, "Birth-Mark" 631–2). Aylmer's ambitions are rendered as competing with religion for he is aiming to create "divinity," "celestial," "purity." Heilman points out that in fact the entire pursuit is described in a way that science itself becomes religion. Hawthorne does not only describe Aylmer's quest in religious terms but also the relationship between Georgiana and Aylmer. Georgiana claims her "worthiness" by how much she "worships" Aylmer using religiously connoted words. The terminology used to describe both science and scientist is, according to Heilman, a sign that science has taken the place of religion. "What Hawthorne has done, really, is to blueprint the course of science in modern imagination, to dramatize its persuasive faith in its omnipotence, and thus is taking on the colors of religion" (Heilman 41). It is not the practices promising security themselves that are religious here but the hope and the belief invested in them which elevates them to a

---

14   The hand has been variously read as humanity that Aylmer does not recognize and therefore destroys. Though it is nature that is imperfect Heilman and others claim that it is not nature but religion that Aylmer is competing with. The mark represents the "hand of God" which connects divine and earthly. The premise is that the "mistake" can be fixed to achieve perfection, or rather divinity. This attempt leads to the recognition that "you have rejected the best the earth could offer" (Hawthorne, "Birth-Mark" 641). Brenda Wineapple has argued that the breach and killing-off of Georgiana is comparable to an abortion, it allows Aylmer to return to his solitary pursuit undistracted by the woman.

force comparable to religion. Hawthorne thus renders the relation of the protagonists to the practice of achieving absolute security as a religious one.

Rather than by facts and empirical proof the scientific practice of security is defined by belief and trust echoing religious faith. And its first amendment is "doubt not" (Hawthorne, "Birth-Mark" 631), "'it cannot fail'" (Hawthorne, "Birth-Mark" 639). Hawthorne lets Aylmer repeat this claim throughout the story: "Do not mistrust me, dearest" (Hawthorne, "Birth-Mark" 635), "have you no trust" (Hawthorne, "Birth-Mark" 638), and "Believe me" (Hawthorne, "Birth-Mark" 633). But rather than the belief in science and the worshipping of scientific means, Hawthorne emphasizes the veneration and faith of the person that Aylmer claims and demands. He does not attempt to prove the power of science to Georgiana but his own command of those powers. In this context Heilman points out that "the story indicates that in the religion of science Aylmer is less a priest than God" (37) because Georgiana considers his aims as "holy" "and with her whole spirit she prayed that, for a single moment, she might satisfy his highest and deepest conception" (Hawthorne, "Birth-Mark" 639). Aylmer as a God figure does not only demand veneration but is worshipped by Georgiana indicating her complicity in this quest. "'Drink, then, though lofty creature.!'" (ibid.) commands the god scientist and she requests "'Give me the goblet . . .'" (ibid). The belief and hope of both, Aylmer and Georgiana, elevate science to a religious faith that seems to be the source of legitimacy of the authoritative voice of science. However, the exclusive focus of the idealization of Aylmer the god-scientist as the arbiter and guardian of security neglects the other side of the coin. It is not only the persuasive belief in the God figure Aylmer but the construction of threat that legitimizes Aylmer's cruel and murderous practice.

Threatening Aspects

The practice and the practitioner promising security from the fatal flaw embodied by the birthmark seem unquestionable. Heilman underlines the construction of science and scientific strive as religion, as faith-based for both Aylmer and Georgiana. But Hawthorne does not simply depict their conviction as a stable status quo governing the plot. Rather, he emphasizes how Aylmer produces the understanding that renders the mark a threat and the scientific practice that potentially threatens Georgiana's life a valid and legitimate attempt and salvational practice. Rather than the reiterative use of religiously associated terminology describing the belief in the power of science Hawthorne emphasizes how the threat is narratively made present. He thus emphasizes the importance of threatening aspects to establish a convincing understanding of security.

There is no event that marks the shift from security, happiness, and good life to the insecurity and threat that Aylmer and Georgiana come to dread. Rather, it is a shift of perception that (re)defines the meaning of the mark on Georgiana's cheek. It was "[o]ne day, very soon after their marriage" (Hawthorne, "Birth-Mark" 628), not a special day that was somehow out of the ordinary. But just one day so indistinguishable that it is not dated or specified. The little mark starts to bother and irritate Aylmer on his otherwise perfect wife. The "visible mark of earthly imperfection'" (ibid.) shocks Aylmer. The construction of insecurity begins with an emotion, and almost more importantly with the communicative act that follows his feeling. When Aylmer asks Georgiana, "'has it never occurred to you that the mark upon your cheek might be removed?'" (ibid.), Hawthorne makes Aylmer the mastermind behind the idea. In the short story the protagonist sets the narrative construction of threat in motion which will determine the understanding of security and threat. With this question Aylmer renders the mark a problem and flaw that should be corrected. However, the meaning of the mark is at that point still not fixed but rather fluctuating: "we hesitate whether to term it a defect or a beauty . . .'" (ibid.).

Initially, Aylmer's opinion of the mark as defect and sign of threat is just one of various attitudes. Georgiana had never considered it a threat but believed her suitors when they told her it was a charm.[15] Aylmer's scientific view is juxtaposed against the romantic mythical understanding of Georgiana's admirers: "Georgiana's lovers were wont to say that some fairy at her birth hour had laid her tiny hand upon the infant's cheek, and left this impress there in token of the magic endowments that were to give her such a sway over all hearts" (Hawthorne, "Birth-Mark" 628). They either loved it or just wished "the semblance of a flaw" away (Hawthorne, "Birth-Mark" 629). Curiously, Aylmer's otherwise distinctively male perspective and gaze aligns him with the women of society who see it as a "bloody hand" (ibid.) that made Georgiana "hideous" (629) and the narrator adds: "But it would be as reasonable to say that one of those small blue stains which sometimes occur in the purest statuary marble would convert the Eve of Powers to a monster" (ibid.). The society surrounding the experiment is only represented in this initial description of ambiguous meanings attached to the mark. The process of fixing the meaning and eradicating the contrasting viewpoints on the meaning of the mark takes place behind closed doors. This process of establishing one unquestionable truth, with no other truths beside it, takes place in the "safe" space of matrimony and is exclusively negotiated between the couple, so between domineering husband Aylmer and his persuadable wife Georgiana.[16] Hawthorne therefore describes how Aylmer's disgust triggered by the little flaw turns her into a *monster* also in her own understanding.

It is not a deeper understanding of the mark that leads to the understanding of the birthmark as a threat, as "the crimson hand." Rather, "selecting it as the symbol of his wife's liability to sin, sorrow, decay, and death, Aylmer's somber imagination was not long in rendering the birthmark a frightful object, causing him more trouble and horror" (Hawthorne, "Birth-Mark" 630). Aylmer does not discern the mark as a sign of a deeper and hidden "truth" but makes it up, imagines it.[17] Hawthorne, thus, indicates a certain degree of non-referentiality to an external truth. Furthermore, it is Aylmer's imagination that causes his affective response and creates the meaning of the mark. It is not reason but an affixation and a rather arbitrarily selected signifier that generates the unfolding of the story. Over time Aylmer "found this one defect grow more and more in-

---

15 Georgiana replies to his inquiry: "'No, indeed,' said she, smiling; but perceiving the seriousness of his manner, she blushed deeply" (Hawthorne, "Birth-Mark" 628). This example indicates Georgiana's affective response to the threatening "feeling" in this situation.

16 In today's terminology of violence, the dynamics between the two would be described as psychological abuse.

17 In feminist readings as well as autobiographical readings of the short story the mark is read as a reference to sexuality and Aylmer's disgust an expression of his fear of female sexual pleasure (Zanger).

tolerable with every moment of their united lives" (Hawthorne, "Birth-Mark" 629). In the beginning the mark is not always there, "now vaguely portrayed, now lost, now stealing forth again and glimmering to and fro with every pulse of emotion that throbbed within her heart" (ibid.).[18] Once Aylmer's mind has constructed the mark as threat, he becomes obsessed. "[I]t became the central point of all. With the morning twilight Aylmer opened his eyes upon his wife's face and recognized the symbol of imperfection; and when they sat together at the evening hearth his eyes wandered stealthily to her cheek" (Hawthorne, "Birth-Mark" 630). The repeated perception of the mark as odious seems to fix the mark in its meaning as well as in its physical appearance. The meaning is thus enforced and stabilized by its iterability. Hawthorne stresses that the performative and reiterative quality of the threat is based on exchange, a communication between the two protagonists. Aylmer's affective response and attachment to the mark circulates between the couple gaining force every time it is perceived. Georgiana "learned to shudder at his gaze" (Hawthorne, "Birth-Mark" 630). By the time they entered the laboratory his repulsion is so strong that "he could not restrain a strong convulsive shudder" (Hawthorne, "Birth-Mark" 633) which causes Georgiana to faint. Hawthorne's rendering of establishing the meaning of the mark rests on the horizontal "communication" of affects. Georgiana does not react to the mark but to her husband's response to it. Hawthorne thus portrays an affective economy in which the mark is attached with meaning that becomes increasingly fixed and unquestionable the more it circulates between the couple. She faints because of the meaning that is attached to Aylmer's expression of disgust, which ultimately signifies the exclusion from her assigned role as adored wife.

The rejection by her husband, or rather his horror and disdain gradually make Georgiana perceive herself, or rather her mark as threatening. It disrupts her domestic life and characterizes her identity and understanding of security as deeply relational. She is taught, so to speak, that her mark is "the fatal flaw of humanity" and that "[t]he crimson hand expressed the ineludible gripe in which mortality clutches the highest and purest of earthly mold, degrading them into kindred with the lowest, and even with the very brutes, like whom their visible frames return to dust" (Hawthorne, "Birth-Mark" 629). The mark becomes the sign of mortality itself, which also Georgiana begins to perceive as a flaw and threat. In this meaning making process, Aylmer is the active part persuading Georgiana of his opinion and instituting the meaning of security. The threat and meaning of the mark is narratively established within the story. Aylmer's behavior and explanations, his thoughts and descriptions dominate the narrative until the threat of the mark is established as fact. Then, "[n]ot even Aylmer now hated it so much as she" (Hawthorne, "Birth-Mark" 636). "Giving in," or being persuaded to hate her own mark makes the healthy young woman ponder that "'methinks I am of all mortals the most fit to die'" (Hawthorne, "Birth-Mark" 639). She becomes a monster in her own understanding, not worthy of life.

---

18   The emphasis on affects not only defines the meaning of threat. They are in the short story also responsible for determining the appearance of the mark: "But if any shifting motion caused her to turn pale there was the mark again, a crimson stain upon the snow, in what Aylmer sometimes deemed as almost fearful distinctiveness" (Hawthorne, "Birth-Mark" 629).

In this affective economy threat and hope circulate, becoming more forceful in their relation to one another. While the threat of the mark makes Georgiana regard her own life as unlivable, the removal of the mark becomes the only hope – promising the return to the security of a good life. "'If there be the remotest possibility of it,' continued Georgiana, 'let the attempt be made at whatever risk. Danger is nothing to me; for life, while this hateful mark makes me the object of your horror and disgust, – life is a burden which I would fling down with joy. Either remove this dreadful hand, or take my wretched life! …'" (Hawthorne, "Birth-Mark" 631). The overemphasis conveyed through the adjectives describes the resolution to attempt the birthmark's removal in predominantly affective terms. Georgiana's fear of rejection and her urge to please and appeal define her understanding of the mark as threat. The threat to security and the desirability of the practices to remove it are thus determined by the fear of having to live with the stigma that the scientific narrative has created rather than the belief in the powers of Aylmer the God-scientist. "There is but one danger—that this horrible stigma shall be left upon my cheek!" cried Georgiana. "Remove it, remove it, whatever be the cost, or we shall both go mad!" (Hawthorne, "Birth-Mark" 638).

Science indeed is "able to provide an ultimate account of reality" (Heilman 37). However, it is not the ultimate account of its power and authority only, but of what is perceived as threat and as security. In the end the experiments that Aylmer performs for Georgiana are only almost "enough to warrant the belief that her husband possessed sway over the spiritual world" (Hawthorne, "Birth-Mark" 633–34). While "the illusion was almost perfect" (Hawthorne, "Birth-Mark" 633) and she is *almost* convinced of the powers, the threat and its affective repercussions are so forceful and real that the feasibility of the practice becomes irrelevant. The practice is the object of "cruel optimism" as Berlant termed it, and represents the cluster of promises that are attached to security. "[T]he fear is that the loss of the object or of the scene of promising itself will defeat the capacity to have any hope about anything" ("Cruel" 94). By performatively creating the threat as an affective reality the practice to remove the mark is legitimated. Not surprisingly, the practice is requested by Georgiana in the end "to save your poor wife from madness" (Hawthorne, "Birth-Mark" 631) not impurity. Hawthorne's use of fear and hope show what the security promised by science really stands for: the return to a normal and normative "good life," rather than the achievement of divinity, purity, or fame, which it represents for Aylmer. It is his disgust and horror that violates the rules of the affective economy that characterizes the gender roles in the 19th century United States. Horror and disgust take the place of admiration and desire destroying the promise of heterosexual nuclear family and of the possibility to please as the underlying and mandatory security practice.

Fiction of Security

Hawthorne does not only foreground the narrative construction and affective force of science as normative power and arbiter of security superseding and replacing the religious grasp on society. He likens the narrative construction of security and threat to fiction. This "allegory of science itself" is an "intricately wrought commentary on the fiction of science" (117) as H. Bruce Franklin points out.[19] Aylmer describes his science "in glowing language of the resources of his art" (Hawthorne, "Birth-Mark" 634) connecting it to "a history of the long dynasty of the alchemists" (ibid.) and the quest for eternal life, the "elixir vitae." Science and its quest for self-empowerment and control is represented as narrative, as stories of scientific geniuses that are housed in the library of the apartment. And Aylmer is part of this narrative materially in form of his book which stands in the same bookshelf as those genealogies of scientists, and as a scientist because he is their successor. Franklin points out that Hawthorne likens science to storytelling (120) as in the scene when Georgiana passes her time in the library. "Georgiana turned over the volumes of his scientific library. In many dark old tomes she met with chapters full of romance and poetry" (Hawthorne, "Birth-Mark" 636). The history of science is read as an aesthetic object, as stories rather than histories or scientific texts. From Georgiana's perspective Hawthorne describes the book of Aylmer's scientific studies as an autobiographic text. "The book, in truth, was both the history and emblem of his ardent, ambitious, imaginative, yet practical and laborious life" (Hawthorne, "Birth-Mark" 636). And reading his text Georgiana has to acknowledge that it is an autobiography of many failed futures. "Much as he had accomplished, she could not but observe that his most splendid successes were almost invariably failures, if compared with the ideal at which he aimed. … The volume, rich with achievements that had won renown for its author, was yet as melancholy a record as ever mortal hand had penned" (ibid.). Hawthorne's narrative establishes Aylmer as the tragic hero through Georgiana's reading, rather than an evil and sadistic murderer (Heilman).[20] More importantly though, the text as literary object is affecting Georgiana, making her cry. The essence of Aylmer's "sorcerer's book" (Hawthorne, "Birth-Mark" 637) is not based on its scientific findings but on melancholy and a longing for something absent and unachievable.

Furthermore, Hawthorne renders science as a form of fiction. Rather than empiric and scientific findings, or the different experiments and approaches to finding a cure, science is represented by illusions. At almost no point is Georgiana or the reader introduced to scientific explanations. Instead, science is represented by illusions and tricks that Aylmer performs to impress Georgiana. "In order to soothe Georgiana, and, as it were, to release her mind from the burden of actual things, Aylmer now put in practice some of the light and playful secrets which science had taught him among its profounder lore" (Hawthorne, "Birth-Mark" 633). Aylmer represents the power of science by creating fiction that is detached from any negative associations. "Airy figures, absolutely bodiless ideas, and forms of unsubstantial beauty came and danced before her" (Hawthorne, "Birth-Mark" 633). Science and its security practices do not show its real face but represent a performance staged for Georgiana as its captive audience.[21]

---

19   Franklin's main point is to argue that Hawthorne can and should be regarded as a Science Fiction writer. However, I find his reading of science as fiction in the short story much more rewarding.

20   This scene also expresses Hawthorne's inclination for irony creating a character defined by his many failures who needs to erase the only little flaw of his otherwise perfect partner.

21   This representation of science reiterates the ambiguous delineation of science and pseudo-science at the end of the 18th and beginning of 19th century as the example of alchemy for instance reveals.

The illusions and tricks are performed to impress Georgiana, but at the same time, they disguise the reality of the security practice. Aylmer's real research, the true treatments and procedures he tries remain hidden from Georgiana as well as from the reader. Only after all his tricks failed, Aylmer discloses a glimpse of "true" science when he resorts to his most prized exhibition. He shows Georgiana an elixir that is reminiscent of Rappaccini's poison. "[H]e showed her a small vial, in which, he remarked, was contained a gentle yet most powerful fragrance, capable of impregnating all the breezes that blow across a kingdom" (Hawthorne, "Birth-Mark" 635). The potion represents both "piercing and invigorating delight" (ibid.) and the power to kill at Aylmer's will. "No king on his throne could keep his life" (ibid.). The potion represents both security and threat and by no means the fiction of pure security Aylmer seeks to construct. It is the first time in the short story that science is perceived as threat. "Why do you keep such a terrific drug?" (ibid.) Georgiana asks. This destabilizing moment of "truth" almost disrupts the fiction of security that the reiterations of belief and trust had formed.

The artificial division of security and threat which Aylmer attempts to maintain by hiding the practices is recreated in the spatial representation Hawthorne offers. The apartment where the story takes place is defined as a space completely secluded from the public.[22] In fact, the society and country surrounding Aylmer and Georgiana are remarkably vague, disappearing outside the closed off apartment the story unfolds in: "They were to seclude themselves in the extensive apartments occupied by Aylmer as a laboratory . . . during his toilsome youth" (Hawthorne, "Birth-Mark" 632). The laboratory is the space of white male discovery, rationality, and conquest of nature's secrets (ibid.). It is the space which harbors the potential of the practices promising security. Science as the pure, intellectual male pursuit is contrasted with the female, love, and emotions that initially represent the rivaling forces introducing the story. Georgiana is described as tempting Aylmer to abandon his higher pursuits and leave his work (-space) for domesticity – threatening his scientific career. While Aylmer literally washes off his work when he "cleared his fine countenance from the furnace smoke, washed the stain of acid from his fingers, and persuaded a beautiful woman to become his wife" (628), the space has to be similarly prepared for Georgiana's arrival. Her entrance into the space of the apartment reiterates the marriage ritual and reveals the true unity formed: that of science and domesticity. Georgiana "is carried over the threshold of the laboratory" (Hawthorne, "Birth-Mark" 632) which accomplishes the performative act of marriage, however, "Georgiana was cold and tremulous" (ibid.). The "intertwining" (Hawthorne, "Birth-Mark" 628) of both passions, domesticity and love of a woman as well as science and pure male intellect is only a semblance. The narrator clarifies from the beginning that the love for Georgiana could only "be by intertwining itself with his love of science" (Hawthorne, "Birth-Mark" 628). Hawthorne's spatial construction of laboratory and abode, however, masks this unity by the artificial separation Aylmer creates.

The apartment is subdivided in laboratory and boudoir, which is the part of the apartment where Georgiana is treated and where she lives. "Aylmer had converted those smoky, dingy, sombre [sic] rooms, where he had spent his brightest years in recondite

---

22   Hawthorne designs a similar reclusive space with Rappaccini's garden, the setting for his other famous short story rendering the scientific experiment of a "mad" scientist.

pursuits, into a series of beautiful apartments not unfit to be the secluded abode of a lovely woman" (Hawthorne, "Birth-Mark" 633). To Georgiana it "looked like enchantment," "a pavilion among the clouds" (ibid.) that feels comfortable. What is represented as the accommodation of a space to the needs of a woman and the creation of a mock domestic sphere is really the careful construction of a space of security which hides the threats and risks contained in scientific practices. In fact, it separates not only the different spaces of domestic and scientific labor but hides the intertwining of both. The room itself represents an experimental set-up that hides its true purpose and characteristic.[23] "Aylmer, excluding the sunshine, which would have interfered with his chemical processes, had supplied its place with perfumed lamps, emitting flames of various hue, but all uniting in a soft, impurpled radiance" (ibid.). The outside is carefully concealed, creating a seemingly completely self-contained artificial space that "appeared to shut in the scene from infinite space" (Hawthorne, "Birth-Mark" 633). It is the stage for the performance of science that is dressed up as domestic, secure space, the proper space for a woman. A safe space, literally as Aylmer "was confident in his science, and felt that he could draw a magic circle round her within which no evil might intrude" (Hawthorne, "Birth-Mark" 633). In this make-believe space not only the appearance is changed but the whole "atmosphere" (ibid.) is created. The "boudoir" is prepared for Georgiana by burning "a pastil" (ibid.) which "had recalled her [Georgiana] from her deathlike faintness" (ibid.). In this simulated space every little bit is a performance put on for Georgiana, a fiction created to hide the underlying reality. Though "Georgiana began to conjecture that she was already subjected to certain physical influences, either breathed in with the fragrant air or taken with her food" (Hawthorne, "Birth-Mark" 636) she could never be sure until Aylmer confesses the failures of all his attempted remedies. Georgiana is held in a naïve, fictional safe space, objectified and secretly experimented on.

The narrative perspective shifts with the entry to the apartment from Aylmer to Georgiana and the boudoir. It is where most of the story takes place, where Aylmer performs his scientific illusions and where he assumes the figure of the God-scientist. The laboratory in contrast remains vaguely alluded to as "an inner apartment" (Hawthorne, "Birth-Mark" 633) that Aylmer and Aminadab appear from or disappear to. "She could hear his voice in the distant furnace room giving directions to Aminadab, whose harsh, uncouth, misshapen tomes were audible in response, more like a grunt and a growl of a brute than human speech" (Hawthorne, "Birth-Mark" 635). As Georgiana is confined to her space, Aminadab is confined to the laboratory reduced to animal grunts. The racism contained in this executer of Aylmer's experiments is striking.[24] More important for the analysis here, however, is that he (as the practitioner of science) and she (as the object of science)

---

23   This "hiding" the true purpose of the room could be compared to high-end hospital or care facilities which are designed to hide the clinical purpose they are built for as much as possible.

24   The description paired with the chosen name indicating the ethnic otherness of Aminadab is a clearly racist depiction reiterated in the lowly "dirty" work of science which has to be executed for Aylmer. In 1987 Thomas Pribek still reiterates the racist imaginary contained in the name "'Aminadab' is an exotic name fitted to a kind of grubby person" (177) when discussing the origin and meaning of the name.

barely come into contact. The two spaces of domestic security and scientific security remain artificially separated, while they are nonetheless connected. The two spaces produce two disparate representations of science, one room of "magic" (Hawthorne, "Birth-Mark" 634) and one of anxiety and threat.

When Georgiana "intruded for the first time into the laboratory" (Hawthorne, "Birth-Mark" 637) "[t]he atmosphere felt oppressively close, and was tainted with gaseous odors which had been tormented forth by the process of science. The severe and homely simplicity of the apartment, with its naked walls and brick pavement, looked strange, accustomed as Georgiana had become to the fantastic elegance of her boudoir" (Hawthorne, "Birth-Mark" 637). Hawthorne renders the boudoir as a "fantastic space" that is opposed to the reality of the working of science. With Georgiana trespassing the boundary to the space of male science Hawthorne grants the first and only view into the work performed in the laboratory representing the promised security. The space is described by the enumeration of laboratory equipment. Rather than the material reality, however, the space reveals an affective shift. Georgiana sees Aylmer hunched over his experiment muttering "'[n]ow, if there be a thought too much or too little, it is all over'" (Hawthorne, "Birth-Mark" 638). Rather than the actual scientific work Hawthorne uses emotions to portray the practice. "How different from the sanguine and joyous man that he had assumed for Georgiana's encouragement!" (ibid.). The repetition of trust, belief and faith that had determined Georgiana's understanding of the practice, had in fact been a charade, a fiction performed for her. With her transgression the seemingly clear affective attachments are threatened as Georgiana exclaims: "'You mistrust your wife; you have concealed the anxiety with which you watch the development of this experiment" (ibid.). The fiction of security represented in the spatial division of the boudoir and the laboratory maintains the division of emotions and their circulation which constitutes the gendered reality of security.

Not surprisingly then, her transgressing the boundary of the gendered security space triggers a strong affective response: when Aylmer sees her "[h]e rushed toward her and seized her arm with a gripe that left the print of his fingers upon it" (Hawthorne, "Birth-Mark" 638). The fiction of domestic security crumbles and reveals the violence that the practice hides, and which represents the real threat to Georgiana as opposed to the mark. The transgression and revelation of the previously secret violence opens up the potential in which Georgiana could assume an autonomous subject position.[25] In the moment of transgression she contradicts Aylmer and his unbroken authority over security. When Aylmer wants to send her away she insists on the truth until Aylmer whispers "there is danger" (ibid.). Georgiana, deeply embedded in the economy of affects that determine the practice as the object of cruel optimism, decides in the end to follow the suicidal practice of removing the mark. The desire of security rendered in the urge to please and appeal for just one moment wins over the reality of threat: "Longer than one moment she well knew it could not be; for his spirit was ever on the march, ever ascending, and each

---

25   This reading also indicates the revelation of the "security practice" to protect and perfect Georgiana as heterosexist violence against a woman, which would also be easily readable as a clear case of domestic violence which started with psychological violence and tragically ended in the woman's death – a common trajectory in many such cases even today.

instant required something that was beyond the scope of the instant before" (Hawthorne, "Birth-Mark" 639). Georgiana realizes long before the narrator tells the reader explicitly that Aylmer and his scientific pursuit to control life and create security "failed to find the perfect future in the present" (Hawthorne, "Birth-Mark" 641). The quest would continue, moving on to the next target, the "next" promise, the next object of study. And again the findings will seem like failures "compared with the ideal at which he aimed" (Hawthorne, "Birth-Mark" 639). This motif of failing to find the perfect future in the present could also be the guiding theme of biological security in *Super Sad True Love Story*, which I will discuss in the next section.

Failed Future in Gary Shteyngart's *Super Sad True Love Story*: The Very Near Future

> The biological invention then tends to begin as a perversion and end as a ritual supported by unquestioned beliefs and prejudices.
> *John B. S. Haldane*

While in Hawthorne's short story the birthmark embodies the threat to Georgiana's and Aylmer's security, in Gary Shteyngart's *Super Sad True Love Story* it is corporeal signs of ageing which represent the clutches of mortality and the obstacle to finding security and happiness for Lenny, the main character. The book is the third of Shteyngart's novels published in 2010 following the *Russian Debutante's Handbook* in 2002 and *Absurdistan* in 2006. With *Super Sad True Love Story* the author appropriates the dystopian genre, which has proliferated since the millennium (Willmett 267), to express his social and political critique of what many scholars call "technocapitalism" (Trapp 71).[26] Shteyngart paints a grim picture of America's future in his "blistering satire of neoliberal society" (Willmetts 271).

The novel tells the story of Lenny's (Leonard Abramovic) and Eunice Park's (aka EUNITARD) relationship set in a future society. The world they live in is marked by illiteracy and digital culture, driven by endless data streams that direct the consumer capitalism of this dystopian future. Society is centered around, shaped and determined by technological and biotechnological developments that facilitate a pervasive digital surveillance "state." In this context, security is not so much embedded in an individual but a collective structure. All that seems to matter is the constant ranking of individuals based on data harvested from the "äppäräti" everybody is wearing around their neck. The story of Lenny's and Eunice's relationship and the destruction of the United States around them is told interchangingly from the perspective of both protagonists. The narrative takes

---

26   In Shteyngart's piece in *The New York Times* promoting the publication of the novel he makes this critique of social media and reliance on smartphones more explicit ("Only Disconnect"). Simon Willmett even asserts that it is "one of the most critically acclaimed examples of this [surveillance based] new wave of dystopian fiction" (286). I would widen the group of dystopian texts that Willmett specifically refers to and include biotechnological (surveillance) dystopias that have similarly gained in number and prominence.

the form of an epistolary novel and each chapter represents either diary entries by Lenny or messages to and from Eunice Park's GlobalTeens Account. Besides the obvious love story between Lenny and Eunice there is another love story: that of Lenny (and his future society) with youth and the hope for eternal life. The novel represents the utopian promise of biosecurity, namely that the consumption of biotechnological services yields the power to efface ageing and death. Lenny's work place "The Post-Human Services," is a company which trades in "eternal life extension" treatments. Both the relationship with Eunice and the love story of Lenny with eternal life end in betrayal and failure. Eternal Life is unachievable for Lenny and turns out to be a fraudulent practice.

Predominantly, the novel is read as a social dystopia compared to George Orwell's *1984*, receiving excessive praise for its treatment of security in the context of a digitalized surveillance state. Many critics focus on the dystopian representation of already existing contemporary practices and developments such as digital surveillance. Brian Trapp calls it "a dystopian political critique, a sort of speculative and satiric worst-case scenario and an indictment of current trends in global technocapitalism" (71). Simon Willmett points out that the novel emphasizes the change of how these surveillance practices – as security practices – have turned from a Foucauldian vision of control of normativity and massification in terms of suppressing difference to a "decentralized, modulating, and 'dividuating' nature of surveillance" (269). Though describing collective structures the practices nonetheless define and impact individual lives. This individualizing form of surveillance, further exacerbates classist, sexist, and racist stereotypes as Trapp and Roy Goldblatt emphasize in their readings on ethnic identity construction in the novel. Though the novel offers a complex construction of a dystopian world, my analysis will focus on the representation of the bio-security promise of eternal life, which is pervaded and governed by the logics of the surveillance state.

Scholars such as Ulla Kriebernegg or Roy Goldblatt also focus their readings on the representation of biotechnology, or more specifically, the representation of age in the novel. In a similar vein as Trapp, however, Kriebernegg emphasizes the similarities of the novel to extradiegetic developments in biogerontology.[27] Though I will turn to the representation of biotechnology in Shteyngart's novel, I will not compare these developments to an extradiegetic present reality.[28] Rather, I will analyze how biosecurity and its promises are represented within the dystopian vision of an excessive digitalized neoliberal capitalism. Shteyngart's text imagines the failure of scientific pursuit to provide control of biological security through continuous biomedical surveillance and intervention. In Shteyngart's novel identity is highly dependent on biosecurity and represents "an 'unfulfilled project' in which the individual is in a permanent state of becoming" (Willmett 272). The permanent state of becoming is marked by the perpetual threat and risk

---

27   Kriebernegg focuses especially on the similarity to the "immortality prophet Aubrey de Grey" (62), who is a British theoretical biogerontologist. Aubrey de Grey, however, is not the only person Joshie and Post-Human services could be modeled on – Bill Fallon and his *Life Extension Foundation* would be another.

28   Nonetheless, I agree with Jameson that "SF does not really attempt to imagine the 'real' future of our social system. Rather, its multiple mock futures serve the quite different function of transforming our own present into the determinate past of something yet to come" ("Progress" 152).

of spiraling downward in the social hierarchy instead of upward as the American Dream would define it. This threat is not exclusive to but especially salient in terms of biosecurity and the possibility of approximating step by step the ultimate security of eternal life. I wish to show how the individual is defined as a biosecurity individual, representing not a passive consenting individual like Georgiana, but an active consumer subject. I will then show how the motivation of this biosecurity subject embodied by Lenny is nonetheless guided by a fiction of biosecurity based on hope and belief. As in Hawthorne, the security practices and the institution promising security take on a religious characteristic. However, in contrast to the 19th century vision of science gone wrong, Shteyngart's strive for absolute biosecurity in immortality is not a higher goal to achieve but a representation of the commodification of risk in which security is for sale.

The Biosecurity Self and Eternal Life

"'I work in the creative economy,' I said proudly. 'Indefinite Life Extension. We're going to help people live forever. I am looking for European HNWIs – that's High Net Worth Individuals – and they're going to be our clients. We call them 'Life Lovers'" (Shteyngart 12). This is how Lenny, the novel's main protagonist, describes his occupation at the start of the novel. While Hawthorne spends a lot of time and detail on how the fact of the fatal threat of the birthmark is established, in Shteyngart's novel the facts are fixed and ingrained in society. Society is not only marked by race, class, and gender but by health and age, producing biosecurity individuals who are intimately defined by security practices. Youth and eternal life represent the promised security for rich individuals provided by Post-Human Services where Lenny works. In this transhuman era, the practice of "dechronification" – a reversal of ageing – represents the pinnacle of the veneration of youth as a mandatory security practice. Here, all diseases seem subsumed under the cipher of ageing, which is understood as an avoidable disease (Kriebernegg).[29] The most minute signs of ageing represent the telltale signs of nearing death and are thus understood as a threat to the biosecurity individual socially as well as existentially. In contrast, indefinite life extension – with its reversal of ageing – embodies the security practice and promise of security.

The youthful and healthy body is not only celebrated but represents the norm of able-bodied security in *Super Sad True Love Story* that defines the individuals in their biosecurity identities. Biological security represents the precondition for a good and successful life as well as the main paradigm of difference. It is continuously determined in biological risk assessment produced by the devices everybody wears and projected publicly for everyone else to see. Any deviation from the ideal of the perfect youthful and healthy body is penalized by exclusion from society. Both corporeal parameters of health and youth determine the position of individuals in the social hierarchy. Lenny, for instance, is an outsider at work and bullied because of his age – he is 39 – and his biological data. "[T]he graffito in the bathroom reads 'Lenny Abramov's insulin levels are whack'" (Shteyngart

---

29   Heike Hartung and Rüdiger Kunow describe this "decline view" with David Gem as a result of the biomedical narrative that dominates the "narrative of old age which depicts the ageing process as completely devoid of positive meaning" (15).

57). Health data and appearance serve to superficially categorize people but also define their access to security in this highly stratified society.

The hierarchization is not rendered as an abstract invisible process imposed from above but as practiced by the people themselves in this data driven world. Lenny is advised by his friends to "'[l]earn to rate everyone around you. Get your data in order" (Shteyngart 70). Constant ranking constitutes a crucial security practice providing people with a sense of belonging and identity which seems equally important to the practices of self-care to improve one's bio-statistics. When Lenny learns how to use the functions of his device in the chapter "RateMe Plus" (Shteyngart 76–96), the app reveals Lenny's life expectancy: "life span estimated at eighty-three (47 percent life span elapsed; 53 percent remaining)" (Shteyngart 90). Health in terms of longevity represents an identity marker that is understood by Lenny as the most important indication of his security status. Health and youth are thus essential components in the stratification of society. Everyone is marked by their biosecurity identity based on health statistics.

Resembling the permanent state of crisis in their country, the protagonist's life is marked by the constantly looming threat of sliding down the ladder of biomedical and consequently financial security. At Lenny's work health ranking is used as a clear hierarchization of the employees, indicating the security of their position within the company.

> [T]he flip board displayed the names of the Post-Human Service employees, along with the results of our latest physicals, our methylation and homocysteine levels, our testosterone and estrogen, our fasting insulin and triglycerides, and, most important, our "mood+stress indicators," which were always supposed to read "positive/play-ful/ready to contribute" but which, with enough input from competitive co-workers, could be changed to "one moody betch today" or "not a team playa this month." (Shteyngart 58).

The biological parameters serve as indicators of a person's worth. The numerical description signifies both the corporeal security status, as well as the social status of the individual. Biosecurity markers designate the position of the individual in the work force and can determine their exclusion from it. Success and therefore class-belonging are thus tied to biological markers since bodily decline directly affects one's social status. Not ranking on the score board could imply the loss of one's job, which for Lenny resembles the exclusion from the source of security. For Lenny, the loss of his position at Post-Human Services would represent "the loss of the object or scene of promising itself" (94) as Lauren Berlant puts it in "Cruel Optimism." This loss "will defeat the capacity to have any hope about anything" (ibid.) revealing the impossibility for Lenny of reaching the desired security. The practice of health ranking and analyzing data contains the promise to approximate total security imagined as eternal life. Though Shteyngart makes clear that Lenny's hope for dechronification treatments are futile, his position in the company nevertheless gives him hope.

"New" biological stratification does not replace old discrimination of class and ethnicity but represents a further intersectional marker. And the intersectionalities determine both the accessibility of security through unlimited life extension as well as the accessibility of this security narrative. Lenny confesses:

but in the end we are still marked for death. I could commit my genome and proteome to heart, I could wage nutritional war against my faulty apo E4 allele until I turn myself into a walking cruciferous vegetable, but nothing will cure my main genetic defect: My father is a janitor from a poor country. (Shteyngart 60)

Shteyngart makes clear that the dream of indefinite life extension and prioritization of self-care is not available to all. When Lenny finds the dead body of an elderly person from his apartment building in the entrance hall he is outraged about the undignified treatment of the corpse. "I backed away. A body badly sheathed in an opaque plastic bag sat in the wheelchair, its head crowned with a pointy pocket of air..." (Shteyngart 79). Lenny's interrogation of the Hispanic undertaker of the "American Medicle [sic] Response," who comes to pick up the corpse, shows that the man is so far removed from Lenny's imaginary of security and world of indefinite life extension that he for one, smokes without caring about its negative impact, and that he regards death as normal: "'It's just death.' 'Happens to everyone, Paco'" (Shteyngart 80). For Lenny as the epitome of a biosecurity individual striving for immortality, the old people that he associates with "the daily carnage of the Death Board by the elevators" (Shteyngart 53) serve as the feared negative horizon to his vision of security. Those unable to compete and deviating from the norm are excluded and left behind.

The security of individuals is marked by their belonging to two groups that are distinguished according to their net worth (High Networth Individuals (HNI) and Low Networth Individuals (LNI)) and their access to biosecurity practice of dechronification (Life Lovers and Impossible to Preserve (ITP)). In the flight lounge Lenny describes the chasm between HNI and ITP. The disgust and amazement about this "one guy who registered *nothing*" reveals the position of those considered "disposable:" "He was at the margins of society, because he was without rank, because he was ITP or Impossible to Preserve, because he had no business being mixed up with real HNWIs in a first-class lounge" (Shteyngart 35). ITPs are not just marginalized; in the biosecurity ideology of Post-Human Services the judgment on those deemed unfit for indefinite life extension is even harsher, clearly categorizing the worth, or rather worthlessness of their lives. The deaths of many rioters, all of them LNI marked by the lack of access to basic medical care, is explained away as Lenny puts it:

We have to remember that our primary obligation is to our clients. We have to remember that all those who died in Central Park over the last few days were, in the long run, ITP, Impossible to Preserve. Unlike our clients, their time on our planet was limited. We must remind ourselves of the Fallacy of Merely Existing, which restricts what we can do for a whole sector of people. Yet, even though we may absolve ourselves of responsibility, we, as technological elite, can set a good example. (Shteyngart 181)

Here people are not only subdivided into High and Low Net Worth Individuals but in the two categories of Life Lovers (the wealthy clients of Post-Human Services), and the Impossible to Preserve (ITPs) as those too poor or too unfit to receive the treatments. People are thus marked in terms of their security potential, so their ability to access biosecurity.

In contrast to the biosecurity individual, the ITPs are marked as "less than human."[30] They are not just at the bottom of society and therefore more at risk but in Lenny's understanding completely excluded from the "we" of the worthy individuals because of their lack of access to eternal life.

Shteyngart's biosecurity individuals expose how much the logics of security inform their self-understanding. Lenny writes in his diary: "A body at the chronological age of thirty-nine already racked with too much LDL cholesterol, too much ACTH hormone, too much of everything that dooms the heart, sunders the liver, explodes all hope" (Shteyngart 5). Lenny's self-description exemplifies the centrality of the biological security parameters for the individual to understand his body. Shteyngart represents the numerical reality defining the security status as an affective response which refers to the future rather than the present. None of the risk markers cited by Lenny is explained as impacting his present state of well-being – Lenny does not suffer any corporeal ailments *yet*. Rather, the present is understood as an indicator for future security determined by risk assessment. And this statistical risk is here represented in affective terms, or what Woodward has termed "statistical panic" (Woodward, *Statistical* 13). The indication of risk markers "explodes all hope" (Shteyngart 5) causing fear and anxiety.

To fit in and to be a successful part of society one has to have perfect health scores as well as look young. This ideal of the youthful and fit body is based on self-care. The successful biosecurity individual has to therefore engage in biosecurity practices to manage their biological parameters and to be able to embody this ideal of a healthy body. Biological security is thus represented not as passive fate but as based on one's own responsibility. Lenny is repeatedly reprimanded to "'Stick with the diet and exercise. Use stevia instead of sugar'" (Shteyngart 126). "Take care of yourself. Go to the Eternity Lounge. Put some Lexin-DC concentrate under your eyes'" (Shteyngart 61). "'You need to detoxify, Len'" (Shteyngart 64). As these examples show, Lenny is not really an ideal example of a responsible biosecurity individual in this society of self-optimization. Nonetheless, the biosecurity promise is central to his identity.

The connection of outward appearance and health shows that also in this data-driven future society the outwards signs of the body are read as indicators of a hidden (and threatening) process within the body. When Joshie comments on Lenny's bald spot he elaborates: "I'm not talking aesthetics here. All that Russian Jewish testosterone is being turned right into dihydrotestosterone. That's killer stuff. Prostate cancer down the road. You will need at least eight hundred milligrams of saw palmetto a day. . . .'" (Shteyngart 65). This scene highlights the reading of the body for signs of risk potential and the associated responsibility of the individual to prevent or minimize that risk. It stresses that prevention and pre-emption dominate the biosecurity thinking of this future. While all ailments and diseases are related to ageing, the cure of distinct disease once they have surfaced is not part of the anticipated goals represented in the novel. Security is not found in an all-encompassing biomedical practice of curing. Rather, the decline of the body has to be preempted before it really starts.

---

30   Shteyngart condenses the attitude of the global North toward problems and human crises in the global South in the representation of the fictive biosecurity classes of the United States.

True security can therefore only be attained with dechronification treatments. "'Eternal life is the only life that matters. All else is just a moth circling the light'" (Shteyngart 275). And to achieve this is the responsibility of the self-reliant biosecurity individual. The blame for letting one's body deteriorate is placed squarely on the individual. For Lenny this represents a chosen and incomprehensible decline, because "Why not keep off drugs and demanding women, spend a decade in Corfu or Chiang Mai, douse his body with alkalines and smart technology, clamp down on the free radicals, keep the mind focused on the work, beef up the stock portfolio, take the tire off the belly, let us fix that aging bulldog's mug?" (Shteyngart 18) Security in *Super Sad True Love Story* is achieved by diverse forms of "technologies of the self" (Foucault). It is not a God-like scientist who subjects an individual to experimental practices but the individual that has to seek out, or rather decide for the security of eternal life by practicing "self-care" – wellness and fitness – paired with biotechnological treatments that represent an informed consumer choice.

The biosecurity clients in Shteyngart's novel are white and male: "Their white, beatific, mostly male faces . . . flashed before me."[31] They are affluent and powerful consumers of security, empowered by their choices and the "privilege of futurity" (Nye 112). The biosecurity subjects – though determined and ranked according to their youthful appearance and biological risk assessments – do not represent a form of biological determinism. To the contrary, nature and biology are understood as fully malleable and controllable if one makes the right choices.[32] Biological security is represented as radical self-empowerment to change and shift one's biological fate if one takes the proper choices of security. The different treatments of dechronification represent a security practice for the wealthy and healthy, while the rest are left with the promise of self-improvement in terms of life-style and discipline. Though the security of eternal life remains unattainable for Lenny, the hope and optimism attached to the security practices enforce their promise as if they were accessible.

Only towards the end does Shteyngart reveal the full extend of what the promise of eternal life looks like and entails when Lenny visits Joshie: "I was looking at dechronification in action. I was looking at Joshie Goldmann himself, his body reverse-engineered into a thick young mass of tendons and forward motion" (Shteyngart 216–7). The true security practice thus goes far beyond sousveillance and the recreational use of surveillance medicine. The promise of eternal life – or the eradication of the ultimate threat of death – is not based on making the biological body as such survive. "Joshie straightened up and I could see the muscle tone, the deep-veined reality of what he was becoming, the little

---

31   The female perspective on security in the novel is very different, for the women in *Super Sad True Love Story* are still dealing with domestic violence and "the politics of idealization" Fetterley pointed out in Hawthorne. Also in other aspects the novel is deeply gendered. While the urge for biosecurity, and its reckless neoliberal elitism is represented almost exclusively by male protagonists, the humane, compassionate side is represented by Eunice, a female. Simon Willmett points out that Eunice is the protagonist that represents hope and autonomy as a subject, one that defies Jameson's critique that dystopian fiction leaves no possibility of imagining an alternative (270).

32   The biosecurity individual is based on biotechnologically facilitated control that relies fully on the self-reliant and responsible individual. The control, however, is here largely described by consumable goods and services.

machines burrowing inside him, clearing up what had gone wrong, rewiring, rededi-cating, resetting the odometer on every cell" (Shteyngart 218). Biosecurity is represented here by the biotechnologically enhanced body which reveals the practice of indefinite life extension as a replacement rather than a healing or enhancement of the ageing body. Shteyngart represents the biosecurity of this future world not as a form of radical self-empowerment in terms of controlling the organic biological make-up, or by altering it. Shteyngart renders future biosecurity as a replacing of vital organs and a re-coding of biological matter echoing the processes of artificial intelligence.

Not surprisingly then, the dechronification process does not only alter the body but the self. As a side effect the treatments alter the personality, "because every moment our brains and synapses are being rebuilt and rewired with maddening disregard for our per-sonalities, so that each year, each month, each day we transform into a different person, an utterly unfaithful iteration of our original selves" (Shteyngart 65).[33] From the perspec-tive of the main protagonist, the promise of security is worth the risk of this potential loss of the self in the post-human future. The hope invested in the security practice by Lenny legitimizes this risk, similar to how Georgiana feels in Hawthorne's story. In fact, beside this one scene describing the material reality of eternal life, Lenny's hope and belief are the main constituents Shteyngart uses to represent immortality.[34] The fervent optimism of both Lenny and Joshie creates the "reality" of the practice, establishing it as an unques-tionable fact.

Hope, Belief, and the Fiction of Security

Shteyngart does not dedicate much detailed explanations to the exact science that pro-vides eternal life. Rather than expounding and developing the details of the biotechnical processes, which is a hallmark of science fiction writing, Shteyngart leaves this rather vague. Within consumer culture not even the representatives of the practice seem to fully know how the security practices work. The knowledge is outsourced to specialized sci-ence teams. Rather, Shteyngart stresses the desires and hopes attached to the security practices establishing the reality of the practices affectively:

> The technology is almost here. As the Life Lovers Outreach Coordinator (Grade G) of the Post-Human Services division of the Staatling-Wapachung Corporation, I will be first to partake of it. I just have to be good and I have to believe in myself. I just have to stay off the trans fats and the hooch. I just have to drink plenty of green tea and alkalized water and submit my genome to the right people. I will need to re-grow my melting liver, replace the entire circulatory system with "smart blood," and find

33   Within the array of practices promising security, writing becomes a security practice in its own right. "Joshie had asked us to keep a diary because the mechanicals of our brains were constantly changing and over time we were transforming into entirely different people" (Shteyngart 193).

34   With this emphasis on hope and belief Shteyngart overcomes the impossibility of representing immortality, which Jameson describes in his chapter about "Longevity and Class Struggle" (*Archae-ologies*). Jameson argues that representations of immortality are representations of a class struggle serving as a "substitute for some more concrete and fundamental worry and fear – some deeper contradiction – at issue in the unconscious" (332).

someplace safe and warm (but not too warm) to while away the angry seasons and
the holocausts. And when the earth expires, as it surely must, I will leave it for a new
earth, greener still but with fewer allergens. (Shteyngart 5)

The descriptions in the quote continue to the end of the universe, indicating early in the
novel the absurdity and fanaticism associated with the quest for immortality. It also describes Lenny's vision of bioscientific security as the belief and the hope he places in the
practices. The hurried list of things he *just* has to do to reach eternal life overtakes the
"almost" that introduces the description and places the practice more firmly in the realm
of future and hope than a present reality. Rather than representing a full-fledged practice Shteyngart stresses the importance of affective attachments to validate the security
practices propagated by Post-Human Services.[35]

It is Lenny's narrative perspective and faith placed in the promise of security that produce the practice as if it was entirely "secure." "'[S]ave money for initial dechronification
treatments; double own lifespan in twenty years and then just keep going at it exponen-
tially until you gain the momentum to achieve Indefinite Life Extension" (Shteyngart 51).
In this description of his quest to achieve the biological and financial status to be eligible
for the treatment promising infinite life the potential is merely related to the ability of
the individual to qualify for the treatment. Lenny's faith placed in the technological fix
turns the possibility of indefinite life extension into fact, though the security practice is
rather a promised security that is *not yet* fully accessible by scientific and technological
means. After all, "[t]he technology is almost here" (Shteyngart 5), meaning *not yet*. The
security is thus not much more than a promise.

While Joshie personifies the security practice of dechronification serving as an idol
of the movement of "Life Lovers," Lenny gives the practice its meaning, its context, and
its force, as it is mainly narrated by him. Lenny anchors the narrative and his navigation
through the thicket of this brave new world provides the narrative guard rails for the
reader. But also intradiegetically it is Lenny's storytelling that gives shape to the security
practice. As the main storyteller he brings the practice to life representing a new version
of a very old tale – immortality.

I painted him a three-dimensional picture of millions of autonomous nanobots inside
his well-preserved squash-playing body, extracting nutrients, supplementing, deliv-
ering, playing with the building blocks, copying, manipulating, reprogramming, replacing blood, destroying harmful bacteria and viruses, monitoring and identifying
pathogens, reversing soft-tissue destruction, preventing bacterial infection, repairing
DNA. . . . "How soon?" Barry asked, visibly excited by *my* excitement. "When will all
this be possible?" "We're almost there," I said. (Shteyngart 123–4)

It is not the mind-blowing biotechnological practices that affect the client's reaction.
Rather, Lenny's hope and belief in the practices and his excitement establish the secu-

---

35   While the hope and belief invested in the security practice of indefinite life extension define its
symbolic capital, it likewise defines its monetary worth. The services sold by Post-Human Services
are in this context venture capital, and an investment in a future in its literal as well as metaphoric
sense.

rity of eternal life as tangible, as "almost here." Shteyngart emphasizes the importance of narrative construction to create a pervasive fiction of security which relies on affective attachments rather than scientific facts. Lenny does not explain scientific procedures but rather "paints a picture." He creates an image of his vision, embodying an artist rather than a salesman of clinical procedures. Lenny's vision of security represents the creation of a science fiction.

The connection between the vision of biotechnologically facilitated security and science fiction is further increased by Shteyngart's description of the posters that adorn Joshie's living room.

> Posters from his youth – science-fiction films . . . – framed conservatively in oak, as if to say they had withstood the test of time and emerged, if not masterpieces, then at least potent artifacts. The name alone. Soylent Green. Logan's Run. Here were Joshie's beginnings. A dystopian upper-class childhood in several elite American suburbs. Total immersion in *Isaac Asimov's Science Fiction Magazine*. The twelve-year-old's first cognition of mortality, for the true subject of science fiction is death, not life. (Shteyngart 217)

With this description of Joshie's home Shteyngart exposes the origin of his vision of dechronification both intra- and extradigetically. The home represents a shrine to 1970s and 1980s sci-fi revealing an origin story of Post-Human Services that clearly underlines the fiction of security. The description thus emphasizes the often-cited connection of biotechnological developments and science fiction. But it also points to science fiction as one of the most important objects circulating different versions of (failed) biosecurity narratives. Since a majority of biotech sci-fi represents dystopian vision, Shteyngart foreshadows with these intertextual references the failure and deconstruction of the security promised by indefinite life extension.

The fiction of security in Shteyngart's novel thus does not only refer to the necessity of creating a pervasive narrative but also to the failure of the promise. The biosecurity promise of Post-Human Services as a successful and promising experiment of radical self-empowerment over the given corporeality represents a thinly veiled fiction. Already early in the novel, descriptions of Joshie's body reveal little glimpses of his age: "Joshie turned away from me. From this angle, I could see another side of him, the slight gray stubble protruding from his perfect egg of a chin – the slight intimations that not *all* of him could be reverse-engineered into immortality. Yet" (Shteyngart 66). In the beginning of the novel, these little glitches are explained by technology not being there yet. However, in post-rupture New York, Lenny informs the reader in a post-scriptum epilogue to the publication of his diary and Eunice Parks GlobalTeens Messages that the treatments turn out to be dangerous and in the end deadly. Lenny reports from an event where a visibly deteriorating Joshie announces the failure of the project: "Onstage, my ersatz papa's face, initially contorted into a serious academic expression, quickly fell apart, and he began to twitch from the recently discovered Kapasian Tremors associated with the reversal of dechronification" (Shteyngart 328). Since Joshie embodies the practice, he also embodies its failure: "Drooling magnificently over his interpreter, he told us, without preamble or apology: 'We were wrong. The antioxidants were a dead end. There was no way to innovate technology in time to prevent complications arising from the application of the old'" (Shteyngart 328). Though the security practices of dechronification failed it is not represented as a failed goal but simply as a failed attempt, the wrong method. The attempt to replace nature, or correct it simply did not work. But instead of a moral of having misunderstood what humanity means and being unable "to enjoy the perfect future in the present," as Hawthorne's narrator puts it, Lenny describes the remorphing of the institution of biosecurity and its practices into something new. "Howard Shu took over Post-Human Services and made of it what he'd always imagined, an enormous lifestyle boutique doling out spa appointments and lip-enhancement surgery" (Shteyngart 329). The failure of the practice does not really represent an end, but a deferral and a new beginning.

Science and Religion

Security is not only depicted as an "affective fact" (Massumi, "Future Birth") produced by a fiction of biosecurity, which ultimately falls apart. Shteyngart represents the hope and belief placed in the security promised by indefinite life extension as a form of religious following of Post-Human Services. As in Hawthorne, the description of the space of security is enticing. With the spatial construction Shteyngart renders the scientific promise of security and self-empowerment as an analogy to religion. The headquarters of Post-Human Services is called the "Life Lover's Outreach division" (Shteyngart 124). It is a public space that has little in common with Aylmer's secluded apartment, and much less with the dungeons of Dr. Frankenstein. Rather, it represents a sanctuary and a place of worship where Life Lovers come to perform the medical rituals obligatory to become immortal.

The analogy with religion is not subtle in Shteyngart's text but constitutes a literal replacing of the old space of security. Echoing the colonial practice of occupying formerly sacred spaces, the headquarter occupies an old and abandoned temple.[36] "The Post-Human Service division of the Staatling-Wapachung Corporation is housed in a former Moorish-style synagogue near Fifth Avenue" (Shteyngart 56). The spatial description is thus reminiscent of a spiritual conquest of another civilization or culture, in this case the religious framework is replaced by the culture of biosecurity.

The company appropriates the space filling it with their own practices of worship as well as the odor of their own security practices.

> The first thing I noticed upon my return was the familiar smell. Heavy use of a special hypoallergenic organic air freshener is encouraged at Post-Human Services, because the scent of immortality is complex. The supplements, the diet, the constant shedding of blood and skin for various physical tests, the fear of the metallic components found in most deodorants, create a curious array of post-mortal odors, of which 'sardine breath' is the most benign. (Shteyngart 57)

---

36   As one example of many, Mexico City was constructed on top of the Aztec temples of Tenochtitlan.

Though familiar, the "smell" of security practices is in fact a stench. Heavy air freshener is used to conceal this uncomfortable side-effect in the otherwise clean and designed space: "Everything bathed in soft colors and the healthy glow of natural wood, office equipment covered in Chernobyl-style sarcophagi when not in use, alpha-wave simulators hidden behind Japanese screens, stroking our overactive brains with calming rays" (Shteyngart 60). As in Hawthorne's story, the scientific space is concealing its true, threatening character. The space of security is altered by smells and design to support the fiction of effortlessness by "hiding" the traces of its practices.

The belief in eternal life by biotechnological means displaces the Jewish tradition that Lenny continuously describes disparagingly as misguided faith. It takes over its space and makes use of the symbolic and spiritual places once assigned to holy objects. "The ark where the Torahs are customarily stashed had been taken out, and in its place hung five gigantic Solari schedule boards" (Shteyngart 58) on which the ranking of the employees is made public. By placing the scoring board of the employees in the position of the holy scripture Shteyngart makes the practice of quantifying the self and statistical risk assessment take the place of the word of God. The practices of assessing individual security statuses is thus likened to a religious practice. Central for the characters to improve their ratings is visiting the Eternity Lounge. This lounge, where the employees practice age prevention techniques as central security practices represents a displacement of a central space within the old synagogue.

> The Eternity Lounge was crammed full of smelly young people checking their äppäräti or leaning back on couches with their faces up to the ceiling, de-stressing, breathing right. The even, nutty aroma of brewing tea snuck a morsel of nostalgia into my general climate of fear. I was there when we first put in the Eternity Lounge, five years ago, in what used to be the synagogue's banqueting hall. (Shteyngart 61)

The spatial continuity of old and new security practices marks the employees more clearly as a community based on faith. It represents a group united by a common belief as well as common practices. Security is thus not only produced by the individual security practices such as "breathing right" but by belonging to the "we" that is produced by the collective practice. And this we represents an exclusive elite whose "lives are worth more than the lives of others" (Shteyngart 165).

Initially, Lenny insists on the difference to the old overcome religious practices: "The truth is, we may think of ourselves as the future, but we are not. We are servants and apprentices, not immortal clients. We hoard our Yuan, we take our nutritionals, we prick ourselves and bleed and measure that dark-purple liquid a thousand different ways, we do everything but pray" (Shteyngart 60). Only at the end does the protagonist himself recognize, or rather acknowledge the spatial continuity. "I stood before one of the stained-glass windows depicting the tribe of Judah, represented here by a lion and crown, and for the first time considered the fact that to several thousand people this had once been a temple" (Shteyngart 255).

Not surprisingly then, Lennie describes Joshie as a form of guru: "And there he was. Younger than before. The initial dechronification treatments – the beta treatments, as we called them – already coursing through him. His face unlined and harmoniously still, . .

. Joshi Goldman never revealed his age" (Shteyngart 63). To Lennie, Joshie appears in this first description of his "ersatz Papa" as a revelation, a spiritual leader. His age reversed and on his way to eternal life Joshie's youthful looks show the material reality of indefinite life extension for the first time to the reader. He lacks any outward signs of ageing and wrinkles that would expose his chronological age and therefore personifies security. But Joshie is not only described as a spiritual leader by Lenny in terms of a connection to and teacher of a higher power. "Joshie's office was on the top floor, the words 'You Shall Have No Other Gods Before Me' still stenciled into the window in English and Hebrew" (Shteyngart 64). Joshie is depicted as a God-figure who is the ultimate judge deciding who is granted access to security and who is not.

However, rather than Joshie, Lenny describes himself and his work analogous to being God "the creator." "I picked out the profiles that appealed the most to me, . . .: I scanned the good cholesterol and the bad, the estrogen buildups and the financial crack-ups," when he is overcome by "an intense desire to set it right" (Shteyngart 123). While Joshie is only represented in his self-centered practice of rejuvenating himself Lenny most closely resembles the urge of his scientific forbears. He wants to correct the mistake nature had build into the human design to improve and help others, if not the worthy part of humanity at large. In Shteyngart's novel the flaw that has to be obliterated is the biological make-up of the human body. And Lenny understands his work to eradicate this flaw and lift the human to a higher level of security as sacred: "Affecting a god-like air – my Eunice-kissed proboscis pointed toward the ceiling, both hands caressing the data in front of me, as if ready to make man out of clay – I scanned the files of our prospective Life Lovers" (Shteyngart 123). Data is represented as the essence and the material a human is made of, and Lenny feels a hubris similar to Aylmer's creationist quest. Like Aylmer's, Lenny's faith in the utopian promise is so strong that he cannot confront the failure leading to a denial of its reality: "Eunice left Joshie even before the decline began. I know little about the young man she left him for . . . After Joshie has finished his warbling, I ran out of the auditorium. I didn't want to ask him what it was like to know that he was about to die. Even at this late date, even after he had betrayed me, the foundation myth between us precluded that question" (Shteyngart 329).

Biosecurity for Sale

As the founder and head of Post-Human Services Joshie represents the part usually associated with the scientist genius – such as Aylmer. However, Joshie is not a scientist, neither is Lenny. They are "'[m]ore like a salesman,'" (Shteyngart 17) as the sculptor in Italy puts it when Lenny boasts to Eunice about his profession in "nanotechnology and stuff'" (ibid.). The biosecurity practice is therefore not only part of a capitalist system and a commodity for sale but is represented by the business delegates rather than the scientists themselves. Not surprisingly then, the headquarters visited by clients is situated in the center of the city, while the scientific practice and research is spatially outsourced to " the ten-story slab of concrete that once served as an adjunct to a large hospital" (Shteyngart 124–5) in a wasteland.[37]

As previously noted, the "frontiers of science and technology" (Shteyngart 22) are an elitist practice only affordable for the wealthy. Lenny's utopia is not based on high principles of equality but is utterly exclusive. It represents a utopian promise for the few that have the "privilege of futurity" (Nye 112). To be eligible "[m]oney equals life. By my estimation, even the preliminary beta dechronification treatments, for example, the insertion of Smart-Blood to regulate my ridiculous cardiovascular system, would run three million Yuan per year" (Shteyngart 77). All the self-improvement and regimen of self-care is thus useless if one does not have the matching wealth to afford the final steps. Or as Vishnu puts it "'Fuck that Immortality bullshit. Ain't going to happen for us anyway. Look at us. We're not HNWIs.' ...We're poster children from Harm Reduction" (95). For the seeker of eternal life such as Lenny, health and wealth are mutually important: "I owed Howard Shu 239,000 yuan-pegged dollars. My first stab at dechronification – gone. My hair would continue to grey, and then one day . . . I would disappear from the earth" (Shteyngart 70). Lenny's pondering makes clear that capital is the first prerequisite to be able to access biological security followed by biological capital. Concerning the cruelty of financial inaccessibility of the treatments to most, Joshie replies: "'Those who want to live forever will find a means of doing so,' Joshie said, a cornerstone of the Post-Human philosophy" (Shteyngart 126). The cornerstone of the "philosophy" thus represents the fervent belief in the U.S. American foundational myth of self-reliance, as well as the neoliberal ideology of self-regulation.

The commodified nature of the security practice is further emphasized when on their way to the subway Lenny discovers a new billboard by the "Staatling-Wapachung Corporation" (Shteyngart 152) for "AN EXCLUSIVE TRIPLEX COMMUNITY FOR NON-U.S. **NATIONALS.**" The offer includes "EXCLUSIVE Immortality Assistance from our Post-Human Service Division" (Shteyngart 152). Lenny is outraged about this offer:

> "EXCLUSIVE Immortality Assistance"? Beg pardon? You had to *prove* you were worthy of cheating death at Post-Human Services. Like I said, only 18 percent of our applicants qualified for our Product. That's how Joshie intended it. . .. Now they were going to bestow immortality on a bunch of fat, glossy Dubai billionaires who bought a Staatling Property "TRIPLEX Living Unit"? (Shteyngart 153)

Eternal Life is here most clearly marked as a commodity, a simple good or service which represents the deflation of the dream and image Post-Human Services and Lenny had propagated. Lenny's representation of the exclusiveness and elite position of the practice that is based on strict rules and tests is contrasted with this adherence to capitalist flows.

---

37   The inner workings of biosecurity are racist and entrenched in neo-colonial practice: "It was time for him to meet our Indians. We have this Cowboy and Indians theme going on at Post-Human Services. At the Life Lovers Outreach division, we call ourselves Cowboys; the 'Indians' are the actual research staff, mostly on loan from the Subcontinent and East Asia, housed at an eighty-thousand-square-foot facility on York and at three satellite locations in Austin Texas; Concord, Massachusetts; and Portland, Oregon." (Shteyngart 124–5)

Furthermore, only the connection of Post-Human Services to capitalism makes it a source of security. Rather than the provided services their belonging to a powerful cooperation provides Joshie with the position of security during the destruction of the United States. In this context eternal life is simply one branch of a big corporation in the business of security.[38] Lenny stresses the connections to security when he describes his employment to the Parks: "'I work for a division of Staatling-Wapachung,' I said.... Property and security and life extension I guess are the three things that we do. All very important in a time of crisis'" (Shteyngart 194). Biotechnology and the hope of controlling the body are part of a diversified investment strategy of a big company which also represents the privatized military force. This merging of biotechnology and security services in one company embodies the ideological fusion of individual and national biosecurity.[39] The corporative link becomes increasingly important as the country around the protagonists slips into crisis. After the first revolts Lenny's äppärät is upgraded to see who of the guards on the streets belongs to Wapachung Contingency. Lenny's employment at Post-Human Services and proximity to Joshie enables him to move relatively unrestricted through the various check points established by the security forces. While the United States is descending into armed conflict the Staatling-Wapachung Corporation, the company that owns Post-Human Services takes over control.

The reliance on and intimate connection to capitalist circulation is established in comments by Joshie throughout the novel. When Lenny initially points out to Joshie that the political and economic situation of the nation is dire Joshie responds: "This is all going to be great for Post-Human Services! Fear of the Dark Ages, that *totally* raises our profile. Maybe the Chinese or the Singaporeans will buy us outright" (Shteyngart 66). Following the first riots in Central Park, which introduce the rupture, Joshie gives a motivational speech to the employees that ends in, "'I say to all the naysayers: The best is yet to come.' / 'Because we are the last, best hope for this nation's future.'/ '[sic]We are the creative economy.'/ '[sic] And we will prevail!'" (Shteyngart 181). Joshie repeatedly stresses in his messages to shareholders and executives that "[t]he expected collapse of the Rubenstein/ ARA/Bipartisan regime presents us with great possibilities" (Shteyngart 240). The violent collapse of the nation and the casualties this produces are reflected by Joshie merely in terms of another business opportunity. Rather than a risk, the insecurity of the rupture is seen as a potential, a possibility that can and should be used. It is not "no more America" as Lenny asks timidly. "'Fuck that. A *better* America'" Joshie replied (Shteyngart 257). But he does not just refer to the potential of new investors. Rather, the insecurity produced by the rupture increased the symbolic capital of Post-Human Services. "The Rupture created a whole new demand for not dying" (ibid.).

While the story of indefinite life extension ends in an apocalyptic event it is not marked by an end. When Lenny goes to an exhibition post rupture he encounters the

---

38   Johannes Völz and Russell A. Berrmann point out that "Liberalism, many critics across the humanities and social sciences now insist, is a type of political rule that employs the logic of security" (4).

39   Donna Haraway's "Cyborg Manifesto" warns against this connection of technology and the military sector. However, the warning is rather against the abuse of power granted by the biotechnological developments (303, 306).

same group of people who were clients at Post-Human Services: "The Staatling-Wa-pachung bigwigs were dressed like young kids, a lot of vintage Zoo York Basic Cracker hoodies from the 2000s, and tons of dechronification, making me think they were actually their own children, but my äppärät informed me that most of them were in their fifties, sixties, or seventies" (Shteyngart 319). Instead of an end, Shteyngart describes a continuation. Äppäräti, data streams, and the practices that determined pre-rupture society continue in the same way as Post-Human Services continues. Though an apoca-lyptic event, the rupture is not an attempt to narrate an ending but rather represents the dystopian and apocalyptic idea in the continuation and iteration of "the same," which marks post rupture America: "Welcome to America 2.0: A GLOBAL Partnership/ THIS Is New York: Lifestyle Hub, trophy City" (Shteyngart 322). New Credit Poles screen "Life Is Richer, Life Is Brighter! Thank You, International Monetary Fund!" (Shteyngart 305) because in post-rupture New York City "'Nothing's changed but the uniforms'" (Shteyn-gart 285). The rupture does not register as the "apocalyptic end" of a nation. Security is simply re-established when connectivity is regained: "at 5:54 p.m. EST, the precise time Telenor, the Norwegian telecommunications giant, restored our communications and our äppäräti started whirring with data, prices, Images, and calumny; 5:54 p.m. EST, a time no one of my generation will ever forget" (Shteyngart 283).

The only security that can console Lenny in this limbo of continuation is the recog-nition and acceptance of his own mortality. The beginning of the last letter mirrors the incipit of the novel: "Today I've made a major decision: *I am going to die*" (Shteyngart 304). These are the same sentences reversed in their meaning. In contrast to the continuation that marks the dystopian narrative of a biosecurity future, *an* end becomes the only hope. Shteyngart thus renders the failure of the commodified practices of biosecurity as an in-dividual recognition that allows the main protagonist to withdraw from the seemingly inescapable consumer's urge to attain biosecurity.

Past – Present – Future

Hawthorne's "The Birth-Mark" and Shteyngart's *Super Sad True Love Story* both represent the utopian promise of ultimate control that is supposed to elevate the human to some-thing more than human – divine or eternal. And both caution against the quest to en-hance or perfect the human body as an ultimately dangerous life-threatening practice. The biosecurity practices in both stories reveal themselves as errant quests, as failures of utopian promises. And both texts formulate the fearful visions that have been attached to science, most recently by scholars of risk. "[C]ertain knowledge and rational control over nature have given way to a permanent sense of anxiety" (S. Hamilton 267), which is tested in the fictional worlds created by Hawthorne and Shteyngart. In a way, both stories represent expressions of emergent risk produced by the (unexpected) side effects of technological and scientific progress, though in both cases the ensuing risk is rather direct and not affecting third parties or places.

Hawthorne devises a clear warning against tinkering with human nature (regardless if understood as nature or as God-given). Shteyngart rather indicates that the pursuit of eternal life – through biotechnological enhancement – is but one more practice, one more consumable good that promises security. Rather than leading to security, however, both practices move the protagonists further away from the "good life" they had hoped for. Georgiana and Joshie die and Lenny is not going to become immortal. The promised security remains out of reach for the protagonists and is as such absent from the narrative. It is represented by the security practices and their promise of security. The practices as stand-ins for security, however, never represent security as such, as Joshie's and Georgiana's fates make clear. Rather, their meaning is fixed by the affective attachments invested in them.

I began this chapter with the question of how the security practices – despite their uncertainty – are made desirable and how they are produced as legitimate and convincing ideas. The literary examples of biosecurity narratives emphasize the centrality of affective attachments that lead to the "solidification" of the understanding of security and its desirability. The position of hope and fear is thus where "the object hovers in its potentialities" (Berlant, "Cruel" 93). In both stories fear of being disgusting and unworthy – because of the mark of the hand or the mark of the body and the data stream – drive the urge and desire for the security practices. The hope attached to eradicating those marks determines the legitimacy and unquestionability of the security practices. Security never just is, but is represented by hope and fear that define the felt proximity, the potentiality, but not the "thing" itself. In both stories affective attachments determine the meaning of the security practice, which turns them into objects of "cruel optimism:" "the condition of maintaining an attachment to a problematic object *in advance* of its loss" (Berlant 94). The practices themselves come to stand in for the promise they reference turning into place holders of the promise of "good life" itself. Berlant describes this "mode" of hovering in a potential with Barbara Johnson's concept of the apostrophe, in which the object/subject is created as a present reality in its absence. Johnson is referring to the representation of an absent lover in a poem, or the representation of a fetus through an ultrasound scan. In the stories the "apostrophe" are the affects attached to the practice of security, which represent security as a present reality.

The focus on threat and hope helps to "track the affective attachments" (Berlant, "Cruel" 97) that define what "good life" is. The fear of not achieving security in purity or eternal life is not really the fear of not being pure or not living eternally but of being barred from the promise of happiness. In both cases the affective attachments reveal a rather normative understanding of security and happiness. For Georgiana it is domestic happiness within the limits of her assigned gender role and division of labor as adored and desired wife. And also Lenny mainly longs for the normative happiness, which is however primarily motivated by fear and meaninglessness.

Security is therefore rather a belief than an actual reality or fixed state. Both stories "dramatize its [the biosecurity practice's] persuasive faith" (41) to borrow Heilman's words one more time. By likening the security practices to religious belief and practice Hawthorne and Shteyngart relate it to a form of dogma that does not allow for an alternative understanding. Taking over the place of religious doctrine both authors underline the nearly blind following of the security individuals. The security practices' basis is faith which hide their risk – the impossibility of achieving security – behind belief and hope. This belief also hides security's complicity in the structures that form what "is for so many a bad life that wears out the subjects who nonetheless, and at the same time, find their conditions of possibility within it" (Berlant, "Cruel" 97). In both cases the security practices promise the protagonist the opportunity to escape their "bad situation" but in both texts the practices and fictions of security hide the real cause of the "bad life:" in Georgiana's case an abusive heterosexist relationship and in Lenny's case, a superficial hyper capitalist society.

Furthermore, both stories emphasize the narrative construction that the security practices are based on. This means that the practices are as much scientific as they are cultural practices of storytelling. They are understood and framed within a cultural narrative that renders their meaning and are embedded in the cultural narrative of their worlds. Georgiana is the meek and mum loyal wife in a misogynist oppressive world in which she can represent the object of experiments dressed up and understood by herself as "pure love." And the constant anxiety of Lenny about being able to receive dechronification treatment only makes sense in the highly stratified world of financial and biological security where youth and health are capital – biological capital. This narrative constructedness is further emphasized by both authors with their explicit references to the role of storytelling and fiction. In Hawthorne's story, Aylmer's narrative power establishes the mark as threat and the scientific promise of providing security is continuously likened to fictional storytelling. Similarly, Lenny as the main narrator constructs the narrative of security which represents immortality as security. The promised security of purity and eternal life are both narratively constructed within the story. They represent fictions of the production of the fiction of security.

What distinctively separates these fictions is their temporality. Hawthorne's story is set in the past, it is a warning of a past failure to affect thoughts and understanding in the present. Shteyngart, however, makes, as Frederic Jameson puts it, the present a determined past. Following Georg Lukács, Jameson proposes in "Progress and Utopia" to understand "genre as a symptom and reflection of historical change" (149). "[T]he emergence of the new genre of SF as a form which now registers some nascent sense of the future, and does so in the space on which a sense of the past had once been inscribed" (150). In both stories the critique of the texts is directed at the present. However, the temporal relation indicates a different understanding of the present that is comparable to the logic of pre-emptive security. The protagonists in *Super Sad True Love Story* are not so much understood as products of their past but are defined by their potential future. This kind of speculative fiction therefore not only circulates fear of science and skepticism toward their messianic biosecurity promise, as I set out in the introduction, but normalizes an understanding of present and future that is fundamental in the understanding of the contemporary biosecurity self. This is an identity that is continuously becoming, continuously under threat like Lenny's, rather than the fixed characterization of Georgiana's identity.

The different structures that the two texts describe also formulate different versions of power and control and different technologies of security. Georgiana represents a "controlled" subject created by the authoritative voice of Aylmer the scientist. He defines her and locks her in her position, quite literally within the space of the boudoir. It represents a power structure where the source of power, those intangible entities floating in most theoretical texts, is fixed and identified. It is the individual scientist and his megalomania that oppresses, transgresses, and exhorts his power. In contrast, Shteyngart describes a broader collective structure. The premises and practices pervade the entire society of the novel. However, collectivization takes a particular form that transcends the imagination of top-down control. The security practices are not imposed by a defined power controlled and surveilled as in Foucault's panopticon. Rather, as Willmett points out, it is individuated. Aylmer and the oppressive state of dystopian novels such as 1984 are replaced here by the seemingly democratic use of data analysis and ranking. This "democratized" or fragmented form of power equally determines, inscribes, and ultimately oppresses. However, its source remains intangible and invisible. As a commodified good, the practices contain the promise of transcending one's "assigned" category. This false sense of possibility that self-quantification simulates represent the same top-down power-relation and fixes individuals in a determined group of belonging. Aylmer's disgust caused by Georgiana's mark is replaced by algorithms, which are based on knowledge produced by science. Though the hope of transcending one's group is built into the narrative of biosecurity in Shteyngart's near future, this hope is a device for fixing identities rather than a real possibility of change.

Furthermore, in Shteyngart's vision the biosecurity practices have moved from the margin to the center symbolized by the space of the security practices. Dystopian biofiction often represents the threat, the beginning of dystopia as a transgression of the boundary due to the scientist's inexhaustible thirst of knowledge. Aylmer's research practice is confined to secrecy and isolation set apart from society. It forms a space of transgression that is mirrored within his laboratory. In contrast to this, Post-Human Services are a public company that is situated prominently and powerfully in the middle of society. While the spatial division of laboratory and boudoir allowed for a transgression of the boundary, Shteyngart does not allow for such a shift. Science is reduced to "the occasional glass cage with mice or some kind of spinning thingamabob" (Shteyngart 124–25) and Lenny's fantastic explanations. The revelation of the "true" working of science is unnecessary as Shteyngart does not formulate a generalized fear of scientific developments. The fear of science has become a fear of commercialized science and corporate interests.[40] This fear of commodified biosecurity, which exacerbates health risks for low-paid individuals, indicates that money and markets instead of higher ideals and ethics create the security narratives represented in the novel. Read together with the temporal logic of Science Fiction that Jameson offers, this constellation describes the biosecurity logic as a logic of the market. The present worth of the individual is based on his or her future potential worth which is predicted by data algorithms. The biosecurity individual of the future can only overcome the biotechnological determination of his identity by accepting death, as Lenny decides that he wants to die after all, abandoning his quest for immortality.

---

40   A historical observation of the narrative construction of science, scientists, and scientific advances is tale-telling in that regard. Frankenstein was created in a secret dungeon, apart from society and literally under ground, and Dr. Moreau is hidden on a pacific island (a place probably as far removed from society as Wells could imagine in the late 19th century). In contrast, contemporary scientists and scientific experiments are "whitewashed" clean laboratories if narrated in James D. Watson's life writing text The Double Helix on the discovery of the structure of the DNA to dystopian narratives of Jurassic Park, Terminator, the Island, etc. (van Dijck, Imagenation 18).

"Know Thyself": Self-Surveillance and Securing the Self in an Age of Digital Biocapitalism

> Es gibt kein richtiges Leben im falschen.
> *Theodor W. Adorno*

The philosophical idea to "know thyself," or γνῶϑι σεαυτόν as the inscription in the ancient Greek Temple of Apollo at Delphi reads, has been central to the idea of what constitutes a "good life." It has inspired thinkers across the centuries, each articulating their own interpretation of this iconic phrase.[1] This maxim has come a long way from ancient Greek philosophy to our current biosecurity culture. Today, knowledge of self does not refer only to a romantic vision of introspection as search for truth, nor does it express the mandate to know one's place, as Aeschylus understood it in *Prometheus Bound*.[2] It more exclusively conveys the desire to improve oneself by self-knowledge gained through self-observation, which also Benjamin Franklin made a principal task to reach the 13 virtues necessary for the "bold and arduous project of arriving at moral perfection" (*Autobiography* 39) and becoming a self-made man. In our own age this self-knowledge includes knowing one's biological body and its potentials. The preceding chapters have shown how much the understanding of self and good life relies on the messianic narrative of medical and scientific salvation whose importance grew in step with the increasing medicalization and biomedicalization of health and life itself during the 19th and 20th century. The biologically inflected knowledge of the self, including the biological make-up of one's body, is crucial for the biosecurity individual and their understanding of self. What ought to be known today is therefore one's future biological security as a necessary precondition to leading a "good life" in the precarious normality dominated by pre-emptive security logics.

---

1 The inscription is the first of the three Delphic maxims in the entrance of the Oracle. Know thyself is the most famous and expresses most prominently the Socratic principle that knowledge must be sought within. In Ralph Waldo Emerson's eponymous poem which expresses his vision of the transcendental self this knowledge is described as the God that is to be found within each person themselves.

2 It expresses the balance between improving oneself and not trespassing set boundaries, which today bioethics committees are concerned with.

The previous chapters have shown that biological security has indeed become a leading paradigm in U.S. American culture, structuring society and decisively influencing individual as well as collective identity formation. Especially Alice Wexler's memoir and the previvor testimonies exemplified how central preventive and pre-emptive security logics, that are usually associated with national security, have become for the understanding of biological security also in non-contagious disease contexts. They showed that health has not been simply redefined in the process of biomedicalization and its shift of focus toward risks, but that this turn has made security concerns rather than health the leading paradigm of understanding the body, life, and identity. The risk of having Huntington's disease or developing breast cancer represent in that context a cessation that marks and redefines life and identity in the same way as actual disease onset. The risk prompted the individuals to reevaluate and retell their life narratives and to establish security narratives to make the ambiguous experiential situation tangible and to fully understand it.

The importance of biomedical risk assessments for the individual indicated how deeply the normative power of experts reaches into people's private lives. The case studies have disclosed how the understanding of security, majorly influenced by the promises of techno-scientific developments, changes our understanding of life, body and self. And the preventive and pre-emptive security logics influence the way the body is understood and encountered, producing new relations between the individual and their body. The possibilities for intervening in the body, from superficial treatments to changes in its make-up have contributed to the rise of a powerful security narrative of radical self-empowerment, which makes health, life and the body appear not as a fateful given fact but as controllable processes. Bodily security becomes in this complex a potential that needs to be managed and pursued actively. Accordingly, the biosecurity individuals produced by biotechnological possibilities and the security logics of pre-emption were represented as self-reliant subjects that fulfilled their responsibility by exercising their citizen rights and duties by choosing the proper way to biological security. This connection of biological security and citizen rights also played an important role at the end of life when the original security promise of survival and cure had failed as exemplified by the representation of physician assisted dying. Rather than a responsibility that individuals are obliged to assume, biosecurity is framed as a "right to choose," a personal freedom the government ought to protect but not intervene in. Individual biosecurity, thus, represents "freedom and liberty" in the analyzed texts and a civil right that is essential for the ability to lead a good life and partake in the promise of the American Dream. This connection was also critically reflected in Shteyngart's dystopian tale, in which biosecurity was a precondition to any form of upward mobility and happiness.

But the new relations forged by the prevalence of biosecurity, especially in its pre-emptive logic, cannot and should not be reduced to the responsibilization of the individual but extend to the intimate ways of knowing one's body and its security status. Especially the logic of pre-emption produces a perpetual state of insecurity as the breeding ground for potential threat. Security practices have therefore proven to be essential for the individual to experience at least a sense of security. And this sense of security is in all four analyses clearly situated beyond the individual experience and outside of the individual body. The understanding of individual risk relies not only on expert reading but on reiterative security practices that fix security temporarily for the present moment of the security performance of, for instance, testing. And the diagnosis, or established official biosecurity narrative is not based on the reading of the body and the feeling of the individual but on risk assessment, on statistics, and on their narrativization.

The different case studies have, however, also shown that this sense of security cannot be simply equated with an idea of perfect health but is a construct which is in need of narrative construction. More importantly than verifying the importance of biosecurity for the understanding of the individual and their position in the biosecurity hierarchy of the United States, all four analyses exemplify the importance of this narrative construction to make a particular understanding of security pervasive and appealing for people to act accordingly to them. All four chapters showed the normative power of the messianic narrative of medical salvation. But they also stressed the importance of individual narrative construction in negotiating the understanding of biological security and individualizing the understanding of biosecurity produced by risk assessment. The analyzed narratives revealed that the individual is held responsible for their biosecurity status as well as for "writing" their own biosecurity narratives negotiating and establishing individual choices of security. They proved not only to be fictions of biosecurity but necessary biosecurity fictions of self which were crucial to understand the "true" self both in corporeal as well as in terms of identity.

While Wexler's memoir exemplified the necessity of the individual to establish her own security narrative to understand her own position and identity, it also revealed how the narrative of security represents not a stable object but a desire, an imaginary that is marked by deferral, receding every time it seems graspable. The previvor testimonies further showed that this imaginary of security depends on performative structures and performances to create a sense of security and self. The security practices performatively make present both risk and security, and the positionality of the individual within this structure. But rather than acknowledging the uncertainty and ambiguity of risk and biological security, the pervasive security scripts in the context of hereditary breast and ovarian cancer omit the uncertainty, which is overwritten by the performance of biosecurity. The testimonies stage a stable image of security which hinges on the ability to perform normalcy and able-bodied femininity as a choice of the responsible self-reliant subject. This emphasis on the body surface and its performance of security is also central in physician-assisted dying. The dominant security narrative of medical salvation, which stresses survival, fails in this context. The documentary represents the negotiation and reconstruction of a new security narrative; one in which survival symbolizes threat while death is turned into the desired security. Besides the necessity of narrative to construct security, the narrative of dying well showed even more clearly the normative understanding of corporeality that underlies the understanding of security. This enforces the dominant biosecurity narrative rather than representing an escape from it: it reiterates total control, the able body, and the absence of suffering. It further revealed the importance of performative structures to establish these meanings, which are contingent on the gaze of the other emphasizing the relationality of security.

The focus on security and its need for narrative thus showed that security is indeed a term that literally slides and shifts. In all analyses, to differing degrees, security narratives represent first and foremost promises whose object – security – continuously recedes and is deferred. The appeal of the promise is not purely based on scientific facts but is based on affective attachment (hope, desire, fear, threat). Sociologists describe the relation of biomedicine and affects as an "economy of hope," which is most obvious in the context of diagnostics, drugs, and pharmaceuticals as exemplified in all cases studied. It is an economy that "sutures together hopeful beliefs that one can recover" (Rose and Novas, "Citizenship" 448). But affects are more fundamental for the security narratives than just representing the hope for survival. Rather, affects are crucial in the "surfacing of bodies" (Ahmed, "Affective" 117) heavily influencing the meaning "recognized" in the materiality of the body. In all analyzed security narratives affects were the most essential constituent in making (in)security felt and real often representing the only form of relating to the techno-scientifically produced futures. Affects make the future tangible *as if* it is present. Genetic disease or dispositions, but also the risk of dehumanizing suffering in dying, or ageing and not meeting standards of bodily perfection were established and made experientially present first and foremost affectively in the interplay of fear and hope. In a perpetual state of becoming the biosecurity individuals are represented as suspended in the ambiguity between feeling secure, healthy and hopeful and the fear, anxiety and shame associated with the non-normative bodily matter. This was crucial in all case studies but especially the literary texts revealed how central the affective attachments are to construct a meaningful narrative and establish the meaning of security and to maintain it. The different discursive formations discussed in the analyses have shown that this dynamic is not exclusive to fiction, nor to a specific perspective on biosecurity but is pertinent in any construction of security. The analyses thus emphasize that biosecurity relies on affective attachments and the creation of "affective fact" rather than objective factual diagnoses. Embedded in a messianic narrative of scientific and medical salvation which claims to "secure the human" they therefore represent narratives of belief and faith.

The biosecurity identities studied in the context of Huntington's disease, hereditary breast cancer risk, and dying as well as in the fictional world of Hawthorne and Shteyngart emphasize that technoscientific innovations aim to facilitate a life that individuals could otherwise not live or participate in. In all chapters the described interventions promised the security necessary to enjoy happiness, and in all instances it was referring to a happy family life where nothing is out of the norm(al). The belief in the promise of "total control" stands in stark contrast to the fearful warnings expressed by dystopian fiction. It also contrasts fields such as disability/CRIP studies (Shakespeare), scholars such as Jürgen Habermas (*Future*), or the parts of posthumanisms warning of a post-human age (Fukuyama, Burfoot). All of these scholars argue for the need to control biotechnological developments and its promise of all-encompassing control.

The knowledge-based identities produced by biosecurity narratives can be enabling, in the sense of Rabinow's biosocialities, such as groups that come together in self-help forums or activism that I have described for breast cancer, Huntington's disease, and physician-assisted dying. But they can also create further paradigms of difference and new forms of discrimination. The advances in genetic testing with its focus on susceptibilities and disease markers produce a group of disposable bodies, or "individuals at risk" that are, though symptom free, perceived as sick. Though this biomedicalized subjectivity (Clarke et. al., "Biomedicalization" 165) is framed as enabling, at the same time it is clearly producing a further category of potentially non-normativity, or "disposable populations" (Giroux 186). Rather then abolishing old categories of discrimination, new genetics, or new biology re-inscribes old binaries in the public understanding of body and self. Weinbaum points out how the "recreational genealogy, race-based medicine, and the new fertility medicine" are rooted in "geneticized ideas of race" (208).[3] Furthermore, biosecurity categories and the technology necessary to establish these categories – be it diagnostic tests or medical interventions – are not simply repeating a cultural and social bias inadvertently as a "mistake." They underlie capital structures, which are more interested in using established systems than criticizing and changing them – unless that would be more profitable.

Biosecurity practices, predominantly advanced by for-profit corporations, can therefore not only be understood as empowering but also as establishing more narrow norms of "human" and good life that individuals are responsible for conforming to. "Increasingly, the emphasis in healthcare is on individuals' 'right to know'" (Petersen, "Governmentality" 195) and the question of testing as raised in Wexler's autobiography and the rejection of the prerogative of testing is today called "ostrich effect" (Fortenbury n.p.) and perceived as an evasion and denial that stand in the way of pursuing security. The idea that biological security is and ought to be a choice and the moral responsibility of the individual, ignores the fact that many people do not have this opportunity, given their biological constitution, their socio-economic position, or their low bioliteracy. Though biosecurity is represented as an empowering choice, it also represents an imperative, which is established in relationality to others, as shown in the different contexts of the case studies: the mothers and ill predecessors, the observing family, the society at large.

The biosecurity practices and developments, though undoubtedly beneficial, threaten to leave no room for non-normative bodies. When the "superior" technomedical culture enhances the body to eradicate nature's mistake, it is instigating a narrower norm rather than broadening the understanding of what is human (Burfoot 69). Deaf culture and the resistance to cochlear implants, which are biotechnological devices that stimulate hearing, is a prime example of this process (Elliott 244). "Many see the widespread use of cochlear implants as a threat to their culture and their collective identity" (ibid. 245).[4] This conflict illustrates the understanding of disability as socially and culturally constructed as proposed in Disability Studies to oppose the purely biomedical model of disability (Linton, Waldschmidt, Davis "Disability," *Disability Studies*). Autism, or Autism Spectrum Disorder, is another example, where the pressure to normalize, and "act" as neurotypicals (Hacking 503), is perceived as an oppression. The claims that a "cure" for autism needs to be found is understood as a violent attack and misconception based on the "situated knowledge" (Haraway) of neurotypicals. To question these norms it is productive and crucial to recognize them as constructions that are established in narrative and performative acts. Because embedded in the sweeping

---

3   This "resurrection" of the biologized understanding of race is similarly discussed in Troy Duster's article "A Post-genomic Surprise" and has found expression in art such as in Paul Vanouse's "Relative Velocity Device" exhibited in the UW Henry Art Gallery.

4   For further discussion on language, implants, and the deaf community see Elaine Gale.

messianic narrative of scientific salvation these "side effects" seem to barely filter in, which is hardly surprising when considering the funding invested in these technologies. According to *statista* (Mikulic, "2022") Johnson & Johnson, as the leading biotech and pharmaceutical company of the U.S. "generated over 95 billion U.S. dollars" in 2022..[5] The aim of deconstructing the truth claim established in the biosecurity narratives is thus not simply to show that there is no stable truth, and that nothing and therefore anything can be constructed as security, but to facilitate the possibility and emphasize the responsibility to critically question what is represented as true and good. It aims to highlight the necessity to establish and decide for the "right," or good, as Adorno asserted in *Minima Moralia* quoted in the epigraph above.

This is especially pertinent as all these developments have undoubtedly benevolent and enabling aspects, however they never come for free, nor from a "interest free" philanthropic entity. Rather they are embedded in a neoliberal market economy that has been formative in the development of the field of biomedicine as Cooper among many others asserts (inter alia 19). Definitions, suggestions, and application of practices are corporatized and commodified. Research, products and services belong to a growing industry dominated by venture capital and multi-national corporations. In studies of biocapitalist structures various scholars have described the production of "biovalue" or "biocapital" (Waldby, Cooper, Sunder Rajan *Biocapital, Lively*). The health sector represents 13 percent of the annual U.S. Gross National Product (Clarke et al., "Biomedicalization" 163), Americans "spent more than $100 billion on drugs in 2000" (Clarke et al., "Biomedicalization" 167). For 2021 *statista* estimated that the spending on medicine in the U.S. "reached approximately 574 billion U.S. dollars" (Mikulic, "Medicine").

In a "stakeholder society" (Petersen, "Governmentality" 194) in which the patient is converted into an active consumer, not only health but the normal has become a choice that is understood in terms of security. Most biotechnological developments are supposed to facilitate a more intimate knowledge about oneself allowing for the proper choice of biosecurity practice. However, the biomedical and biotechnological developments that emphasize the "somatic individuality" (Rose and Novas, "Genetics" 487) distance the person from an autonomous "subjective" perception of the self. The felt reality of the individual relies on a network of linkage since this form of self-knowledge is highly mediated through visualization technologies, specialist readings, culture, and the televised mantra of direct to consumer marketing. All those agents that supposedly "help" to know the self are represented as natural fact rather than interpretations negotiated by multiple agents. But more importantly, they are supposed to "help" the individual to make the right choice. This choice, however, is not the choice Enlightenment thinkers had in mind but a consumer choice that disguises the imperative of biosecurity.[6]

Furthermore, health has been commodified to such an extent that diagnostic technology, or the "new medical gaze" of surveillance medicine becomes an integral part of everyday life. Examples of the recreational use of biomedical information are abundant and range from genetic testing and biohacking to biointelligent watches and walking

---

5   The NIH invests $37,3 billion annually in medical research (NIH "Budget") at least $6.5 billion of which go directly to biotech research (NIH "Estimates of Funding").

6   I am rephrasing Deborah Lupton's title *Imperative of Health*.

apps.[7] Today, the phrase "know thyself" is the slogan of the "Quantified Self" movement. Their philosophy proposes self-tracking – large parts of it health related – as a necessary and useful way of life.[8] This movement, among other developments, makes clear that biosecurity is fundamental in medical practice and a securitized form of health; but it also epitomizes how deeply the logics of biosecurity pervade everyday life. Pre-emptive logics of biosecurity have moved from the professionalized space of medicine to the private individual life without an explicit relation to medical practice.

Biosecurity logics not only pervade the public in form of medical practice, advertising, media reports, life writing and speculative fiction but enter it in a more intimate manner in everyday performances that are often not necessarily associated with biomedicine, biotechnology, and much less with biosecurity. The hype and widespread use of health-tracking shows that the economy of hope and fear surrounding biosecurity is so strong that its logics have become an integral part of society. Furthermore, the health-monitoring practices reveal that it is not really the possible interventions that represent the 'object' of hope but rather the knowledge of the body (and its promises for a potential future self).

The broad adoption of health surveillance in the private and most intimate spaces of people's lives shows that practices of biosecurity have turned into everyday practices. The digitalization that majorly influences also the process of biomedicalization, which Clarke et al. describe, has infiltrated life by being integrated in it. "In the current technoscientific revolution, 'big science' and 'big technology' can sit on your desk, reside in a pillbox, or inside your body. That is, the shift to biomedicalization is a shift from enhanced control over external nature (i.e., the world around us) to the harnessing and transformation of internal nature (i.e., biological processes of human and nonhuman life forms), often transforming 'life itself'" (Clarke et al., "Biomedicalization" 164). Health apps and health-trackers play a bigger role in most people's life than genetic tests and represent a more and more normal and normalized understanding of and access to the body. They extend the logic of diagnostics to the everyday and turn cultural and social practices into security practices. These practices show how the logic of biosecurity also pervades many parts of society and culture that are usually not regarded as medical. The biomedical self-surveillance is no longer restricted to a patient-doctor relationship, nor to a designated space but infiltrates all aspects and spaces of life.[9] And this form of health monitoring at every step also counts as what Rose has termed "biological identity practices" ("Politics" 18) or "digital bio-citizenship" (Rose and Novas, "Citizenship" 442).

The field of mobile Health (mHealth) is big and diverse. In its widest sense it describes the use of mobile and digital devices in healthcare. The term also includes devices and applications that have diagnostic functions and can be used as proper diagnostic tools – however, here I will focus on self-quantification in its "recreational" use. This form of health-tracking is not a minor practice of dispersed individuals but a proper movement,

---

7   For a discussion of biohacking see *Biohacking, Bodies, and Do it Yourself* by Mirjam Grewe-Salfeld.

8   Gary Wolf titled his first article in Wired "Know Thyself: Tracking Every Facet of Life, from Sleep to Mood to Pain, 24/7/365" (qtd. in Lupton "Your Data" 64).

9   Gísli Pálsson argues in "Decode Me!" that the boundary between "experts and lay persons has blurred and refashioned" (185) in reference to personal genomics such as 23andMe.

as I have noted before. What started as a practice of "computer nerds" has reached mainstream and websites such as MedHelp, which register "30,000 new tracking projects a month" according to Gary Wolf ("Data Driven"). Wolf is the creator of MedHelp and is often represented as the founder of the Quantified Self Movement, which has grown into a global phenomenon. In addition, the use of more casually oriented self-tracking makes health monitoring a mainstream practice. The practices are widely subsumed under the term "lifelogging" (Selke *Lifelogging*, Selke "Introduction")[10] and describe the collecting and analyzing of biometric data, so the monitoring of health and life practices. Though the use of self-surveillance can be all-encompassing, in most cases it is limited to selective practices focused on specific health conditions such as blood pressure or oxygen levels, monitoring sleep rhythm or body posture, or geared toward fitness and diet. The list of available products is long, from personal genomics in the form of take-home tests such as 23andMe to activity trackers such as step counter, pulse apps, sleep apps, UV sensor apps, blood sugar apps, diet and weight apps, mood apps. All these apps represent security practices that promise more control and ultimately more security. The difference between these and a normal scale or stopwatch and the like is that apps and trackers are always around and collect personal data at every step for ready comparison, rating, and sharing. The fitness app iBody, just one example of many data monitoring systems, combines the different readings of biometric data and offers fitness and health improvement suggestions. For pregnancy and early parenthood, apps promise security by managing biometric and behavioral data to assure that the unborn child progresses as prescribed by the statistics of biosecurity. And with the iStetoscopePro or BabyScope the parents can even monitor the baby's heartbeat at home, both a practice of security and a performance of personhood of a future biosecurity individual. This self-surveillance for the home turns security practices into normal everyday performances. And as Crawford already pointed out in relation to the movement of healthism, this ritualization of security practices also emphasizes the responsibility of the individual and "risks fostering the illusion that individual responsibility is sufficient" (Crawford 377).

This extension of biosecurity practice to the everyday can be understood as a further "colonization" of life by biomedical norms, as theories of medicalization would categorize it. However, most of the focus in research is, for obvious reasons, directed at the collection and use of personal data, as for instance Deborah Lupton's article "You are your Data" makes clear. The complex dangers of uncontrollable data mining by corporations, breaches of privacy, warnings of further stratification of society, to concerns about individuals controlled by algorithms are especially in the post-Snowden, post-Facebook Analytica times, most prevalent and obvious. The practices and devices are regularly discussed in volumes such as Stefan Selke's anthology *Lifelogging*, which is dedicated to the increasing growth, use and importance of self-surveillance. Similarly, in his 2014 monograph Selke warns that these practices enforce social pressure and lead to a loss of es-

---

10   Selke differentiates different types of lifelogging according to their aim: *"monitoring health"* (Selke, "Introduction" 5) are practices which "enable preventive lifestyle" (6). Further categories are human tracking, human Digital Memory, Digital Immortality (ibid.).

sential part of understanding human existence (23).[11] And also the project "Probing the Limits of the Quantified Self" at the University of Mannheim investigates the influences on identity and identity construction.

Another obvious point of concern is the embeddedness of the technologies in neoliberal market structures: These products are part of a big market with a stable growth, though Forbes still judged in 2014 that the "hype is a year ahead of the market," and therefore ahead of its promise. Mainstream health trackers are still mainly fitness-based. Nonetheless, already their promises harvested huge investments: "Fitbit raised $43 million in venture funding in August [2014]" (Guglielmo and Olson). Not surprisingly, the leading tech companies have included health-related tools and gadgets in their production portfolio, such as Apple's Healthkit or Google's research on smart contact lenses that can detect glucose levels. According to tech expert Stephen Oesterle, Google spends $8 billion a year on research and development (Farr n.p.). Facebook has also ventured into healthcare already since 2014 (Farr and Oreskovic).

Similar to biomedicine, the practices of self-surveillance and their development are deeply connected and intertwined with the neoliberal market economy. But they are an expression of "bioeconomics" (Rose, "Politics" 15) also in a different way. Sundar Rajan identifies biocapital as "new and particular forms of currency, such as biological material and information" (*Biocapital* 17) mainly focusing on patenting, genomics and the worth of organic material. He stresses, as noted at the beginning, that the symbolic capital of biotechnology is generated by the field's promise to save lives (*Biocapital* 19).[12] Furthermore, this process translates back into symbolic capital based on the promise of biosecurity which is extended to health-tracking as a recreational practice. Technical evangelists represent their technological developments as closely related to the messianic narrative of scientific and medical salvation and its promise of self empowerment and improvement. Selke points out that the leading technical evangelists Gordon Bell, Jim Gemmell, Gary Wolf, and Mark Zuckerberg all represent the belief and faith that digital health-tracking will help to improve the body (*Lifelogging* 33). Though the term technical evangelist has its roots in a more superficial indication of the person responsible for promoting technology, its resonance with religion underlines the structures of belief and hope – of faith – that dominate these promises.

The practices of self-surveillance, as their medical counterparts, show how the promise of healing and cure has been partially replaced by a logic of prevention and pre-emption in which information becomes the true currency necessary to improve one's own biovalue, as worker, as lover, as friend, as scholar, as parent, as a person. As in the field of biotechnology, the hopes and promises relate to both health improvement and financial growth. In fact, the promises of mHealth and specifically wearables are astonishingly wide-ranging, from improving health to reducing healthcare costs, fixing infrastructural problems of healthcare, empowering and emancipating the users, and facilitating a better and happier life. The promises and hopes attached to the use of

---

11   Likewise, Anita L. Allen's article "Dredging up the Past" formulates such privacy concerns and potential dangers of the practice in a legal context.

12   Sunder Rajan stresses Marx's emphasis on the "mystical" or "magical" the "[t]he 'theological' character of the commodity becomes a central symptom of its fetish" (*Biocapital* 18).

wearables and other practices of quantification show that it is not only the actual inter-ventions but the knowledge of the biological make-up that is seen as the requirement for the access to security, and therefore "good life."

Most discussions regarding biocapitalism focus on medical knowledge, applications, and possibilities, all of which are controlled and regulated by the FDA. The field of health-tracking, however, is not necessarily supervised by the FDA and most devices are not un-derstood as medical practice as such.[13] They therefore enter the market comparatively unmonitored and unregulated. Though the FDA theoretically would have oversight over many applications and devices it wants to direct its oversight to what it terms "mobile medical apps" ("Mobile" 4). They have put this in practice for now by categorizing apps as "low risk" and therefore not enforcing their requirements (FDA "Mobile"). Health apps and wearables are part of the fitness and health movements and are as such part of the wider trend of healthism that Robert Crawford describes as a movement based on "holis-tic health" and "self-care" already for the 70s and 80s (366). But even though the devices cannot be categorized as medical devices the trackers nonetheless normalize a medi-calized understanding of life. Though these technologies might hide their relation to diagnostic tools they are still based on the reading and analysis of biometric data and therefore rely on biomedical knowledge. Cortez et al. point out that mHealth based on medically developed algorithms is designed to produce a diagnosis and treatment op-tions (327). And though Nils Heyen rightfully argues that self-trackers should also be understood as "prosumers," so as people that do not simply consume knowledge, "but (also) produce their own knowledge" (285), first and foremost they reproduce and reit-erate biosecurity logics. Every use produces a "self diagnosis" and every "self-diagnosis" produces a potential patient and consumer. Furthermore, the majority of casual users, who are not part of the "professionalized" Quantified Selfers, "prefer a rather compre-hensible and tangible display" over "scientifically valid and precise data" (Meißner 236).

Wearables do not really sell the actual improvement of the body but "just" knowl-edge about the body. In prepared data graphs security becomes tangible and the body appears controllable. The self-produced knowledge of one's body represents a calculable, optimizable, and controllable life that is comparable to a business plan as Sunder Rajan has pointed out in the context of genetic tests (*Lively* 150). What is primarily marketed is hope and fear attached to the messianic promise of science echoed in the symbolic cap-ital of wearables. The devices are possessions that promise better and easier access to biological security. What is actually purchased, though, is information. The value of the practice is thus based on the promise that the information represents – the promise of a material change in reality. The devices are an expression of the mantra that one has to "know and manage" (Rose and Novas, "Citizenship" 441) one's biological identity. In their clear reliance on biomedical knowledge production, wearables thus reproduce medical knowledge and the logic of understanding the body and life.

Health-tracking, as sousveillance in general was conceived as a countermovement to surveillance. Stephen Mann, a long time self tracker, explains that it is the "logical demo-

---

13   "Mobile Medical Applications: Guidance for Industry and Food and Drug Administration Staff" is-sued February 2015 is preceded by a warning that the FDA is challenging the definition of "device" amended by "the 21st Century Cures Act."

cratic answer to external surveillance: they [the tracker] provide a means for sousveillance or watching from beneath" (qtd. in Ward 48). Lifelogging was conceived as an emancipation against nature as much as against the paternalistic model of medicine. But the knowledge generated by mHealth products is not a counter-knowledge to the dominant narrative but relies on it and therefore reiterates it. The widespread use of health-tracking therefore normalizes biosecurity logics as an additional part of the self, reinforcing biosecurity identities.

The circulation of these digitalized "technologies of the self" and the hope placed in them are not just produced by companies that sell wearables, but are also supported by political, academic, and public institutions (Cortez et al. 372). Many researchers place their hopes in wearables as a way to "reduce the cost . . . and capture more reliable, valid, and responsive ratio-scaled outcome measures" (Dobkin and Dorsch 788). Health monitoring practices thus promise better and more efficient research as well as functioning potentially as "lifestyle behavior change catalyst" (Doherty et al. 323). Furthermore, mHealth is heralded as having the potential to fix infrastructural problems of healthcare, and facilitate easier access to normal forms of healthcare. This belief is also shared by the WHO: "The use of mobile and wireless technologies to support the achievement of health objectives (mHealth) has the potential to transform the face of health service delivery across the globe" (WHO "mHealth"). And ultimately, mHealth promises to improve health. The messianic promise of biotechnological research thus also surrounds these apps and the field of digital health. These hopes set in mHealth products and health monitoring increase the circulation and lend authority to the practices.

Another major and not surprising player in the circulation of affects that reinforce the truth value or authority of the security narratives are insurance companies. They are for obvious reasons interested in the biometric data of their clients and therefore also in the further development of technologies. The knowledge of one's own body can now be turned into capital by the individual themselves. It is a trade: Fitbit advertised that using their product would allow customers to "earn up to $1,500 for Healthy Behavior with Fitbit's New Healthcare Integration" (staff, Fitbit et al. n.p.). The commodification of health has thus turned health practices into labor. Their support and user incentives through monetary rewards elevate the health tracker to official biosecurity practices.[14] Every step becomes a security practice. But Fitbit also targets employers and researchers with their promise. Fitbit sells software to companies for their employees with the promise of reducing healthcare costs for their employees (Guglielmo and Olson). An important part of Fitbit health solution (staff, Fitbit et al.) are "challenges" to "generate excitement and drive engagement with a variety of individual and team challenges" to keep employees healthy and efficient, complementing the financial incentive.

The effortless adoption of health-tracking as beneficial security practices might also be explained because the conclusions seem so instinctive, so natural. The person who constantly controls their heart rhythm can hardly be surprised by a heart attack. And if the individual is connected via the internet, as Gordon Bell and Jim Gemmell, the

---

14   In the state of West Virginia, the app "Go365," a wellness reward program, was supposed to be made a mandatory program for teachers in order to access health insurance. Strong resistance and a state-wide strike halted the program (Bidgood).

founders of MyLifeBit envision it, help can reach the individual sooner. "Depending on the severity or risk, they will e-mail us alerts to follow up with our doctors as soon as possible, or immediately connect us to our doctor's office, or even dial 911 and send for an ambulance" (Bell and Gemmell, *Total Recall* 104). However, the conclusion that an all-encompassing control of the body automatically leads to better health is questionable as Jennifer Ruth Fosket shows with the example of mammography prevention screenings. In contrast to all these promises of security and enhancements stand the categories which the FDA applies to the devices of self-tracking. Cortez et al. discuss that "Congress created three classes of devices on the basis of their risk" (374) rather than their benefits. The FDA uses these risk categories in their 2014 report (6). It reveals the emancipatory promise of bottom-up knowledge production as yet another fiction of security. The imaginary of this kind of security narrative has reverberated throughout my analyses, pointing out the necessity of narrative and the constructedness of security.

Furthermore, this health-tracking has been marketed as producing a better understanding of the self, improving and thereby further replacing an intimate relation to one's body. I do not wish to imply that this digitized version of the body replaces the actual experience of the body. It does not eradicate or dissolve the body. Though an app can quantify my run and analyze my data producing a shareable reward in a postable graph, it does not replace the feeling of shortness of breath, of heat creeping up the body, of lightheaded exhaustion. A concentration app might record my attention span correlating it with my other data, but it obviously does not replace the feeling of desperation when the thought keeps escaping the pen. Nonetheless, the quantifiable data shapes how we understand each of these moments – as surmountable, optimizable processes that are just a question of will. The security practices of lifelogging reveal how deep the logics of biosecurity have pervaded the most intimate spaces of U.S. culture, reiterating and reproducing biosecurity logics in their understanding of the self.

Furthermore, lifelogging and self-quantification do not just promise the creation of a better understanding of body. The Quantified Self Movement makes the claim not just to facilitate the view inwards to monitor and learn about bodily functions but the self. In "The Data Driven Life" Gary Wolf asserts that self-quantification is not just about efficiency. "Trackers are exploring an alternate route. Instead of interrogating their inner worlds through talking and writing, they are using numbers. They are constructing a quantified self." In his Ted Talk "The Quantified Self" he makes this even more clear when he describes tracking as a route to deeper "self knowledge" (4:40). In this understanding the self is represented in numbers instead of writing and reflection. Lifelogging in its more all encompassing recording of everything makes similar claims. It originally describes the recording of an entire life as in the research project MyLifeBits by Gordon Bell and Jim Gemmell. In this self experiment Gordon Bell's entire life since 1998 is recorded. His digitalized memory can be read as an autobiographic text of a paranoid reader. Their vision was published in *Total Recall*, (republished as *Your Life Uploaded*). Though very few people use the comprehensive representation of the self as in lifelogging, the practice indicates nonetheless a new form of self-representation and understanding that becomes increasingly common and may be paradigmatic for our time and the biosecurity individual as the portrait and biography once were. Many scholar such as Pablo Abend and

Matthias Fuchs wonder: "What kind of a subject does a society produce when its members translate their bodies into discrete numerical objects?" (13).

Deborah Lupton asserts that "[c]ontemporary self-tracking tools and records are the latter-day versions of the paper diary or journal, photo album, keepsake and memento box or personal dossier" ("Your Data" 74). Anita L. Allen has compared lifelogging to Andy Warhol's "time capsule." Many other texts seem to find a historic predecessor for the practices in Benjamin Franklin's autobiography and his meticulous collection of his life. However, the self that is produced in this kind of self representation is not akin to the self that emerges out of life writing texts. Traditionally the act of writing life is understood as creating the self in the present of the reflection (so the narrative now) (Bruner 38). Though usually written in a retrospective form, life writing texts are always directed toward the future. This is on the one hand the "known future outcome" of most life writing texts according to Folkenflik ("Self"). On the other hand, it is the represented self that is to shine forth and survive the author as an immortal image. The self represented in the biometric data of self-trackers is similarly a retrospective representation that defines the narrative present, if one can call the moment of analysis that. However, they are future-directed in a different way. They create –numerically – mini individualized utopian tales, producing a future version of an improved self as Lupton asserts. It describes in that sense rather a practice of reading than of writing, a hermeneutic reading that can be linked back to the Puritan understanding of life and security. The temporality echoes a Puritan understanding of predetermination rather then of biological determinism in which the body represents an unchangeable fate. The self is predetermined by the body and its biological constitution, which we need to work on to really know it and be able to facilitate its true potential. If the reading shows that the coffee intake is actually reducing my attention span I cut it out (one of Wolf's examples) determined by biometric data.

The biosecurity subject that is represented in all these apps can be seen as paradigmatic for the biosecurity individual. It shows how deeply biosecurity logics have pervaded society. But if "self-tracking data practices can be understood as self-narrative and as performative selfhood" ("Your Data" 68), as Lupton suggests, we are indeed departing from the understanding of the human as a subject with a free will as imparted to us from Enlightenment thought. Stefan Danter, Wilfried Reichert, and Regina Schober suggest that it is not just an identity but a "concept of the human which is based on numerical and statistical models" (55). So what does it mean to understand and intellectually accept numbers and information condensed in security narratives as the main constituents of identity formation? In part this "data driven life" mirrors the identity discourse of certain parts of posthumanisms. The subject is not constructed in language but in numbers embodying the idea of life as a correctable code representing the contemporary posthuman condition, or posthuman "predicament," as Braidotti identified it.[15] Hayles, who is most closely associated[16] with this disembodied vision of posthumanism writes:

> But the posthuman does not really mean the end of humanity. It signals instead the end of a certain conception of the human, a conception that may have applied, at best, to that fraction of humanity who had the wealth, power, and leisure to conceptualize themselves as autonomous beings exercising their will through individual agency and choice. (Hayles 286)

And Cary Wolfe, too, expresses reservations against this form of humanism urging us to "rethink the underlying models of subjectivity that ground the dominant" (xxx) commenting on Disability Studies as an example of decentering the "human" that has been envisioned and defined by agency and autonomy. In the face of such a forceful biotechnological overdetermination posthuman critique seems both promising as well as dangerous. The theoretical approaches think beyond the narrow confines of "the human" to find a way to include individuals – humans, other than humans, non-humans – that are excluded from the concept of the autonomous subject, such as someone with Alzheimer's Disease. And though this cultural critique of the biosecurity individual is indebted to and based on theories of deconstruction and performativity and shares the critique on normative understandings of the human and what is human, I cautious in sharing the techno-scientific belief underlying the theories and their seeming hostility to "human choice and the power of the human to transform the social world" (533) as Brennan puts it in "Post-Human." Or rather, I do not share their optimism in facilitating new ways of conviviality by relying on technologies developed by neoliberal market interests. This seems impossible and naïve in a time when the possibilities granted by the field of biomedicine bear the threat to facilitate more narrow norm(ativity) instituted by the very same technologies that are perceived as freeing us from those normativities.

Supposedly, the information produced by biotechnological practices as well as trackers should enable us to question what is human and become better humans of a post-anthropocentric world.[17] However, the supposedly neutral information free from cultural biases is, as science itself, based on biases which are reproduced. Simon Schaupp shows that the quantified self movement is with 80% of the participants being men not only representatively more male but that "self-tracking discourses are male-dominated"

---

15   Braidotti establishes in *The Posthuman* her theory of post-anthropocentrism and her critique of Cartesian/Kantian subject. She proposes the dissolution of the distinction between animal and human: "the human has exploded under the double pressure of contemporary scientific advances and global economic concerns" (1) emphasizing the need for a new concept of conviviality.

16   She represents the vision that the essence of the human is code, which means it will be replaceable and overcomable. She formulates her vision explicitly against forms of "the antihuman and the apocalyptic" (291).

17   "Although some current versions of the posthuman point toward the antihuman and the apocalyptic, we can craft others that will be conducive to the long-range survival of humans and of the other life-forms, biological and artificial, with whom we share the planet and ourselves" (Hayles 291).

(260). Biases are programmed into algorithms as the dangerous shortcomings of various face recognition technologies have made obvious. The structural racism underlying the production of these practices became clear as the technologies failed to recognize black skin (Lohr). This, like many other examples, not only demonstrates the cultural biases imparted into scientific analysis but also shows how far we are from a post-human future.

The posthuman condition (as methodology and as reality) is very exclusive. And while the media provides circulation and normalization of images of "biomedicalized subjectivities," large parts of the U.S. population (as well as large parts of the world) are barred from access to this form of knowledge of the self. They are positioned outside the force field of the security promise. Though a reconceptualization of what is traditionally understood as "human" seems promising in its attempts to include formerly excluded individuals, it also risks providing a philosophical basis for a further biomedicalization that serves economic and political interests, in line with the neoliberal agenda of individualized responsibilities.

Works Cited

ABC Health Report. "Huntington's Disease." Created by Lynn Malcolm, ABC.net, 29 March 2010, https://abc.net.au/radionational/programs/healthreport/huntingtons-disease-part-one-of-a-two-part-feature/3112964.

Abend, Pablo and Mathias Fuchs. "Introduction: The Quantified Self and Statistical Bodies." *Quantified Selves / Statistic Bodies. Special Issue of Digital Culture and Society*, edited by Pablo Abend and Mathias Fuchs. vol. 2, no. 1, 2016, pp. 5–21, https://doi.org/10.14361/dcs-2016-0102.

Adams, Henry. *The Education of Henry Adams*. Boston: Houghton Mifflin Co., 1918; Oxford UP, Reissue Edition, 2008.

Adams, John Quincy. "American Principles" 1821. *The American Soul: The Contested Legacy of the Declaration of Independence*, edited by Justin Buckley Dyer, Rowman and Littlefield Publishers, Inc., 2012, pp 30–33.

Adams, Rachel. *Raising Henry: A Memoir of Motherhood, Disability, and Discovery*. Yale UP, 2013.

Adorno, Theodor Wiesengrund. *Minima Moralia: Reflexionen Aus Dem Beschädigten Leben*. 1951. Suhrkamp, 2011.

Aeschylus. *Prometheus Bound and Other Plays: Prometheus Bound, The Suppliants, Seven Against Thebes, The Persians*. Translated by Philip Vellacott, Penguin, 1961.

Agus, David B. "The Outrageous Cost of a Gene Test" *The New York Times Magazine*. May 20 2013, https://nytimes.com/2013/05/21/opinion/the-outrageous-cost-of-a-gene-test.html.

Ahmed, Sara. *The Promise of Happiness*. Duke UP, 2010.

Ahmed, Sara. "Open Forum Imaginary Prohibitions: Some Preliminary Remarks on the Founding Gestures of the 'New Materialism.'" *European Journal of Women's Studies*, vol. 15, no. 1, 2008, pp. 23–39, https://doi.org/10.1177/1350506807084854.

Ahmed, Sara. "The Politics of Bad Feeling." *Australian Critical Race and Whiteness Studies Association Journal*, vol. 1, 2005, pp. 72–85, https://static1.squarespace.com/static/58ad660603596eec00ce71a3/t/58becb77893fc0f72747d4e8/1488898936274/The+Politics+of+Good+Feeling.pdf.

Ahmed, Sara. *The Cultural Politics of Emotion*. Edinburgh UP, 2004.

Ahmed, Sara. "Affective Economies." *Social Text*, vol. 79, no. 22, 2004, pp. 117–139, https://muse.jhu.edu/article/55780.

Ahmed, Sara. "Communities that Feel: Intensity, Difference and Attachment." *Affective Encounters: Rethinking Embodiment in Feminist Media Studies*, edited by Anu Koivunen and Susanna Paasonen. University of Turku, 2000, pp. 10–24.

Ahmed, Sara. "Beyond Humanism and Postmodernism: Theorizing a Feminist Practice." *Hypatia*, vol. 11, no. .2, 1996, pp. 71–93, https://jstor.org/stable/3810265.

A.I. Artificial Intelligence. Directed by Steven Spielberg, Warner Bros, 2001.

Alice's Restaurant. Directed by Arthur Penn, United Artists, 1969.

Allen, Anita L. "Dredging up the Past: Lifelogging, Memory, and Surveillance." *The University of Chicago Law Review*, vol.75, no. 1, 2008, pp. 47–74, https://jstor.org/stable/20141900.

Almeling, Rene, and Shana Kushner Gadarian. "Reacting to Genetic Risk: An Experimental Survey of Life between Health and Disease." *Journal of Health and Social Behavior*, vol. 55, no.4, 2014, pp. 482–503, https://jstor.org/stable/43187071.

Alperen, Martin J. *Foundations of Homeland Security: Law and Policy*. John Wiley & Sons, 2011.

American Cancer Society. "Cancer Facts and Figures 2019." Atlanta: American Cancer Society, 2019, https://cancer.org/content/dam/cancer-org/research/cancer-facts-and-statistics/annual-cancer-facts-and-figures/2019/cancer-facts-and-figures-2019.pdf.

American Pregnancy Org. "Keepsake Ultrasounds Or Sonograms." *American Pregnancy Association*, June 2015, https://americanpregnancy.org/pregnancy-health/keepsake-ultrasound/.

American Pregnancy Org. "Birth Defects Prevention Campaign." *American Pregnancy Association*, July 2015, https://americanpregnancy.org/healthy-pregnancy/birth-defects/birth-defects-prevention-campaign-70941/.

Amoore, Louise. *The Politics of Possibility: Risk and Security Beyond Probability*. Duke UP, 2013.

Amyes, Sebastian. *Magic Bullets, Lost Horizons: The Rise and Fall of Antibiotics*. Taylor and Francis, 2001.

Ana. "Ana." *Voices of FORCE*, facingourrisk.org, https://facingourrisk.org/get-involved/HBOC-community/voices-of-FORCE/voices-individual.php?voice=583.

Anderson, Ben. "Preemption, Precaution, Preparedness: Anticipatory Action and Future Geographies." *Progress in Human Geography*, vol. , 9.April 2010, 1–22, https://doi.org/10.1177/0309132510362600.

Anderson, Ben. "Hope for Nanotechnology: Anticipatory Knowledge and the Governance of Affect." *Area*, vol. 39, no. 2, 2007, pp. 156–165. jstor.org/stable/40346022.

Anderson, Benedict. *Imagined Communities: Reflections on the Origin and Spread of Nationalism*. 1983. Verso, 1991.

Anker, Susanne, Dorothy Nelkin. *The Molecular Gaze: Art in the Genetic Age*. Cold Spring Harbor Laboratory, 2003.

Anzaldúa, Gloria. *Borderlands – La Frontera: The New Mestiza*. Aunt Lute Books, 1987.

Apple, Rima. "Constructing Mothers: Scientific Motherhood in the Nineteenth and Twentieth Centuries." *Social History of Medicine*, vol. 8, no. 2, 1995, pp. 161- 178, https://shm.oxfordjournals.org/.

Ariès, Philippe. *The Hour of Our Death*. Translated by Helen Weaver, New York: Vintage Books, 1981.

Ariès, Philippe. "The Reversal of Death: Changes in Attitudes toward Death in Western Society." *Death in America*, edited by David E. Stannard, U of Pennsylvania P, 1975, pp. 134–158.

Ariès, Philippe. *Western Attitudes toward Death: from the Middle Ages to the Present*. Translated by Patricia M Ranum, John Hopkins UP, 1974.

Ariès, Philippe. *Centuries of the Child: A Social History of Family Life*. 1960. Translated by Robert Baldick. Knopf, 1962.

Aristotle. *The Poetics of Aristotle*, edited and translated by S.H. Butcher, Macmillan, 1898, h ttps://archive.org/details/poeticsofaristoooaris.

Armitage, David. *The Declaration of Independence: A Global History*. 2007. Harvard UP, 2008.

Armour, Ellen T., and Susan M. St. Ville. "Judith Butler in Theory." *Bodily Citation: Religion and Judith Butler*, edited by Ellen T. Armour, and Susan M St. Ville. Columbia UP, 2006, pp. 1–14.

Armstrong, David. "The Rise of Surveillance Medicine." *Sociology of Health and Illness*, vol. 17, no. 3, 1995, pp. 393–404, https://doi.org/10.1111/1467-9566.ep10933329.

Aronsson, Carin Andrén, and TEDDY Study Group. "Use of Dietary Supplements in Pregnant Women in Relation to Sociodemographic Factors – A Report from the Environmental Determinants of Diabetes in the Young (TEDDY) Study." *Public Health Nutrition*, vol.16, no. 8, 2013, pp 1–25, https://doi.org/10.1017/S1368980013000293.

Asimov, Isaac. *Fantastic Voyage*. Perma Bound, 1966.

Atwood, Margaret. *Oryx and Crake: a Novel*. Doubleday, 2003.

Atwood, Margaret. *The Handmaid's Tale: a Novel*. 1986, Anchor Books, 1998.

Aufderheide, Patricia. *Documentary Film: A Very Short Introduction*. Oxford UP, 2007.

Austin, John Langshaw. *How to Do Things with Words*. 1962. Harvard UP, 1975.

Baldwin, David A.. "Concept of Security." *Review of International Studies*, vol. 23, 1997, pp. 5–26, https://jstor.org/stable/20097464.

Barbot, Oxiris. "Order of the Commissioner." New York City Department of Health and Mental Hygiene. April 9, 2019, https://www1.nyc.gov/assets/doh/downloads/pdf/pr ess/2019/emergency-orders-measles.pdf.

Bc31. "Bc31's Story." Breastcancer.org, July 14, 2016. breastcancer.org/community/acknowledging/genetic-testing/bc31.

Beall, Otho T. Jr. and Richard H. Shryock. *Cotton Mather: First Significant Figure in American Medicine*. Baltimore MD, 1954.

Beatty, John. "Origins of the U.S. Human Genome Project: Changing Relationships between Genetics and National Security." *Controlling Our Destinies: Historical, Philosophical, Ethical, and Theological Perspectives on the Human Genome Project*, edited by Phillip R. Sloan, U of Notre Dame P, 2000, pp. 131 – 154.

Beck, Ulrich. *Risikogesellschaft: Auf dem Weg in eine andere Moderne*. Suhrkamp Verlag, 1986.

Beck, Ulrich. *World Risk Society*. Polity, 1999.

Becker, Carl. *The Declaration of Independence: A Study on the History of Political Ideas*. Harcourt, Brace and Company, Inc., 1922.

Beecher Stowe, Harriet. *Uncle Tom's Cabin*, edited by Elizabeth Ammons, *Uncle Tom's Cabin: Authoritative Text, Background and Context, Criticism*. W. W. Norton & Company, 1994.

Behling, Laura L. *Gross Anatomies: Fictions of the Physical in American Literature*. Susquehanna UP, 2008.

Belkin, Lisa . "How Breast Cancer Became this Year's Hot Charity." *New York Times Magazine*, 22. Dec. 1996, pp. 40–46, 52, 55–56.

Bell, Carlos Gordon, and Jim Gemmell. "Erinnerung Total." *Spektrum der Wissenschaft*, vol. 5, 2007, pp. 84–92.

Bell, Carlos Gordon, and Jim Gemmell. *Your Life Uploaded: The Digital Way to Better Memory, Health, and Productivity*. Plume, 2010.

Belling, Catherine. "Narrating Oncogenesis: The Problem of Telling When Cancer Begins." *Narrative*, vol. 18, no. 2, 2010, pp. 229–247.

Belling, Catherine. "Hypochondriac Hermeneutics: Medicine and the Anxiety of Interpretation." *Literature and Medicine*, vol. 25, no. 2, 2006, pp. 376–401.

Benjamin, Walter. "On the Concept of History." 1940. *Selected Writings Volume 4 1938–1940*. Translated by Edmund Jephcott et al., edited by Howard Eiland and Michael W. Jennings. Harvard UP, 2003.

Benjamin, Walter. "Artwork in the Age of Mechanical Reproduction." 1935. *Illuminations: Essays and Reflections*, edited by Hannah Arendt, Translated by Harry Zohn, 1968, Schocken Books, 2007, pp. 217–252.

Bentham, Jeremy. "A Short Review of the Declaration of Independence." 1826. *The American Soul: The Contested Legacy of the Declaration of Independence*, edited by Justin Buckley Dyer, Rowman and Littlefield Publishers, Inc., 2012, pp. 16–18.

Berchick, Edward R., Emily Hood, and Jessica C. Barnett. "Health Insurance Coverage in the United States: 2017 – Current Population Reports." *Census.gov*, 12 Sept. 2018, https://census.gov/library/publications/2018/demo/p60-264.html.

Bercovitch, Sacvan. *The American Jeremiad*. Wisconsin: U of Wisconsin P, 1978.

Berlant, Lauren. "Cruel Optimism" *The Affect Theory Reader*, edited by Melissa Gregg and Gregory J. Seigworth. Duke UP, 2010, pp. 93–117.

Biddinger, Paul D, Elena Savoia, Sarah B. Massin-Short, Jessica Preston, and Michael A. Stoto. "Public Health Emergency Preparedness Exercises: Lessons Learned." *Public Health Reports*, vol. 125, no. 5, 2010, pp. 100–6, https://jstor.org/stable/41557943.

Bidgood, Jess. "'I Live Paycheck to Paycheck': A West Virginia Teacher Explains Why She's on Strike." *The New York Times*, 1 March 2018, https://nytimes.com/2018/03/01/us/west-virginia-teachers-strike.html.

Bieber Lake, Christina. *Prophets of the Posthuman: American Fiction, Biotechnology, and the Ethics of Personhood*. U of Notre Dame P, 2003.

Bingham, Nick, and Steve Hinchliffe. "Mapping the Multiplicities of Biosecurity." *Biosecurity Interventions: Global Health and Security in Question*, edited by Andrew Lakoff and Stephen J. Collier. Columbia UP, 2008, pp. 173–193.

Bioshock. 2K Games, 2007.

Black Mirror. Charlie Brooker, creator, season 1–5, Channel 4 Television Corporation, Netflix, 2011/2013/2017/2018.

Blade Runner. Directed by Ridley Scott, Warner Bros. 1982.

Blade Runner 2049. Directed by Denise Villeneuve, Warner Bros. 2017.

Boesky, Amy. *What We Have: A Memoir, One Family's Inspiring Story About Love, Loss, and Survival*. Gotham Books, 2010.

Boesky, Amy. "'This is How We Live': Witnessing and Testimony in BRCA Memoirs." *Tulsa Studies in Women's Literature*, vol. 32/33, No2/1, *Theorizing Breast Cancer: Narrative, Politics, Memory*, 2013/2014, pp. 89–105, https://jstor.org/stable/43653278.

Bostrom, Nick. "A History of Transhumanist Thought." *Journal of Evolution and Technology*, vol. 14, April 2005, pp.1-25, https://www.nickbostrom.com/papers/history.pdf.

Bouwsma, William J., "From History of Ideas to History of Meaning." *The Journal of Interdisciplinary History*, vol. 12, no.2, *The New History: The 1980s and Beyond (II)*, 1981, pp. 279–291, https://jstor.org/stable/203030.

Braidotti, Rosi. *The Posthuman*. Polity, 2013.

Brandt, Allan M. "Racism and Research: The Case of the Tuskegee Syphilis Study." *The Hasting's Center Report*, vol. 8, no. 6, 1978, pp. 21–29, https://doi.org/10.2307/3561468.

Breast Cancer Organization. "U.S. Breast Cancer Statistics." *Breastcancer.org*, 25 June 2020, https://breastcancer.org/symptoms/understand_bc/statistics.

Breast Cancer Organization. "Genetic Testing Facilities and Costs." *Breastcancer.org*, 23 June 2016, https://breastcancer.org/symptoms/testing/genetic/facility_cost.

Breast Cancer Organization. "Members Share Their Genetic Testing Stories." *Breastcancer.org*, 25 Feb. 2019, https://breastcancer.org/community/acknowledging/genetic-testing.

Brennan, Teresa. *The Transmission of Affect*. Cornell UP, 2004.

Brennan, Timothy. "The Problem with Post-humanism." *Crossroads of American Studies: Transnational and Biocultural Encounters*, edited by Frederike Offizier, Marc Priewe, and Ariane Schröder. Winter, 2016, pp.529- 551. American Studies – A Monograph Series vol. 269.

Bright Pink. "Personal Stories of Prevention." *Bright Pink*, https://brightpink.org/bright-stories/.

Bright Pink. "One-on-One Support." *Bright Pink*, https://brightpink.org/1on1support/.

Broad, William J. "Nobel Prize in Chemistry Awarded to Tomas Lindahl, Paul Modrich and Aziz Sancar for DNA Studies." *The New York Times*, 7 Oct. 2015, https://nytimes.com/2015/10/08/science/tomas-lindahl-paul-modrich-aziz-sancarn-nobel-chemistry.html.

Brodsky, Phyllis L. "Where Have All the Midwives Gone?" *Journal of Perinatal Education*, vol. 17, no. 4, 2008, pp. 48–51, https://doi.org/10.1624/105812408X324912.

Brodwick, Caitlin, Creator. "Screw You Cancer." season 1, Glamour, https://video.glamour.com/series/screw-you-cancer.

Brown, Phil. "Naming and Framing: The Social Construction of Diagnosis and Illness." *Journal of Health and Social Behavior*, vol. 35, 1995, pp. 34–52, https://jstor.org/stable/2626956.

Brumberg, Joan Jacobs. *The Body Project: An Intimate History of American Girls*. Vintage Books, 1998.

Bruner, Jerome. "The Autobiographical Process." *The Culture of Autobiography: Constructions of Self-Representation*, edited by Robert Folkenflik. Stanford U.P., 1993, pp. 39–56.

Brunner, Otto, Werner Conze, and Reihardt Koselleck. "Sicherheit, Schutz." 1994, *Geschichtliche Grundbegriffe: Historisches Lexikon zur politisch-sozialen Sprache in Deutschland*. Band 5, Pro –Soz. Klett-Cotta, 2000, pp. 831–862.

Bryan, Elizabeth. *Singing the Life: A Family in the Shadow of Cancer*. Vermillion, 2007.

Buchanan, Ian. "Metacommentary on Utopia, or Jameson's Dialectic of Hope," *Utopian Studies*, vol. 9, no. 2, pp.18-30, https://jstor.org/stable/20719759.

Bud, Robert. *The Uses of Life: A History of Biotechnology*. Cambridge UP, 1993.

Buhr, Shawn. "To Inoculate of Not to Inoculate?: The Debate and the Smallpox Epidemic of Boston in 1721." *Constructing the Past*, vol.1, no.1, 2000, pp. 61–67, https://digitalco mmons.iwu.edu/constructing/vol1/iss1/8.

Bullocks, Christopher. *The Cobbler of Preston: a Farce. As it is acted at the Theatre-Royal in Drury-Lane. By His Majesty's servants*. W. Wilkins, and sold by W. Hinchcliffe, 1716, https://ar chive.org/stream/coblerofprestonfoobull?ref=ol.

Burgess, J.Peter. "Introduction." *The Routledge Handbook of New Security Studies*, Routledge, 2010, pp. 1–4.

Burfoot, Annette. "Human Remains: Identity in the Face of Biotechnology." *Cultural Critique*, vol. 53, 2003, pp. 47–71, https://jstor.org/stable/1354624.

Burri, Regula Valérie, and Joseph Dumit, editors. *Biomedicine as Culture: Instrumental Practices, Technoscientific Knowledge, and New Modes of Life*. Routledge, 2007.

Bury, Michael. "Chronic Illness as Biographical Disruption." *Sociology of Health and Illness*, vol. 4, no. 2, 1982, pp. 167–182, https://doi.org/10.1111/1467-9566.ep11339939.

Bush, George W. "Remarks by the President on Smallpox Vaccination." *The White House: President George W Bush*, 13 Dec. 2002, https://georgewbush-whitehouse.archives.go v/news/releases/2002/12/20021213-7.html.

Bush, George W. "President Outlines On Pandemic Influenza Preparedness and Response." *The White House: President George W. Bush*. Nov. 1, 2005, https://georgewbus h-whitehouse.archives.gov/news/releases/2005/11/20051101-1.html.

Bush, George W. "President Bush Delivers Graduation Speech at Westpoint." *The White House: President George W Bush*, 1 June 2002, https://georgewbush-whitehouse.archiv es.gov/news/releases/2002/06/20020601-3.html.

Butler, Judith. "Performative Acts and Gender Constitution: An Essay in Phenomenology and Feminist Theory." *Theatre Journal*, vol. 40, no. 4, 1988, pp. 519–531, https://jstor.or g/stable/3207893.

Butler, Judith. *Gender Trouble: Feminism and the Subversion of Identity*. 1990. Routledge, 1999.

Butler, Judith. *Bodies that Matter: On the Discursive Limits of "Sex"*. Routledge, 1993.

Butler, Judith. *Precarious Life: The Power of Mourning and Violence*. Verso, 2004.

Butler, Sandra, and Barbara Rosenblum. *Cancer in Two Voices*. 1991, Login Publisher Consortium, 1996.

Caduff, Carlo. "Anticipations of Biosecurity." *Biosecurity Interventions: Global Health and Security in Question*, edited by Andrew Lakoff, and Stephen J. Collier. Columbia UP, 2008, pp.256-277.

Cagle, Chris. "Postclassical Nonfiction: Narration in the Contemporary Documentary." *Cinema Journal*, vol. 52, no. 1, 2012, pp. 45–65, https://doi.org/10.1353/cj.2012.0115.

Calgary 002. "Calgary 002's Story." *Breastcancer.org*, 30 Nov. 2017, https://breastcancer.or g/community/acknowledging/genetic-testing/calgary002.

Calhoun, Craig. *Social Theory and Politics of Identity*. Blackwell, 1994.

Campbell, Christopher. "Review: How to Die in Orgon" *Sundance*, 3 Feb. 2011, https://blo g.moviefone.com/2011/01/27/how-to-die-in-oregon-review-sundance/.

Campbell, Courtney, and Jessica Cox. "Hospice and Physician-Assisted Death: Collaboration, Compliance, and Complicity." *Hasting's Center Report*, vol. 40, 2010, pp. 26–35, https://doi.org/10.1353/hcr.2010.0016.

Campos, Paul, Abigail Saguy, Paul Ernsberger, Eric Oliver, and Glenn Gaesser. "The Epidemiology of Overweight and Obesity: Public Health Crisis or Moral Panic?" *International Journal of Epidemiology*, vol. 35, 2006, pp. 55–60, https://doi.org/10.1093/ije/dyi 254.

Cancer Treatment Center of America. "Can Playing Video Games Help Cancer Patients?" *Cancer Center*, 14 Feb 2017, https://cancercenter.com/discussions/blog/can-playing-v ideo-games-help-cancer-patients/.

Canguilhem, Georges. *The Normal and the Pathological*. Translated by Carolyn R. Fawcett. Zone Books, 1991.

Canguilhem, Georges. *Writings on Medicine*. 1989, Translated by Stefanos Geroulanos and Todd Meyers. Fordham UP, 2012.

Carroll, Lewis. "The Walrus and the Carpenter." *Alices Adventures in Wonderland and Through the Looking Glass*. 1871, edited by Peter Hunt, Oxford UP, 2006, pp.162-166.

Carter, Thatcher. "Body Count: Autobiographies by Women Living with Breast Cancer." *Journal of Popular Culture*, vol. 36, no.4, 2003, pp. 653–668, https://doi.org/10.1111/1540 -5931.00039.

Cassell, Eric J. *The Nature of Suffering and the Goal of Medicine*. Oxford UP, 1991.

CellCraft. CellCraft Team, 2015.

Center for Disease Control and Prevention. "Breast Cancer Statistics." *CDC*, 8 June 2020, https://cdc.gov/cancer/breast/statistics/index.htm.

Center for Disease Control and Prevention. "State School and Vaccination Law." *CDC*, 28 April 2017, https://cdc.gov/phlp/publications/topic/vaccinations.html.

Center for Disease Control and Prevention. "Death and Mortality." *CDC*, 21 Nov. 2020, h ttps://cdc.gov/nchs/fastats/deaths.htm.

Center for Disease Control and Prevention. "United States Life Tables, 2014." *National Vital Statistics Report*, vol. 66, no. 4, 2017, pp. 1–63, https://cdc.gov/nchs/data/nvsr/nvsr 66/nvsr66_04.pdf.

Center for Disease Control and Prevention." Pregnancy Mortality Surveillance System." *CDC*, 7 August 2018, https://cdc.gov/reproductivehealth/maternalinfanthealth/preg nancy-mortality-surveillance-system.htm.

Center for Disease Control and Prevention. "Attention-Deficit/ Hyperactive Disorder: Data and Statistics About ADHD." *CDC*, 16 Nov. 2020, https://cdc.gov/ncbddd/adh d/data.html.

Center for Disease Control and Prevention. "Celebrating the Fourth of July: Be Healthy, Be Prepared." *CDC*, 1 July 2015, https://blogs.cdc.gov/publichealthmatters/2015/07/c elebrating-the-fourth-of-july-be-healthy-be-prepared/.

Center for Disease Control and Prevention. "Opioid Overdose: Understanding the Epidemic." *CDC*, 19 March 2020, https://cdc.gov/drugoverdose/epidemic/index.html.

Center for Disease Control and Prevention. "Chronic Disease in America." *CDC*, 23 Oct 2019, https://cdc.gov/chronicdisease/resources/infographic/chronic-diseases.htm.

Center for Disease Control and Prevention. "Disability Impacts All of Us." *CDC*, 16 Sept. 2020, https://cdc.gov/ncbddd/disabilityandhealth/infographic-disability-imp acts-all.html.

Center for Disease Control and Prevention. "National Intimate Partner and Sexual Violence Survey: 2015 Data Brief." *CDC*, Nov. 2018, https://cdc.gov/violenceprevention/ pdf/2015data-brief508.pdf.

Charon, Rita. *Stories Matter: The Role of Narrative in Medical Ethic.* Routledge, 2002.

Chilton, Paul. "The Meaning of Security." *Post-Realism: The Rhetorical Turn in International Relations*, edited by F. A. Beer and R. Hariman, Michigan State U.P., 1996, pp. 193–216.

Clark, Ronald. *J.B.S.: The Life and Work of J.B.S. Haldane.* 1968. Bloomsbury, 2013.

Clarke, Adele E., Janet K. Shim, Laura Mamo, Jennifer Ruth Fosket, and Jennifer R. Fishman. "Biomedicalization: A Theoretical and Substantive Introduction." *Biomedicalization: Technoscience, Health, and Illness in the U.S.*, edited by Adele E. Clarke, Laura Mamo, Jennifer Ruth Fosket, Jennifer R. Fishman, and Janet K. Shim, Duke UP, 2010, pp. 1–44.

Clarke, Adele E., Jennifer Ruth Fosket, Laura Mamo, Jennifer R. Fishman, and Janet K. Shim. "Charting (Bio)medicine and (Bio)medicalization in the United States 1890-Present." *Biomedicalization: Technoscience, Health, and Illness in the U.S.*, edited by Adele E. Clarke, Laura Mamo, Jennifer Ruth Fosket, Jennifer R. Fishman, and Janet K. Shim, Duke UP, 2010, pp. 88–103.

Clarke, Adele E., Janet K. Shim, Laura Mamo, Jennifer Ruth Fosket and Jennifer R. Fishman. "Biomedicalization: Technoscientific Transformations Of Health, Illness, and U.S. Biomedicine." *American Sociological Review*, vol. 68, no. 2, 2003, pp. 161-194, https ://jstor.org/stable/1519765.

Clayton, Jay. "The Ridicule of Time: Science Fiction, Bioethics, and the Posthuman." *American Literary History*, vol. 25, no. 2, 2013, pp. 317–340, https://muse.jhu.edu/journals/ alh/summary/v025/25.2.clayton.html.

Clayton, Jay. "Convergence of the Two Cultures: A Geek's Guide to Contemporary Literature." *American Literature*, vol 74, no. 4, 2002, pp.807-831, https://muse.jhu.edu/articl e/38213.

Cloud Atlas. Directed by Tom Tykwer, Lana Wachowski, and Lilly Wachowski, Cloud Atlas Production, 2012.

Clough, Patricia T., and Craig Willse, editors. *Beyond Biopolitics: Essays on the Governance of Life and Death.* Duke UP, 2011.

Clough, Patricia T. "The Affective Turn: Political Economy, Biomedia, and Bodies." *The Affect Theory Reader*, edited by Melissa Gregg and Gregory J. Seigworth, Duke UP, 2010, pp. 206–227.

Cohen, Wilbur J. "Reflecting on the Enactment of Medicare and Medicaid." *Health Care Financial Review*, 1985, pp. 3–11. ncbi.nlm.nih.gov/pmc/articles/ PMC4195078/pdf/hcfr-85-supp-003.pdf.

Cohen, Sheldon, and Sarah D. Pressman. "Positive Affect and Health." *Association of Psychological Science*, vol 15, no. 3, 2006, pp. 122–125, https://doi.org/10.1111/j.0963-7214.2 006.00420.x.

Colbert, Marcella. "The Medicalization of Death and Dying." *Life and Learning. XIV*, University Faculty for Life. Conference, 2005, pp. 227–238.

Collier, Stephen J., and Andrew Lakoff. "The Problem of Securing Health." *Biosecurity Interventions: Global Health and Security in Question*, edited by Stephen J. Collier and Andrew Lakoff. Columbia UP, 2008, pp. 7–32.

Collier, Stephen J., Andrew Lakoff, and Paul Rabinow. "Biosecurity: Toward and Anthropology of the Contemporary." *Anthropology Today*, vol. 20, no. 5, 2004, pp. 3–7, https://jstor.org/stable/3695224.

Collins, Sara R., Munira Z. Gunja, and Michelle M. Doty. "How Well Does Insurance Coverage Protect Consumers from Health Care Costs: Finding from the Commonwealth Fund Biennial Health Insurance Survey, 2016." *Commonwealthfund.org*, 18 Oct. 2017, https://commonwealthfund.org/publications/issue-briefs/2017/oct/how-well-does-insurance-coverage-protect-consumers-health-care.

Cole, Thomas R. *The Journey of Life: A Cultural History of Aging*. Cambridge UP. 1992.

Compassion and Choice. "History of the End-of-Life Choice Movement." *Compassionandchoice.org*, https://compassionandchoices.org/resource/history-end-life-choice-movement/.

Compassion and Choice. "News: Brittany Maynard Family, Compassion & Choices Making End of-Life Care Progress." *Compassionandchoice.org*, 10 March 2015, https://compassionandchoices.org/brittany-maynard-family-compassion-choices-making-end-of-life-care-progress/.

Compassion and Choice. "Brittany Maynard's Legacy: One Year Later." *Youtube*, uploaded by Compassion and Choice, 5 Oct. 2015, https://www.youtube.com/watch?v=uzpotp8Fzio&feature=emb_logo.

Connolly, William E. "The Complexity of Intention." Critical Inquiry, vol. 37, no. 4, 2011, pp. 791-798, https://jstor.org/stable/10.1086/660993.

Conrad, Peter. *The Medicalization of Society: On the Transformation of Human Condition into Treatable Disorder*. John Hopkins UP, 2007.

Conrad, Peter. "Shifting Engines of Medicalization." *Journal of Health and Social Behavior*, vol. 46, no. 1, 2005, pp. 3–14, https://jstor.org/stable/4147650.

Conrad, Peter. "Use of Expertise: Sources, Quotes, and Voice in the Reporting of Genetics in News." *Public Understanding of Science*, vol. 8, 1999, pp. 285–302, https://doi.org/10.1088/0963-6625/8/4/302.

Conrad, Peter. "Public Eyes and Private Genes: Historical Frames, News Constructions, and Social Problems." *Social Problems*, vol. 44, no. 2, 1997, pp. 139–154. jstor.org/stable/3096939.

Contagion. Directed by Stephen Soderbergh, Warner Bros. Pictures, 2011.

Cooper, Melinda. *Life as Surplus: Biotechnology and Capitalism in the Neoliberal Era*. U of Washington Press, 2008.

Cooper, Melinda. "Resuscitations: Stem Cells and the Crisis of Old Age." *Body and Society*, vol. 12, no. 1, 2006, pp. 1–23, https://doi.org/10.1177/1357034X06061196.

Cortez, Nathan G., Glenn Cohen, Aaron S. Kesselheim. "FDA Regulation of Mobile Health Technologies." *The New England Journal of Medicine. Health Law, Ethics, and Human Rights*, vol. 371, no. 4, 2014, pp. 372–379, https://doi.org/10.1056/NEJMhle1403384.

Corvellec, Hervé. "The Narrative Structure of Risk Accounts." *Risk Management*, vol. 13, no. 3 2011, pp. 101–121, https://jstor.org/stable/41289349.

Crane, Stephen. *Maggie: A Girl of the Streets*. 1893. W.W. Norton & Company, 1979.

Crawford, Robert. "Healthism and the Medicalization of Everyday Life." *International Journal of Health Services*, vol. 10, no. 3, 1980, pp. 365–388, https://doi.org/10.2190/3H2H-3XJN-3KAY-G9NY.

Crick, Francis. "Nobel Lecture: On the Genetic Code." *NobelPrize.org.*, 11 Nov. 1962, https://nobelprize.org/prizes/medicine/1962/crick/lecture/.

Crile, George. *What Women Should Know about the Breast Cancer Controversy*. Macmillan, 1993. Digitalized 2008.

Culler, Jonathan. "Philosophy of Literature: The Fortunes of the Performative." *Poetics Today*, vol. 21, no. 3, 2000, pp. 503–519, https://muse.jhu.edu/article/27834/pdf.

Curran, Charles A. "Death and Dying." *Journal of Religion and Health*, vol. 14, no. 4, 1975, pp. 254–264, https://jstor.org/stable/27505312.

Danter, Stefan, Wilfried Reichardt and Regina Schober. "Theorizing the Quantified Self: Self-Knowledge and Posthumanist Agency in Contemporary US-American Literature." *Quantified Selves / Statistic Bodies. Special Issue of Digital Culture and Society*, edited by Pablo Abend and Mathias Fuchs. vol. 2, no. 1, 2016, pp. 53–70, https://doi.org/10.14361/dcs-2016-0105.

Davenport, Charles B. "Huntington's Chorea in relation to Heredity and Eugenics." *American Journal of Insanity*, vol. 73, 1916, pp. 283–285. Published online 1 April 2006, https://doi.org/10.1176/ajp.73.2.195.

Davenport, Charles B., and Arthur H. Estabrook. *The Nam Family: A Study in Cacogenics*. Long Island, N.Y.: Cold Spring Harbor, 1912, https://digitized scholarworks.iupui.edu/handle/1805/1148.

Davis, Tracy C. "Between History and Event: Rehearsing Nuclear War Survival." *TDR*, vol. 46, no. 4, 2002, pp. 11–45. Web. 13 June 2015, https://jstor.org/stable/1146976.

Davis, Tracy C. *Stages of Emergency: Cold War Nuclear Civil Defense*. Duke UP 2007.

Davis, Lennard J. "Disability: The Next Wave or Twilight of the Gods?" *PMLA*, vol. 120, no. 2, 2005, pp. 527–532. jstor.org/stable/25486179.

Davis, Lennard J. "Visualizing the Disabled Body: The Classical Nude and the Fragmented Torso." *The Body: A Reader*, edited by Mariam Fraser and Monica Greco. Taylor & Francis, 2004, pp. 167–181.

Davis, Lennard J., editor. *The Disability Studies Reader*. Routledge, 2nd Edition, 2006.

Davis, Lennard J., and David B. Morris. "Biocultures Manifesto." *New Literary History*, vol. 38, no. 3, 2007, pp. 411–418, https://jstor.org/stable/20058015.

Dean, Tim. "The Biopolitics of Pleasure." *South Atlantic Quarterly*, vol. 111, no. 3, 2012, pp. 477–496, https://doi.org/10.1215/00382876-1596245.

Death with Dignity. "Terminology of Assisted Dying." *Death with Dignity.org*, https://deathwithdignity.org/terminology/.

de Chadarevian, Soraya. "Portrait of a Discovery: Watson, Crick, and the Double Helix." *Isis*, vol. 94, no. 1, 2003, pp. 90–105, https://doi.org/10.1086/376100.

DelVecchio Good, Mary-Jo. "The Biotechnical Embrace." *Culture, Medicine and Psychiatry*, vol. 25, 2001, pp. 395–410, https://doi.org/10.1023/a:1013097002487.

De Melo-Martín, I. "Firing up the Nature/Nurture Controversy: Bioethics and Genetic Determinism." *Journal of Medical Ethics*, vol. 31, no. 9, 2005, pp. 526–530, https://doi.org/10.1136/jme.2004.008417.

Deny, Martina, and Elaine Morley. "Editorial: The Aesthetics of Security in Literature and Visual Media." *eTransfer*, vol. 2, 2012, pp. 1–4.

Derrida, Jacques. *Specters of Marx: The State of the Debt, the Work of Mourning and the New International*. 1993, Translated by Peggy Kamuf, 1994, Routledge Classics, 2006.

Derrida, Jacques. "Signature, Event, Context." *Limited Inc*. Translated by Samuel Weber, and Jeffrey Mehlman. Northwestern UP, 1ed. 1988, pp. 1–24.

Derrida, Jacques. "Declaration of Independence." *New Political Science*, vol. 15, 1986, pp. 7–15, https://doi.org/10.1080/07393148608429608.

Derrida, Jacques. *Writing and Difference*. 1967, Translated by Alan Bass. 1978 Routledge Classics. 2001.

Derrida, Jacques. "Différance." 1968, *Margins of Philosophy*, 1972, Translated by Alan Bass, 1982, U of Chicago P, 1972, pp. 278–310.

DeShazer, Mary K.. *Mammographies: The Cultural Discourses of Breast Cancer Narratives*. U of Michigan P, 2015.

DeShazer, Mary K. and Anita Helle. "Theorizing Breast Cancer: Narrative, Politics, Memory." *Tulsa Studies in Women's Literature*, vol. 32, no. 2/ vol. 33, no. 1, Fall 2013/Spring 2014, pp. 7–23, https://muse.jhu.edu/article/550195.

Diagnostic and Statistical Manual of Mental Disorders: Dsm-5. Arlington, VA: American Psychiatric Association, 2013.

Dick, Philip Kindred. *Do Androids Dream of Electric Sheep?*. 1968, Del Rey, Reprint 2017.

Didion, Joan. *We Tell Ourselves Stories in Order to Survive: Collected Nonfiction*. Everyman's Library, 2006.

Dillon, Michael. "Biopolitics of Security." *The Routledge Handbook of New Security Studies*, edited by J. Peter Burgess, Routledge, 2010, pp. 61–71.

Dillon, Michael. "Virtual Security: A Life Science of (Dis)order." *Millennium –Journal of International Studies*, vol. 32, 2003, pp. 531–558, https://doi.org/10.1177/03058298030320030901.

Dillon, Michael. "Specters of Biopolitics: Finitude, Eschaton, and Katechon." *South Atlantic Quarterly*, vol. 110, no. 3, 2011, pp. 780–792.

Dillon, Michael, and Luis Lobo-Guerrero. "Biopolitics of Security in the 21st Century: An Introduction." *Review of International Studies*, vol. 34, 2008, pp. 265–292, https://doi.org/10.1017/S0260210508008024.

Djabi53. "Djabi53's Story." *Breastcancer.org*, 14 July 2016, https://breastcancer.org/community/acknowledging/genetic-testing/djabi53.

Dobkin, Bruce H., Andrew Dorsch. "The Promise of mHealth: Daily Activity Monitoring and Outcome Assessments by Wearable Sensors." *Neurorehabilitation and Neural Repair*, vol. 25. no.9, 2011, pp.788-798, https://doi.org/10.1177/1545968311425908.

Doherty, Aiden R., Steve E Hodges, Abby C King, Alan F Smeaton, Emma Berry, Chris J A Moulin, Siân Lindley, Paul Kelly, and Charlie Foster. "Wearable Cameras in Health: The State of the Art and Future Possibilities." *American Journal of Preventive Medicine*, vol. 44, no. 3, 2013, pp. 320–323, https://doi.org/10.1016/j.amepre.2012.11.008.

Douglas, Mary. *Risk and Blame: Essays in Cultural Theory*. London, Routledge, 1992.

Douglass, Frederick. "What to a Slave is the Fourth of July?: An Address Delivered in Rochester, New York, on 5 July 1852." 1852, *Norton Anthology: African American Litera-*

ture, edited by Henry Louis Gates Jr and Nellie Y. McKay. W.W. Norton & Company, 1997, pp. 379–391.

Do You Really Want to Know?. Directed by John Zaritsky, Knowledge Network, 2013.

Draper, Janet, and Jenny Hockey. "Beyond the Womb and the Tomb: Identity, (Dis)embodiment and the Life Course." *Body and Society*, vol. 11, no. 41, 2005, pp. 41–57, https://doi.org/10.1177/1357034X05052461.

Dreiser, Theodor. *Sister Carrie*. 1900, Signet Classics, 2009.

Drescher, Jack. "Out of DSM: Depathologizing Homosexuality." *Behavioral Sciences*, vol. 5, 2015, pp. 565–575, https://doi.org/10.3390/bs5040565.

Drum, Charles E., Glen White, Genia Taitano, and Willi Horner-Johnson. "The Oregon Death with Dignity Act: results of a Literature Review and Naturalistic Inquiry." *Disability and Health Journal*, vol. 3, 2010, pp. 3–15, https://doi.org/10.1016/j.dhjo.2009.10.001.

Duffy, John. *The Sanitarians: A History of American Public Health*. U of Illinois P, 1990.

Dugdale, Lydia. "The Art of Dying Well." *Hasting's Center Report*, vol. 40, no. 6, 2010, pp. 22–24, https://doi.org/10.1002/j.1552-146X.2010.tb00073.

Duster, Troy. "A Post-Genomic Surprise. The Molecular Reinscription of Race in Science, Law, and Medicine." *British Journal of Sociology*, vol. 66, no. 1, 2015, pp.1-27, https://doi.org/10.1111/1468-4446.12118.

Dyer, Justin Buckley, editor. *The American Soul: The Contested Legacy of the Declaration of Independence*. Rowman and Littlefield Publishers, Inc., 2012.

Dylan, Bob. "Song to Woody." *Bob Dylan*, Columbia/Capitol, 1962.

Dylan, Bob. "Last Thoughts on Woody Guthrie." *Bootleg Series vol.1-3*, Columbia, 1991.

Eades, Charlotte. "Brain Cancer: Dying to Live, Living to Die." *Youtube*, Uploaded by Charlotte Eades. 2014–2016.

Eakin, John Paul. "Introduction: Mapping the Ethics of Life Writing." *Ethics of Life Writing*, edited by John Paul Eakin, Cornell UP, 2004.

Eakin, John Paul, editor. *The Ethics of Life Writing*. Cornell UP, 2004.

Earle, Sarah, Pam Foley, Carol Komaromy, Cathy E. Lloyd. "Health Medicine and Surveillance in the 21st Century." *Surveillance and Society*, vol. 6, no. 2, 2009, pp. 96–100, https://doi.org/10.24908/ss.v6i2.3250.

Edelman, Lee. "The Future is Kid Stuff: Queer Theory, Disidentification, and the Death Drive." *Narrative*, vol. 6, no. 1, 1998, pp. 18–30, https://jstor.org/stable/20107133.

Edson, Margaret. *Wit*. Faber and Faber. 1999.

Ehrenreich, Barbara. "Welcome to Cancerland: A Mammogram Leads to a Cult of Pink Kitch." *Harper's Magazine*, Nov. 2001, pp. 43–53.

Ehrenreich, Barbara. *Natural Causes: An Epidemic of Wellness, the Certainty of Dying, and Killing Ourselves to Live Longer*. Hachette Book Group, 2018.

Ehrenreich, Barbara and Deirdre English. *For Her Own Good: Two Centuries of Experts' Advice to Women*. 1978, Anchor Books, 2005.

Elliott, Carl. *Better Than Well: American Medicine Meets the American Dream*. W.W. Norton & Company, 2003.

Emerson, Ralph Waldo. "Gnothi Seauton." 1831, archive.vcu.edu, https://archive.vcu.edu/english/engweb/transcendentalism/authors/emerson/poems/gnothi.html.

Engs, Ruth Clifford. *The Progressive Era's Health Reform Movement: A Historical Dictionary*. Praeger, 2003.

Esterianna, Leah. "Dancing Mania." *Letters of Dance*, pp. 4, https://www.pbm.com/~lindahl/lod/vol3/dancing_mania.html#n1.

Esposito, Roberto. "The Enigma of Biopolitics." *Bios: Biopolitics and Philosophy*, Translated by Timothy Campbell, U of Minnesota P, 2008, pp. 13–44.

Eternal Sunshine of the Spotless Mind. Directed by Michel Gondry, Focus Features, 2004.

Fantastic Voyage. Directed by Richard Fleischer, Twentieth Century Fox, 1966. Film.

Farr, Christina. "Apple, Google, Samsung Vie to Bring Health Apps to Wearables." *Reuters.com*, 23 June 2014, https://reuters.com/article/us-tech-healthcare-mobilephone-insight/apple-google-samsung-vie-to-bring-health-apps-to-wearables-idUSKBN0EY0BQ20140623.

Farr, Christina, and Alexei Oreskovic. "Exclusive: Facebook Plots First Steps Into Healthcare." *Reuters.com*, 3 Oct. 2014, https://reuters.com/article/idUSKCN0HS0972014100 3.

Fausto-Sterling, Anna. "Refashioning Race: DNA and the Politics of Health Care." *Differences: Journal of Feminist Cultural Studies*, vol. 15, no. 3, 2004, pp. 1–37, https://muse.jhu.edu/article/174488.

FBI. "Amerithrax or Anthrax Investigation." *fbi.gov*, https://fbi.gov/history/famous-cases/amerithrax-or-anthrax-investigation.

Fearnley, Lyle. "Redesigning Syndromic Surveillance for Biosecurity." *Biosecurity Interventions: Global Health and Security in Question*, edited by Andrew Lakoff and Stephen J. Collier, Columbia UP, 2008, pp. 61- 88.

Fears, J. Rufus. "Freedom: The History on an Idea." *Footnotes: The Newsletter of FPRI's Watchman Center*, vol. 12, no. 19, 2007, np, https://www.fpri.org/docs/media/fn1219-lwf-fears.pdf.

Federal Emergency Management Agency. "America's PrepareAthon." *FEMA*, 30 Sep. 2015. community.fema.gov.

Felman, Shoshana. *The Scandal of the Speaking Body: Don Juan, J.L. Austin, or Seduction in Two Languages*, Translated by Catherine Porter. Stanford UP, 2003.

Felski, Rita. "Nothing to Declare: Identity, Shame, and the Lower Middle Class." *PMLA*, vol. 115, no. 1, 2000, pp. 33–45, https://jstor.org/stable/463229.

Ferraro, Susan. "The Anguished Politics of Breast Cancer." *The New York Times*. 15 Aug. 1993, section 6, page 25, column 1, https://beautyoutofdamage.com/nytimesaug151993.pdf.

Fetterley, Judith. *The Resisting Reader: A Feminist Approach to American Fiction*. Indiana UP, 1978.

Fischer-Lichte, Erika. *Ästhetik des Performativen*. Suhrkamp, 2004.

Fitzgerald, Francis Scott. *The Great Gatsby*. 1925, Wordsworth Classics, 1993.

Fluck, Winfried. *Das Kulturelle Imaginäre. Eine Funktionsgeschichte des Amerikanischen Romans 1790–1900*. Suhrkamp, 1997.

Fluck, Winfried. "Funktionsgeschichte und Ästhetische Erfahrung." *Funktionen von Literatur: Theoretische Grundlagen und Modellinterpretationen*, edited by Marion Gymnich and Ansgar Nünning. Wissenschaftlicher Verlag Trier, 2005, pp. 29–53.

Folkenflik, Robert. "Introduction: The Institution of Autobiography." The Culture of Autobiography: Constructions of Self-Representation. Stanford UP, 1993, pp. 1–20.

Folkenflik, Robert. "The Self as Other." *The Culture of Autobiography: Constructions of Self-Representation*. Stanford UP, 1993, pp. 215–236.

Foner, Eric. *The Story of American Freedom*. W.W. Norton & Company, 1998.

FORCE. "Facing Hereditary Cancer Empowered Home Page." *FORCE*, https://facingour risk.org/index.php.

FORCE. "Angelina Jolie and BRCA 1." *FORCE Message Board*. May 2013, https://facingourr isk.org/messageboard/viewtopic.php?f=3&t=46837&hilit=angelina+Jolie.

Ford, Betty. "First Lady Betty Ford's Remarks to the American Cancer Society." New York City, 7 Nov. 1975, Speech, *fordlibrarymuseum.org*, https://fordlibrarymuseum.gov/libr ary/bbfspeeches/751107.asp.

Forster, Edward Morgan. *Aspects of the Novel*. 1927, Harvest Book, 1985.

Fortenbury, Jon. "When Health Ignorance is Bliss: Why so Many People Avoid Taking Medical Tests?" *The Atlantic*, 21 Oct. 2014, https://theatlantic.com/health/archive/20 14/10/when-health-ignorance-is-bliss/381370/.

Fosket, Jennifer Ruth. "Breast Cancer Risk as Disease: Biomedicalizing Risk." *Biomedicalization: Technoscience, Health, and Illness in the U.S.*, edited by Adele E. Clarke, et al. Duke U, pp. 331–352.

Foucault, Michel. *The Birth of the Clinic: An Archeology of Medical Perception*. Translated by A. M. Sheridan Smith, Vintage Books, 1994.

Foucault, Michel. "Technologies of the Self." *Technologies of the Self: A Seminar with Michel Foucault*, edited by Luther H. Martin, Huck Gutman, Patrick H. Hutton, Univ. of Massachusetts Press, 1988, pp. 16–49.

Foucault, Michel. *Security, Territory, Population: Lectures at the Collége de France 1977–78*. Translated by GrahamBurchell, edited by Michel Senellart, Francois Ewald, and Alessandro Fontana, Palgrave, 2007.

Foucault, Michel. "11 Lecture: 17 March 1976." *Society Must Be Defended*, Translated by David Macey, edited by Mauro Bertani, Alessandro Fontana, and Francois Ewald, Picador, pp. 239–263.

Foucault, Michel. "The Subject and Power." *Critical Inquiry*, vol. 8, no. 4, 1982, pp. 777–795, https://jstor.org/stable/1343197.

Foucault, Michel. *Discipline and Punish: The Birth of the Prison*. 1975, Translated by Alan Sheridan. Random House, 1995.

Fox, Susannah, and Maeve Duggan. "Mobile Health 2012." *Pew Research Center*, 2012, https://pewinternet.org/files/old-media/Files/Reports/2012/PIP_MobileHealt h2012_FINAL.pdf.

Frank, Arthur. *The Wounded Storyteller: Body, Illness, and Ethics*. U of Chicago Press, 1995.

Franklin, Benjamin. "Letter to Joseph Priestly." 1780, *The Private Correspondence of Benjamin Franklin – Comprising a Series of Letters on Miscellaneous, Literary, and Political Subjects, 1753–1790. Volume 1*, edited by William Temple Franklin and Henry Colburn, 1917, pp. 52–53.

Franklin, Benjamin. *The Autobiography of Benjamin Franklin*. edited by John Bigelow, J.B. Lippincott & Co. 1868, GoogleBooks.

Franklin, Bruce H. "Hawthorne and Science Fiction." *The Centennial Review*, vol.10, no.1, 1966, pp.112-130.

Freemon, Frank R. "Pretesting for Huntington's Disease: Another View." *The Hasting's Center Report*, vol. 3, no. 4, 1973, pp. 13, https://jstor.org/stable/3561533.

Freud, Sigmund. "Thoughts for the Time of War and Death." 1915, *The Standard Edition of the Complete Psychological Works of Sigmund Freud. 1957, vol. XIV (1914–1916)*. Translated by James Strachey, Anna Freud, Alix Strachey, and Alan Tyson. The Hogarth Press, 1973, pp. 273–302.

Friedan, Betty. *Feminine Mystique*. 1963, Dell, 1974.

Friedman, Sue, Rebecca Sutphen, and Kathy Steligo. *Confronting Hereditary Breast and Ovarian Cancer: Identify Your Risk, Understand Your Options, Change Your Destiny*. John Hopkins U.P., 2012.

Frisby, Cynthia M. "Messages of Hope: Health Communication Strategies that Address Barriers Preventing Black Women from Screening for Breast Cancer." *Journal of Black Studies*, vol. 32, no.5, 2002, pp. 489–505, https://jstor.org/stable/3180949.

Fromm, Harold. "Muses, Spooks, Neurons, and the Rhetoric of 'Freedom'." *New Literary History*, vol. 36, no. 2, 2005, pp. 147–159, https://jstor.org/stable/20057886.

Fulda, Kimberly G., and Kristine Lykens. "Ethical Issues in Predictive Genetic Testing: A Public Health Perspective." *Journal of Medical Ethics*, vol. 32, Nr. 3, 143–147, https://doi.org/10.1136/jme.2004.010272.

Fukuyama, Francis. *Our Posthuman Future. Consequences of the Biotechnology Revolution*. Farrar, Straus and Giroux, 2002.

Funk, Kristi. "A Patient's Journey: Angelina Jolie." *Pink Lotus Breast Center*, 14 May 2013, https://pinklotusbreastcenter.com/breast-cancer-101/2013/05/a-patients-journey-angelina-jolie/.

Fuss, Diana. "Last Words." *ELH*, vol. 76, no. 4, 2009, pp. 877–910, https://jstor.org/stable/27742966

Gaddis, John Lewis. *Surprise, Security, and the American Experience*. Harvard UP, 2004.

Gale, Elaine. "Exploring Perspectives on Cochlear Implants and Language Acquisition within the Deaf Community." *The Journal of Deaf Studies and Deaf Education*, vol. 16, no. 1, 2011, pp. 121–139, https://doi.org/10.1093/deafed/enq044.

Garland-Thomson, Rosemarie. "Feminist Disability Studies." *Signs: Journal of Women in Culture and Society*, vol. 30, no. 2, 2005, pp. 1557–1587, https://jstor.org/stable/10.1086/423352.

Gattaca. Directed by Andrew Niccol, *Columbia Pictures*, 1997.

Genette, Gérard. *Narrative Discourse Revisited*. 1983. Translated by Jane E. Lewin. UP, 1988.

Gessen, Masha. *Blood Matters: From Inherited Illness to Designer Babies, How the World and I Found Ourselves in the Future of the Gene*. Houghton Miflin Harcourt, 2008.

Giddens, Anthony. "Risk and Responsibility." *The Modern Law Review*, vol. 62, no. 1, 1999, pp. 1–10, https://jstor.org/stable/1097071.

Gilroy, Paul. *Between Camps: Nations, Culture, and the Allure of Race*. Harvard UP, 2000.

Gilroy, Paul. "A Response." *Ethnicities*, vol. 2, no. 4, 2002, pp. 554–560, https://jstor.org/stable/23890193.

Gin, Brian R. "Genetic Discrimination: Huntington's Disease and the Americans with Disabilities Act." *Columbia Law Review*, vol. 97, no. 5,1997, pp. 1406–1434, https://doi.org/10.2307/1123439.

Giroux, Henry A. "Reading Hurricane Katrina: Race, Class, and the Biopolitics of Disposability." *College Literature*, vol. 33, no. 3, 2006, pp. 171–196, https://jstor.org/stable/25115372.

Gloyna, Tanja. "Versprechen." *Historisches Wörterbuch der Philosophie Online*, edited by Joachim Ritter, Karlfried Gründer, and Gottfried Gabriel. Schwabe AG, https://doi.org/10.24894/HWPh.4617.

Goffman, Erving. *Stigma*. London: Penguin, 1963.

Goldberg, Matt. "Sundance 2011: How to Die in Oregon – Review." *Collider*. 27 Jan. 2011, https://collider.com/how-to-die-in-oregon-review/.

Goldblatt, Roy. "Trying to Be 'Forever Young' and the Reality of Old Age in Gary Shteyngart's Super Sad True Love Story." *Crossroads of American Studies: Transnational and Biocultural Encounters*, edited by Frederike Offizier, Marc Priewe, and Ariane Schröder. Winter, 2016, pp.507-523. American Studies – A Monograph Series vol. 269.

Good Morning America. "One Woman's Choice Defies Breast Cancer Destiny." *Youtube*. 25 April 2008, uploaded by Doubleday Publishing, https://youtube.com/watch?v=NAteUqDt4Bk

Grady, Denise, Tara Parker-Pope, and Pam Belluck. "Jolie's Disclosure of Preventive Mastectomy Highlights Dilemma" *The New York Times*. 14 May 2013, https://nytimes.com/2013/05/15/health/angelina-jolies-disclosure-highlights-a-breast-cancer-dilemma.html.

Grady, Denise. "Haunted by a Gene." *The New York Times*. 10 March 2020, https://nytimes.com/2020/03/10/health/huntingtons-disease-wexler.html.

Grewe-Salfeld, Mirjam. *Biohacking, Bodies, and Do it Yourself: The Cultural Politics of Hacking Life Itself*. transcript, 2020.

Gu, Yoe. "Narrative, Life Writing, and Healing: The Therapeutic Functions of Storytelling." *Neohelicon*, no.45, 2008, pp.479-489, https://doi.org/10.1007/s11059-018-0459-4.

Guglielmo, Connie and Parmy Olson. "The Case Against Wearables, Or Why We Won't All Look Like The Borg This Year" *Forbes*. 3 March 2014, https://forbes.com/sites/connieguglielmo/2014/02/12/the-case-against-wearables/.

Gutierrez, Alberto. "Warning Letter: Document Number: GEN1300666." *FDA*, 22 Nov. 2013, https://fda.gov/ICECI/EnforcementActions/WarningLetters/2013/ucm376296.htm.

Habermas, Jürgen. *The Future of Human Nature*. 2001. Translated by William Rehg, Max Pensky, and Hella Beister. Polity Press, 2003.

Hacking, Ian. "How We Have Been Learning to Talk about Autism: A Role for Stories." *Cognitive Disability and Its Challenge to Moral Philosophy*, Special Issue in *Metaphilosophy*, vol. 40, no. 3/ 4, 2009, pp. 499–516, https://jstor.org/stable/24439798.

Haldane, John Burdon Sanderson. *Daedalus, or Science and the Future: A Paper Read to the Heretics, Cambridge, on February 4th*. London: Kegan Paul, Trench, Trubner & Co., LTD., https://static.torontopubliclibrary.ca/da/pdfs/37131068273747d.pdf.

Hall, Stuart. "Ethnicity: Identity and Difference." *Becoming National: A Reader*, edited by Geoff Eley and Ronald Grigor Suny, Oxford UP, 1996, pp. 339–351.

Hamilton, Sheryl N. "Traces of the Future: Biotechnology, Science Fiction, and the Media." *Social Science Fiction*, special issue in *Science Fiction Studies*, vol. 30, no. 2, 2003, pp. 267–282, https://jstor.org/stable/4241173.

Hamilton, John T. "Procurators: On the Limits of Caring for Another." Telos, no. 170, 2015, pp. 7–22, https://doi.org/10.3817/0315170007.

Hamilton, John T. *Security: Politics, Humanity, and the Philology of Care*. Princeton UP, 2013.

Hansen, Randall, and Desmond King. *Sterilized by the State: Eugenics, Race, and the Population Scare in Twentieth-Century North America*. Cambridge UP, 2013.

Haraway, Donna. "A Cyborg Manifesto: Science, Technology and Socialist-Feminism in the Late Twentieth Century." 1985. *The Cybercultures Reader*, edited by David Bell and Barbara M. Kennedy, Routledge, 2000, pp. 291–324.

Hardwig, John: "Going to Meet Death: The Art of Dying in the Early Part of the Twenty-First Century." *Hasting's Center Report*, vol. 39, no. 4, 2009, pp. 37 -45, https://doi.org/10.1353/hcr.0.0151.

Hartman, Stephanie. "Reading the Scar in Breast Cancer Poetry." *Feminist Studies*, vol. 30., no.1, 2004, pp. 155–177, https://jstor.org/stable/3178563.

Hartung, Heike, and Rüdiger Kunow. "Introduction: Age Studies." *Amerikastudien/ American Studies*, vol. 56, no.1, 2011, pp. 15–22.

Hawthorne, Nathaniel. *The Scarlet Letter*. 1850. Penguin, 2003.

Hawthorne, Nathaniel. "Rappaccini's Daughter" 1844. *Mosses from an Old Manse*. 1846. Modern Library Classics, 2003, pp. 71 – 99.

Hawthorne, Nathaniel. "The Birth-Mark." 1843. *The Norton Anthology of Short Fiction. 3rd Ed.*, edited by R.V. Cassill, W.W. Norton & Company, 1986, pp. 628–641.

Hayles, N. Katherine. *How We Became Posthuman: Virtual Bodies in Cybernetics, Literature, and Informatics*. U of Chicago P, 1999.

Heidegger, Martin. *Being and Time*. 1927. Translated by John Macquarrie, and Edward Robinson, Harper and Row Publishers, 1962.

Heilman, Robert Brechthold. "Hawthorne's 'The Birthmark:' Science as Religion." 1949. *Literary Theories in Praxis*, 1987, edited by Shirley F. Staton, U of Pennsylvania P. 4th Ed. 1993, pp. 35–41.

Hemmings, Clare. "Invoking Affect: Cultural Theory and the Ontological Turn." *Cultural Studies*, vol. 19, no. 5, 2005, pp. 548 -567, https://doi.org/10.1080/09502380500365473 .

Henry, Katherine. *Liberalism and the Culture of Security: Nineteenth-Century Rhetoric of Reform*. U of Alabama P, 2011.

Herndl, Diane Price. "Our Breasts, Our Selves: Identity, Community, and Ethics in Cancer Autobiographies." *Signs*, vol. 32, no.1, 2006, pp. 221–245, https://jstor.org/stable/10.1086/505542.

Herndl, Diane Price. "Virtual Cancer: BRCA and Posthuman Narratives of Deleterious Mutation." *Theorizing Breast Cancer: Narratives, Politics, Memory*, special issue in *Tulsa Studies in Women's Literature*, vol.32/33, no.2/1, 2013/ 2014, pp.25-45, https://jstor.org/stable/43653275.

Hesiod. *Works and Days*. Translated and Edited by A.E. Stallings, Penguin Books, 2018.

Heyen, Nils B. "Self-Tracking as Knowledge Production: Quantified Self Between Prosumption and Citizen Science." *Lifelogging: Digital Self-tracking and Lifelogging–Between Disruptive Technology and Cultural Transformation*, edited by Stefan Selke, Springer, 2016, pp. 283–304.

Hirsch, Jenny. "Race, Genetics, and Scientific Integrity" *Journal of Health Care for the Poor and Underserved*, vol. 2, no. 3, 1991, pp. 331–334, https://doi.org/0.1353/hpu.2010.0046.

History of Vaccines. "All Timelines Overview." *History of Vaccines.org*, The College of Physicians of Philadelphia, https://www.historyofvaccines.org/timeline/all.

Hoffman, Margaret, and Di Cooper. "Healthwatch: Breast Cancer: A Stitch in Time Saves Nine." *Agenda: Empowering Women for Gender Equity*, vol. 28, 1996, pp. 108–112, https://doi.org/10.1080/10130950.1996.9675509.

Holloway, Karla F.C. "Editor's Afterword: Private Bodies/Public Texts: Literature, Science, and States of Surveillance." *Literature and Medicine*, vol. 26, no. 1, 2007, pp. 269–276, https://doi.org/10.1353/lm.2008.0004.

Holloway, Karla F.C. *Private Bodies, Public Texts: Race, Gender, and a Cultural Bioethics.* Duke UP, 2011.

Horwitz, Allan V., and Gerald N. Grob. "The Checkered History of American Psychiatric Epidemiology." *The Milbank Quarterly*, vol 89, no. 4, 2011, pp. 628–657, https://doi.org/10.1111/j.1468-0009.2011.00645.x.

Howarth, Glennys. *Death and Dying. A Sociological Introduction.* Oxford: Polity Press, 2007.

How To Die in Oregon. Directed by Peter Richardson, performances by Harry Bruton, Ray Carnay, Cody Curtis, Docurama, Jan. 2011.

Howe, Susan. *The Birthmark: Unsettling the Wilderness in American Literary History.* Wesleyan U.P., 1993.

Hughes, Kate, and DonnaWyatt. "The Rise and Sprawl of Breast Cancer Pink: An Analysis." *Visual Studies*, vol. 30, no.3, 2015, pp. 280–294, https://doi.org/10.1080/1472586X.2015.1017351.

Hughes, Langston. "Harlem." 1951, 1959. *Norton Anthology: African American Literature*, Edited by Henry Louis Gates and Nellie Y McKay, W.W. Norton & Company,1997, pp. 1267.

Humphrey, Derek. "Liberty and Death: A Manifesto Concerning an Individuals's Right to Choose to Die." *Finalexit.org.*, April 8. 2007, https://finalexit.org/liberty_and_death_manifesto_right_to_die_by_derek_humphry.html

Huntington, George. "On Chorea." 1872. *Neuropsychiatry Classics*, vol. 15, no.1, 2003, pp.109-112, https://doi.org/10.1176/jnp.15.1.109.

Huxley, Aldous. *Brave New World.* 1932. Harper Perennial Modern Classics, 1998.

Igoe, Katherine. "The 'Angelina Jolie' Effect." *News and Research.* Havard Medical School Website. 14 Dec. 2016, https://hms.harvard.edu/news/angelina-jolie-effect.

Illich, Ivan. "The Medicalization of Life." *Journal of Medical Ethics*, vol. 1, no. 2, 1975, pp. 73–77, https://jstor.org/stable/27715497.

Illich, Ivan. *Medical Nemesis: The Expropriation of Health.* 1975. Pantheon Books, 1976.

"Immigration Act" 1891. U.S. Congress. "Chapt. 551. An Act in Amendment to the Various Acts Relative to Immigration and the Importation of Aliens Under Contract or Agreement to Perform Labor." 51st Congress, Sess. II, Chap. 551; 26 Stat. 1084.; 3 March 1891, https://library.uwb.edu/Static/USimmigration/26%20stat%201084.pdf.

"Immigration Act" 1907. U.S. Congress. "Chap. 1134. An Act To Regulate the Immigration of Aliens into the United States." Fifty-Ninth Congress, Session 11, Ch. 1134. 1907: 898–911, https://loc.gov/law/help/statutes-at-large/59th-congress/session-2/c 59s2ch1134.pdf.

Inception. Directed by Christopher Nolan, Warner Bros. Pictures, 2010.

Infectonator. Toge Productions, 2017.

In Time. Directed by Andrew Niccol, New Regency Productions, 2011.

Iser, Wolfgang. "The Current Situation of Literary Theory: Key Concepts in the Imaginary." *New Literary History*, vol. 11, 1979, pp. 1–20, https://doi.org/10.2307/468868.

Ishiguro, Kazuo. *Never Let Me Go*. 2005, Vintage Books, 2006.

Jackson, Charles O., editor. *Passing: The Vision of Death in America*. Greenwood Press, 1977.

Jacobson v Massachusetts. 197 US 11–39. Supreme Court of the US. 1905. *U.S. Reports: Volume 197 (55)*. Library of Congress, https://cdn.loc.gov/service/ll/usrep/usrep197/usre p197011/usrep197011.pdf.

James, William. "What is an Emotion?" *Mind*, vol. 9, no. 34, 1884, pp. 188–205, https://jst or.org/stable/2246769.

Jameson, Frederic. *Postmodernism or the Cultural Logic of Late Capitalism*. Duke UP, 1991

Jameson, Frederic. *The Seeds of Time*. Columbia UP, 1994.

Jameson, Frederic. "Progress Versus Utopia: or, Can We Imagine the Future?" *Utopia and Anti-Utopia*, special issue in *Science Fiction Studies*, vol. 9, no. 2, 1982, pp. 147–158, http s://jstor.org/stable/4239476.

Jameson, Frederic. *Archeologies of the Future: The Desire Called Utopia and Other Science Fictions*. Verso, 2005.

Jayne, Allen. *Jefferson's Declaration of Independence: Origins, Philosophy, and Theology*. U of Kentucky P., 1998.

Jefferson, Thomas. "A Tribute of Gratitude (letter) to Edward Jenner." Monticello, 14. May, 1806. *The Letters of Thomas Jefferson: 1743–1826*, https://iupui.edu/ ~histwhs/h364.dir/jeffjenner.html.

Jefferson, Thomas. "The American Mind." 1825. *The American Soul: The Contested Legacy of the Declaration of Independence*, edited by Justin Buckley Dyer, Rowman and Littlefield Publishers, Inc., 2012, pp. 19.

Jefferson, Thomas. "Fifty Years Later." 1826. *The American Soul: The Contested Legacy of the Declaration of Independence*, edited by Justin Buckley Dyer, Rowman and Littlefield Publishers, Inc., 2012, pp. 34–35.

Johnson, Barbara. "Apostrophe, Animation, and Abortion." *Diacritics*, vol. 16, no.1, 1986, pp.28-47, https://doi.org/10.2307/464649.

Jolie, Angelina. "My Medical Choice" *The New York Times*. Opinion Pages. 14 May 2013, htt ps://nytimes.com/2013/05/14/opinion/my-medical-choice.html.

Jolie Pitt, Angelina. "Angelina Jolie Pitt: Diary of a Surgery." *New York Times Magazine*. 24 March, 2015, https://nytimes.com/2015/03/24/opinion/angelina-jolie-pitt-diary-of-a-surgery.html.

Jones, Colin, and Roy Porter, editors. *Reassessing Foucault: Power, Medicine, and The Body*. Routledge, 1994, 2001.

Kahn, Jennifer. "The CRISPR Quandary." *The New York Times*, 9 Nov. 2015, https://nytimes .com/2015/11/15/magazine/the-crispr-quandary.html.

Kaltofen, Carolin. "Engaging Adorno: Critical Security Studies After Emancipation." *Security Dialogue*, vol. 44, no.1, 2013, pp.37-51, https://doi.org/10.1177/0967010612470392.

Kass, Leon R. *Human Cloning and Human Dignity: The Report of the President's Council on Bioethics*. New York: Public Affairs, 2002.

Kass, Leon R. "Welcome and Opening Remarks." *President's Council on Bioethics*, session 18 Jan. 2002, https://bioethicsarchive.georgetown.edu/pcbe/transcripts/jan02/jan18 open.html.

Kasper, Anne S., Susan J. Ferguson, editors. *Breast Cancer: Society Shapes an Epidemic*. Palgrave, 2002.

Kellehear, Allan. "On Dying and Human Suffering." *Palliative Medicine*, vol. 23, 2009, pp. 388–397, https://doi.org/10.1177/0269216309104858.

Kellehear, Allan. *Social History of Dying*. Cambridge UP, 2007.

Kemp, Martin. "The Mona Lisa of Modern Science." *Nature*, vol. 421, 2003, pp. 416–420, https://doi.org/10.1038/nature01403.

Kemp, Martin. *Visualizations. The Nature Book of Art and Science*. Oxford U P, 2000.

Kennerly, David Hume. "First Lady Betty Ford's Breast Cancer Surgery." Photographed 2 Oct. 1974. *Gerald R. Ford Library*, https://fordlibrarymuseum.gov/images/avproj/pop -ups/A1170-18A-BBF.html.

Khatib, Sami. "The Messianic Without Messianism: Walter Benjamin's Materialist Theology." *Anthropology and Materialism*, vol. 1, 2013, pp. 1–17, https://doi.org/10.4000/am. 159.

"King James Bible." King James Bible Online, 2016, https://kingjamesbibleonline.org.

King, Martin Luther Jr. "I Have a Dream..." 28 Aug. 1963. Address Delivered at the Civil Rights March on Washington D.C. for Jobs and Freedom, Washington D.C., https://kinginstitute.stanford.edu/king-papers/documents/i-have-dream-ad dress-delivered-march-washington-jobs-and-freedom.

King, Samantha. "Pink Ribbons Inc: Breast Cancer Activism and the Politics of Philanthropy." International Journal of Qualitative Studies in Education, vol. 17, no.4, 2004, pp. 473–492, https://doi.org/10.1080/0951839041000-1709553.

King, Samantha. "Pink Diplomacy: On the Uses and Abuses of Breast Cancer Awareness." *Health Communication*, vol.25, no.3, 2010, pp. 286–289, https://doi.org/10.1080/10410 231003698960.

Kingston, Maxine Hong. *Tripmaster Monkey: His Fake Book*. 1987. Random House, 1990.

Klawiter, M. "From Private Stigma to Global Assembly: Transforming the Terrain of Breast Cancer." *Global Ethnography: Forces, Connections and Imaginations in a Postmodern World*, edited by M. Blum Burawoy et al., U of Californa P., 2000, Pp. 299–334.

Klawiter, Maren. *The Biopolitics of Breast Cancer: Changing Cultures of Disease and Activism*. U of Minnesota P, 2008.

Klaver, Elizabeth: "A Mind Body Flesh Problem: The Case of Margaret Edson's Wit." *Contemporary Literature*. vol XLV, no. 4, 2004, pp. 659–682, https://doi.org/10.2307/35935 45.

Kleinman, Arthur. *The Illness Narratives: Suffering, Healing, and the Human Condition*. Perseus Book Group. 1988.

Kluger, Jeffrey. "The Angelina Effect: TIME's New Cover Image Revealed." *Time.com*, 15 May 2013, https://healthland.time.com/2013/05/15/the-angelina-effect-times-new-cover-image-revealed/.

Koblentz, Gregory D. "Biosecurity Reconsidered: Calibrating Biological Threats and Responses." *International Affairs*, vol. 34, no. 4, 2010, pp. 96–113, https://jstor.org/stable/40784563.

Koblentz, Gregory D. "From Biodefense to Biosecurity: The Obama Administration's Strategy for Countering Biological Threats." *International Affairs*, vol. 88, no. 1, 2012, pp. 131–48, https://jstor.org/stable/41428545.

Koch, Erin. "Disease as Security Threat." *Biosecurity Interventions: Global Health and Security in Question*. edited by Andrew Lakoff and Stephen J. Collier, Columbia UP, 2008, pp. 121- 146.

KOMEN. "2019 Susan G. Komen Twin Cities Race for the Cure: Minutes." https://awinmn.org/events/2019-race-for-the-cure/.

Kriebernegg, Ulla. "Ending Aging in the Shteyngart of Eden: Biogerontological Discourse in a Super Sad True Love Story." *Journal of Ageing Studies*, vol. 27, 2013, pp. 61–70, https://doi.org/0.1016/j.jaging.2012.10.003.

Kübler-Ross, Elisabeth. "On the Fear of Death." *Passing: The Vision of Death in America*, edited by Charles O. Jackson, Greenwood Press, 1977, pp. 210–218.

Kübler-Ross, Elisabeth. *On Death and Dying: What the Dying Have to Teach Doctors, Nurses, and Their Own Families*. 1967. Touchstone, 1997.

Kunow, Rüdiger. "The Biology of Community: Contagious Disease, Old Age, Biotech, and Cultural Studies." *Communicating Disease: Cultural Representations of American Medicine*, edited by Carmen Birkle and Johanna Heil, Winter, 2013, pp. 265–287.

Kunow, Rüdiger. "Coming of Age." *Representation and Decoration in a Postmodern Age*, edited by Alfred Hornung and Rüdiger Kunow. Winter, 2009, pp. 295–308.

Kunow, Rüdiger. *Material Bodies: Biology and Culture in the United States*. Winter, 2018. [Series: *American Studies: A Monograph Series*].

Kushner, Rose. *Breast Cancer: A Personal History and an Investigative Report*. Harcourt Brace Jovanovich, 1974.

Lakhtakia, Ritu. "A Brief History of Breast Cancer: Part I, Surgical Domination Reinvented." *Sultan Qaboos University Medical Journal*, vol. 14, no. 2, 2014, pp. 166–169. Epub 2014 Apr 7. PMID: 24790737; PMCID: PMC3997531.

Lakoff, Andrew. "From Population to Vital System: National Security and the Changing Object of Public Health." *Biosecurity Interventions: Global Health and Security in Question*, edited by Andrew Lakoff and Stephen J. Collier, Columbia UP, 2008, pp. 33–60.

Lane, Harlan. "Construction of Deafness" *Disabilities Studies Reader*, edited by Lennard Davis, Routledge, 2006, pp. 79–92.

Latour, Bruno. "Why Has Critique Run out of Steam? From Matters of Fact to Matters of Concern." *Critical Inquiry*, vol. 30, no. 2, 2004, pp. 225–248, https://jstor.org/stable/10.1086/421123.

Latour, Bruno. "The More Manipulation the Better." *Representation in Scientific Practice Revisited*, edited by Catelijne Coopmans, Janet Vertesi, Michael Lynch, and Steve Woolgar, MIT Press, 2014, pp. 343–350.

Lederberg, Joshua. "Biological Future of Man." *Man and His Future*, edited by Gordon Wolstenholme, Little, Brown and Co., 1963, pp. 263–273.

Lejeune, Philippe. *On Autobiography*. 1975. Translated by Katherine Leary, edited by Paul John Eakin. U of Minnesota P., 1989.

Lepore, Jill. "It's Spreading: Outbreaks, Media Scares, and the Parrot Panic of 1930." *The New Yorker*, 1 June 2009, pp. 46–50.

Lerner, Baron H. *Breast Cancer Wars: Fear, Hope and the Pursuit of a Cure in Twentieth-Century America*. Oxford UP, 2001.

Lerner, Baron H. "Inventing a Curable Disease: Historical Perspectives on Breast Cancer." *Breast Cancer: Society Shapes an Epidemic*, edited by Anne S. Kasper and Susan J. Ferguson, Palgrave, 2002, pp. 25–49.

Levin, Miles. *Keep Fighting, Stop Struggling: The Miles Levin Story*, edited by Dianne Rice, Kindle Edition, 2012.

Levinas, Emmanuel. *Alterity and Transcendence*. Translated by Michael B Smith. Columbia UP, 1995.

Levinas, Emmanuel. *Time and Other*. Translated by Richard A. Cohen, Duquesne UP, 1987.

Levitas, Ruth. "Discourses of Risk and Utopia." *The Risk Society and Beyond: Critical Issues for Social Theory*. Sage Publication, 2000, pp. 198–211, https://doi.org/10.4135/9781446 219539.n11.

Levitas, Ruth. *Utopia as Method: The Imaginary Reconstitution of Society*. Palgrave, 2013.

Leys, Ruth. "The Turn to Affect: A Critique." *Critical Inquiry*, vol. 37, 2011, pp. 434–472, https://doi.org/10.1086/659353.

Lilypond. "Lilypond's Story." *Breastcancer.org*, 7 May 2018. https://breastcancer.org/community/acknowledging/genetic-testing/Lilypond.

Lincoln, Abraham. "Gettysburg Address." 19 Nov. 1863. *The American Soul: The Contested Legacy of the Declaration of Independence*, edited by Justin Buckley Dyer, Rowman and Littlefield Publishers, Inc., 2012, pp 83–84.

Linton, Simi. "What is Disability Studies?" *PMLA*, vol. 120, no. 2, 2005.pp. https://jstor.org/stable/25486177.

Lisa J. "Lisa J." *Voices of FORCE*. Facingourrisk.org, https://facingourrisk.org/get-involved/HBOC-community/voices-of-FORCE/voices-individual.php?voice=575.

Locke, John. "Two Treatises of Government." 1689. *Two Treatise of Government and a Letter Concerning Toleration*, edited by Ian Shapiro. Yale UP, 2013, pp. 1–210.

Locke, Margaret. "Breast Cancer: Reading the Omens." *Anthropology Today*, vol. 14, no. 4, 1998, pp. 7–16, https://doi.org/10.2307/2783351.

Lohr, Steve. "Facial recognition is Accurate, if You're a White Guy." *The New York Times*, 9 Feb. 2018, https://nytimes.com/2018/02/09/technology/facial-recognition-race-artificial-intelligence.html.

Lombardo, Paul A. *A Century of Eugenics in America: From the Indiana Experiment to the Human Genome Era*. Indiana UP, 2011.

Long, Susan Orpett "Cultural Scripts for a Good Death in Japan and the United States: Similarities and Differences." *Social Science and Medicine*, vol. 58, 2004, pp. 913–928, https://doi.org/10.1016/j.socscimed.2003.10.037.

Lorde, Audre. *The Cancer Journals*. 1980. Sheba Feminist Publishers, 1985.

Lowry, Lois. *The Giver*. 1993. Harper Collins, 2014.

Luhmann, Niklas. *Risk: A Sociological Theory*. Translated by Rhodes Barrette. De Gruyter, 1993.

Lupton, Deborah. *Imperative of Health: Public Health and The Regulated Body*. 1995. Sage Publications, 1997.

Lupton, Deborah. "You are Your Data: Self-Tracking Practices and Concepts of Data." *Lifelogging: Digital Self-tracking and Lifelogging– Between Disruptive Technology and Cultural Transformation*, edited by Stefan Selke, Springer, 2016, pp. 61–79.

MacKay, Charles R. "Ethical Issues in Research Design and Conduct: Developing a Test to Detect Carriers of Huntington's Disease." *Ethics and Human Research*, vol. 6, no. 4, 1984, pp 1–5. PMID: 11649560.

Maloney, William James. *The Medical Lives of History's Famous People*. Bentham, 2014.

Marcum, James A. "Reflections of Humanizing Biomedicine." *Perspectives in Biology and Medicine*, vol. 51, no. 3, 2008, pp. 392–405, https://doi.org/10.1353/pbm.0.0023.

Marelli, Giana D., and Rae A. Moses. "Obituaries and the Discursive Construction of Dying and Living." *Texas Linguistic Forum*, vol. 47, 2003, pp. 123–130.

Marketwatch. "Ultrasound Devices Market to Reach US $ 7.0 Billion by 2022." *Marketwatch.com*, 16 Oct. 2018, https://marketwatch.com/press-release/ultrasound-devices-market-to-reach-us-70-billion-by-2022-2018-10-16.

Markvoort, Eva. "65 Red Roses." 65_Red Roses, https://65redroses.livejournal.com

Mason, Bobbie Ann. *Spence And Lila*. 1988. Ecco, 1998.

Massumi, Brian. "Potential Politics and the Primacy of Preemption." *Text and Critique*, vol. 10, no.2, 2007, pp. 1–9, https://doi.org/0.1353/tae.2007.0066.

Massumi, Brian. "The Future Birth of the Affective Fact." *radicalempiricism.org*, Oct. 2005, pp. 1–11.

Massumi, Brian. "Fear (The Spectrum Said)." *Positions: East Asia Cultures Critique*, vol. 13, no. 1, 2005, pp. 31–48, https://muse.jhu.edu/article/185296.

Massumi, Brian. "The Autonomy of Affect." *Cultural Critique*, vol. 31, no. 2, 1995, pp. 83–109, https://jstor.org/stable/1354446.

Mather, Cotton. *Parentator: Memoirs of Remarkables in the Life and the Death of the Ever-Memorable Dr. Increase Mather. Who Expired, August 23.* 1724. Ann Arbor, MI: Text Creation Partnership, 2007-01. *Evans Early American Imprint Collection*, name.umdl.umich.edu/N02149.0001.001.

Matuschka. "Beauty out of Damage." 1993. Cover *The New York Times Magazine*, 13 Aug. 1993, https://nytimes.com/2018/08/15/insider/breast-cancer-mastectomy-photo.html.

Mayer, Michelle Lyn. "Portrait of a Dying Mom." *Blogspot*, 2008, https://diaryofadyingmom.blogspot.com/.

Maynard, Brittany. "Brittany Maynard's Legislative Testimony." *Youtube*, uploaded by Compassion and Choice, 31. March 2015, https://youtube.com/watch?v=Mi8AP_EhM94.

Maynard, Brittany. "A Video for All My Friends." *Youtube*, uploaded by Compassion and Choice, 30 Oct. 2014.

McCabe, Linda L. and Edward R. McCabe. "Are We Entering a 'Perfect Storm' for a Resurgence of Eugenics? Science, Medicine, and Their Social Context." *A Century of Eugenics in America: From the Indiana Experiment to the Human Genome Era*. Edited by Paul A. Lombardo, Indiana UP, 2011, pp. 193–218.

McFarland, Sara. "How Much Does Pregnancy Cost Each Trimester?" *Parasil.com*, 30 March 2017, https://parasail.com/2017/03/30/pregnancy-cost-trimester-chart/.

Meadows, Donella H., et al. *The Limits of Growth: A Report of the Club of Rome's Project on the Predicament of Mankind*. Universe Books, 1972.

Meißner, Stefan. "Effects of Quantified Self Beyond Self-Optimization." *Lifelogging: Digital Self-tracking and Lifelogging– Between Disruptive Technology and Cultural Transformation*, edited by Stefan Selke, Springer, 2016, pp. 235–248.

Melville, Herman. "Bartleby: The Scrivener." 1853. *Billy Budd, Bartleby, and Other Stories*. 1986. edited by Peter Coviello, 2013, pp. 17–54.

Merleau-Ponty, Maurice. *Phenomenology of Perception*. 1945. Translated by Donald A. Landes, Routledge, 2012.

Metzger, Deena. "Warrior Poster." 1979, https://cdn.jwa.org/sites/default/files/mediaobjects/warrior_poster.jpg.

Metzl, Jonathan. "'Mother's Little Helper': The Crisis of Psychoanalysis and the Miltown Resolution." *Gender and History*, vol.15, no.2, 2003, pp. 240–267, https://doi.org/10.1111/1468-0424.00300.

Meyer, Adolf. "The Mental Hygiene Movement." *The Canadian Medical Association Journal*, vol. 8, no. 7, 1918, pp. 632–634, https://doi.org/10.2307/368156.

Meyer, Dan. "A Brief History of Medicine and Statistics." *Essential Evidence Based Medicine*. Cambridge UP, 2009, pp. 1- 10.

Middleton, Katrina L. "Mastectomy." 1988. *Her Soul Beneath the Bone: Women's Poetry on Breast Cancer*, edited by Leatrice Lifshitz, U of Illinois P, 1991, pp. 39.

Mikulic, Matej. "2022 list of top U.S. Biotech and Pharmaceutical Companies Based on Revenue." *statista*, 14 Oct. 2022, https://statista.com/statistics/257436/top-global-biotech-and-pharmaceutical-companies-based-on-revenue/.

Mikulic, Matej. "U.S. total medicine spending 2002–2021." *statista*, 8 June 2022, statista.com/statistics/238689/us-total-expenditure-on-medicine/.

Milburn, Colin. *Nanovision: Engineering the Future*. Durham: Duke UP, 2008.

Mitchell, Pita. *Contagious Metaphors*. Bloomsbury, 2012.

Mitford, Jessica. *The American Way of Death Revisited*. Alfred A. Knopf, 1998.

Mitford, Jessica. *The American Way of Birth*. Penguin Books, 1992.

Mizruchi, Susan. "Risk Theory and the Contemporary American Novel." *American Literary History*, vol. 22, no. 1, 2010, pp. 109–135, https://muse.jhu.edu/journals/alh/summary/v022/22.1.mizruchi.html.

Moses, Michele. "What Drives Doomsday Preppers." *The New Yorker*, 13 Nov. 2018, https://newyorker.com/culture/culture-desk/what-drives-doomsday-preppers.

Moynihan, Ray, and Alan Cassels. *Selling Sickness: How Drug Companies Are Turning Us All into Patients*. Allen and Unwin, 2005.

Mukherjee, Siddartha. The Emperor of All Maladies: A Biography of Cancer. Fourth Estate, 2011.

Nash, Meredith. "From 'Bump' To 'Baby': Gazing at the Foetus in 4D." *Philament Surveillance*, vol. 10, 2007, pp. 1–25, https://philamentjournal.com/wp-content/uploads/2019/06/Nash_Article_Bump.pdf.

National Institute of Neurological Disorders and Stroke. "Huntington's Disease: Hope Through Research." *NINDS*, 18 Nov. 2019, https://catalog.ninds.nih.gov/pubstatic//2 0-NS-19/20-NS-19_508.pdf.

National Institute of Health. "Biennial Report of the Directors, National Institute of Health: Fiscal Year 2006 &2007." *NIH*, 2008/09, https://report.nih.gov/biennialrep ort0607/.

National Institute of Health. "Budget." *NIH*, 29 June 2020, https://nih.gov/about-nih/w hat-we-do/budget.

National Institute of Health. "Strategic Vision for The Future: From Curative to Preemptive." Biennial Report of the Director. *NIH*, 2008, https://rarediseases.info.nih.gov/f iles/nihbreport_admincopy_may22congress[1].pdf.

National Institute of Health. "Revitalization Act of 1993, Public Law 103–43." *Institute of Medicine (US) Committee on Ethical and Legal Issues Relating to the Inclusion of Women in Clinical Studies*, edited by A.C. Mastroianni, R. Faden, and D. Federman. "Women and Health Research: Ethical and Legal Issues of Including Women in Clinical Studies: Volume I." Washington (DC), National Academies Press (US), 1994, https://ncbi.nlm. nih.gov/books/NBK236531/.

National LGBT Cancer Network. "Queer Women Breast Cancer Survivors and Reconstruction Decisions." *Cancer Network*, https://cancer-network.org/cancer-informati on/lesbians-and-cancer/queer-women-breast-cancer-survivors-reconstruction-de cisions/.

Nelkin, Dorothy, and M. Susan Lindee. *The DNA Mystique: The Gene as Cultural Icon*. 2004. U of Michigan P, 2007.

Nelkin, Dorothy. *Selling Science: How the Press Covers Science and Technology*. W.H. Freeman, 1995.

Never Let Me Go. Directed by Mark Romanek, Fox Searchlight Pictures, 2010.

Newman, William R. *Promethean Ambitions: Alchemy and the Quest to Perfect Nature*. New of Chicago P, 2004.

New York Department of Health. "Advice to Those Who have Colds: Grip Influenza or Pneumonia." 1929. *The New York Academy of Medicine*, 11 Dec 2013, https://nyamcenterf orhistory.files.wordpress.com/2013/12/advice_1_watermark.jpg.

Ngai, Sianne. *Ugly Feelings*. Harvard UP, 2005.

Nichols, Bill. "The Voice of the Documentary." *Film Quarterly*, vol. 36, no.3. 1983, pp. 17–30, https://jstor.org/stable/3697347.

Nichols, Bill. *Introduction to Documentary*. 2001, Indiana UP, 2010.

Nie, Jing-Bao, et a. "Healing Without Waging War: Beyond Military Metaphors in Medicine and HIV Cure Research." *American Journal for Bioethics*, vol. 16, no. 10, 2016, pp. 3–11, https://doi.org/10.1080/15265161.2016.1214305.

Nixon, Richard. "State of the Union Address, January 22, 1971". *Public Papers of The Presidents of the United States: Richard M. Nixon 1971*. University of Michigan Library, 2005, pp. 50–58, https://Name.umdl.umich.edu/4731800.1971.001.

Nixon, Richard. "Remarks to the American Medical Association's House of Delegates Meeting in Atlanta City, New Jersey June 22 1971." *Public Papers of The Presidents of the United States: Richard M. Nixon 1971*. University of Michigan Library, 2005, pp. 761–770, https://Name.umdl.umich.edu/4731800.1971.001.

Nixon, Richard. "Proclamation 4120—Cancer Control Month, 1972." April 4, 1972, *Public Papers of The Presidents of the United States: Richard M. Nixon 1972.* University of Michigan Library, 2005.

Nixon, Richard. "Special Message to Congress: Proposing a Comprehensive Health Insurance Plan." 6 Feb 1974. *The Nixon Foundation*, https://issuu.com/richardnixonfoundation/docs/nixonchipspeech.

Nobel Prize.Org. "All Nobel Prizes in Physiology or Medicine." *The Nobel Prize*, https://nobelprize.org/prizes/lists/all-nobel-laureates-in-physiology-or-medicine/.

Novas, Carlos. "The Political Economy of Hope: Patients' Organizations, Science and Bio-value." *Biosocieties*, vol. 1, no. 03, 2006, pp. 289–305, https://doi.org/10.1017/S1745855206003024.

Nussbaum, Martha C. "Compassion: The Basic Social Emotion." *Social Philosophy and Policy*, vol. 13, no. 1, 1996, pp. 27–58, https://doi.org/10.1017/S0265052500001515.

Nye, Coleman. "Cancer Previval and the Theatrical Fact." *The Drama Review*, vol. 56, no. 4, 2012, pp. 104–120, https://jstor.org/stable/i23362379.

Obama Barack. "Remarks by the President on Ebola." 2014. *The White House: President Barack Obama*, 28 Oct. 2014, https://go.wh.gov/pV8swn.

O'Brien, Sharon: "The Country of the Ill" (Review). *American Quarterly*, vol. 52, no. 4, 2000, pp. 765–774, https://doi.org/10.1353/aq.2000.0051.

Oh, Sam S., Neeta Thakur, et al. "Diversity in Clinical and Biomedical Research: A Promise Yet to Be Fulfilled." *PloS Med*, vol. 12, no. 12, 2015, pp. 1–9, https://doi.org/10.1371/journal.pmed.1001918.

O'Neil, Luke. "$50 Could Have Saved Him, But His GoFundMe pitch Didn't Get the Clicks." *Boston Globe*, 7 March 2019. WEB, https://bostonglobe.com/ideas/2019/03/07/could-have-saved-him-but-his-gofundme-pitch-didn-get-clicks/44416UyhloXUf-DRIxE5SlI/story.html.

Oregon Public Health Division. "Oregon Death with Dignity Act: 2014 Data Summary." 2 Feb. 2015, https://oregon.gov/oha/PH/PROVIDERPARTNERRESOURCES/EVALUATIONRESEARCH/DEATHWITHDIGNITYACT/Documents/year17.pdf.

Orenstein, Peggy. "Our Feel-Good War on Breast Cancer." *New York Times Magazine.* 25 April 2013, https://www.nytimes.com/2013/04/28/magazine/our-feel-good-war-on-breast-cancer.html?_r=0&pagewanted=print.

Orenstein, Peggy. "Reacting to Angelina Jolie's Breast Cancer News." *The New York Times.* 15 May 2013, https://6thfloor.blogs.nytimes.com/2013/05/15/reacting-to-angelina-jolies-breast-cancer-news/.

Orphan Black. created by Kim Coghill et al., seasons 1–5, BBC America, 2013–2017.

Orwell, George. *Nineteen Eighty-Four (1984).* 1949. Penguin, 2000.

Pálsson, Gísili, and Paul Rabinow. "Iceland: The Case of a National Human Genome Project." *Anthropology Today*, vol. 15, no. .5, 1999, pp. 14–18, https://doi.org/10.2307/2678370.

Pálsson, Gísili. "Decode Me! Anthropology and Personal Genomics." *Current Anthropology*, vol. 53, no. S5, 2012, pp.185-195, https://doi.org/10.1086/662291.

Parker, Andrew, and Eve Kosofsky Sedgwick. "Introduction: Performativity and Performance." *Performativity and Performance*, edited by Andrew Parker and Eve Kosofsky Sedgwick. New York: Routledge, 1995, pp. 1–18.

Parsons, Talcott. "The Sick Role and the Role of the Physician Reconsidered." *Health and Society*, special issue in *Milbank Memorial Fund Quarterly*, vol. 53, no. 3, 1975, pp. 257–78, https://doi.org/10.2307/3349493.

Pathway Genomics. "OmeCare: Home Page." https://omecare.co/.

Patterson, James T. *The Dread Disease: Cancer and Modern American Culture.* Harvard U.P., 1987.

Person, Leland S. *The Cambridge Introduction to Nathaniel Hawthorne.* Cambridge UP, 2007.

Petersen, Alan. "Governmentality, Critical Scholarship, and the Medical Humanities." *Journal of Medical Humanities*, vol. 34, no. 3/4, 2003, pp. 187–201, https://doi.org/10.1023/A:1026002202396.

Pfaelzer, Jean, and R.M.P. "Parody and Satire in American Dystopian Fiction of the Nineteenth Century." *Science Fiction on Women, Science Fiction by Women*, special issue in *Science Fiction Studies*, vol.7, no 1, 1980, pp. 61–72.

Philips, Elizabeth M., Adebola O. Odunlami, and Vence L. Bonham. "Mixed Race: Understanding Difference in the Genome Era." *Social Forces*, vol. 86, no. 2, 2007, pp. 795–820, https://doi.org/10.1093/sf/86.2.795.

Picoult, Jodi Lynn. *My Sister's Keeper: A Novel.* Pocket Books, 2004.

Pildes, Richard H., and Bradley A. Smith. "The Fifteenth Amendment: Common Interpretation." *Interactive Constitution*, https://constitutioncenter.org/interactive-constitution/interpretation/amendment-xv/interps/141.

Pivar, David J. *Purity and Hygiene: Women, Prostitution, and the ,American Plan,' 1900–1930.* Greenwood Press, 2002.

PlagueInc. Ndemic Creations, Miniclip Ltd., 2012.

Plato. "Apology." *The Last Days of Socrates: Euthyphro, Apology, Crito, Phaedo.* Translated by Hugh Tredennick and Harold Tarrant. Penguin, 1969, pp. 37–67.

Port, Dina Roth. *Previvors: Facing the Breast Cancer Gene and Making Life Changing Decisions: A Groundbreaking Guide with the Stories of Five Courageous Women.* Penguin, 2010.

Powell, Betty. "Descartes' Machines." *Proceedings of the Aristotelian Society New Series*, vol. 71, 1970/71, pp. 209–222.

"Previvor's Story." *Breastcancer.org*, 14 July 2016, https://breastcancer.org/community/acknowledging/genetic-testing/previvor.

Pribek, Thomas. "Hawthorne's Aminadab: Sources and Significance." *Studies in the American Renaissance*, 1987, pp.177–186, https://jstor.org/stable/30228133.

Probyn, Elspeth. "Writing Shame". *The Affect Theory Reader*, edited by Melissa Gregg, and Gregory J. Seigworth. Duke UP, 2010, pp. 71–92.

Prometheus. Directed by Ridley Scott, Twentieth Century Fox, 2012.

"Promises." *Stanford Encyclopedia of Philosophy.* 10 Oct. 2008, https://plato.stanford.edu/entries/promises/.

Prucher, Jeff. *Brave New Words: The Oxford Dictionary of Science Fiction.* Oxford UP, 2006.

Queller, Jessica. "Cancer and the Maiden." *The New York Times*, 5 March 2005, https://nytimes.com/2005/03/05/opinion/cancer-and-the-maiden.html.

Queller, Jessica. *Pretty is What Changes: Impossible Choices, the Breast Cancer Gene, and How I Defied My Destiny.* Spiegel & Grau, 2009.

Rabin, Roni Caryn. "No Easy Choices on Breast Reconstruction." *The New York Times*, 20 May 2013, https://well.blogs.nytimes.com/2013/05/20/no-easy-choices-on-breast-reconstruction/.

Rabinow, Paul, and Nikolas Rose. "Biopower Today." *BioSocieties*, vol. 1, 2006, pp. 195–217, https://doi.org/10.1017/S1745855206040014.

Rabinow, Paul. "Episodes or Incidents: Seeking Significance." *Biosecurity Interventions: Global Health and Security in Question*, edited by Andrew Lakoff and Stephen J. Collier, Columbia UP, 2008, pp. 279–284.

Rabinow, Paul. *Essays on the Anthropology of Reason*. Princeton UP, 1996.

Ranji, Usha, and Alina Salganicoff. "State Medicaid Coverage of Perinatal Services: Summary of State Survey Findings." Nov. 2009. *The Kaiser Family Foundation*, pp. 1–28. kff.org/wp-content/uploads/2013/01/8014.pdf.

Rapp, Rayna. *Testing Women, Testing Fetus: The Social Impact of Amniocentesis in America*. 1999. Routledge, 2005.

Reibstein, Janet. *Staying Alive: A Family Memoir*. Bloomsbury, 2002.

Reid, John Phillip. *The Concept of Liberty in the Age of the American Revolution*. U of Chicago P, 1988.

Rhodes, Colbert, and Clyde B. Vedder. *An Introduction to Thanatology: Death and Dying in American Society*. Charles C. Thomas, 1983.

Rich, Adrienne. "A Woman Dead in Her Forties." *The Dream of a Common Language*. W.W. Norton & Company, 1978, pp. 53–58.

Ricoeur, Paul. *Time and Narrative, vol. 1*. Translated by Kathleen McLaughlin and David Pellauer. University of Chicago Press, 1984.

Ricoeur, Paul. "Narrative Identity." *Philosophy Today*, vol. 35, no. 1, 1991, pp.73-81, https://doi.org/10.5840/philtoday199135136.

Rieder, John. "On Defining SF, or Not: Genre Theory, SF, and History." *Science Fiction Studies*, vol. 37, no. 2, 2010, pp.191-209, https://jstor.org/stable/25746406 .

Ritter, Joachim, and Karlfried Gründer, editors. "Sicherheit." *Historisches Wörterbuch der Philosophie*. Schwabe and Co Ag, 2007, vol. 9 Se-Sp, pp. 745–750.

RNN. "Fighting Huntington's Disease." *Youtube*, uploaded by RFL, 1 Dec. 2010, https://youtube.com/watch?v=YzBvDIClDSI.

Robin31. "Robin 31's Story." *Breastcancer.org*, 4 July 2016, https://breastcancer.org/community/acknowledging/genetic-testing/robin31.

Rolling Stones. "Mother's Little Helper." *Aftermath*. Decca Records, 1966.

Roosevelt, Theodore. "T. Roosevelt Letter to C. Davenport About 'Degenerates Reproducing'." 1913. *American Philosophical Society*, https://eugenicsarchive.org/html/eugenics/static/images/1242.html.

Rose, Nikolas, and Carlos Novas. "Biological Citizenship." *Global Assemblage: Technology, Politics, and Ethics as Problems of Anthropology*, edited by Aihwa Ong and Stephen J. Collier. Blackwell. 2003, pp. 439–463.

Rose, Nikolas, and Carlos Novas. "Genetic Risk and the Birth of the Somatic Individual." *Economy and Society*, vol. 29, no. 4, 2000, pp.485-513, https://doi.org/10.1080/03085140050174750.

Rose, Nikolas. "The Politics of Life Itself." *Theory, Culture and Society*, vol. 18, no. 6, 2001, pp. 1–30, https://doi.org/10.1177/02632760122052020.

Rose, Nikolas. *The Politics of Life Itself: Biomedicine, Power, and Subjectivity in the Twenty-First Century*. Princeton UP, 2007.

Rose, Nikolas. "The Human Sciences in a Biological Age." *ICS Occasional Paper Series*, vol. 3, no. 1, 2012, pp. 1–24, https://doi.org/0.1177/0263276412456569.

Rose, Dael A. "How Did the Smallpox Vaccination Program Come About? Tracing the Emergence of Recent Smallpox Vaccination Thinking." *Biosecurity Interventions: Global Health and Security in Question*, edited by Andrew Lakoff and Stephen J. Collier, Columbia UP, 2008, pp. 89- 119.

Rosen, George. "Benjamin Rush on Health and the American Revolution." *AJPH*, vol. 66, no. 4, 1976, pp. 397–398, https://doi.org/10.2105/ajph.66.4.397.

Rosenberry, Edward H. "Hawthorne's Allegory of Science: 'Rappaccini's Daughter'." *American Literature*, vol. 32, no. 1., 1960, pp.39-46. jstor.org/stable/2922800.

Rosenfeld, Albert. "At Risk for Huntington's Disease: Who Should Know What and When?" *The Hasting's Center Report*, vol. 14, no. 03, 1984, pp. 5–8, https://doi.org/10.2307/3561179.

Rothschild, Emma. "What is Security?" *Daedalus*, vol. 124, no. 3, 1995, pp. 53–98, https://jstor.org/stable/20027310.

Rucker, Mary E. "Science and Art in Hawthorne's 'The Birth-Mark'." *Nineteenth-Century Literature*, vol. 41, no.4, 1987, pp.445-461, https://jstor.org/stable/3045227.

Rush, Benjamin. "Observations on the Duties of a Physician, and the Methods of Improving Medicine." Delivered in the University of Pennsylvania, February 7, 1789. *American Journal of Medicine*, vol.11, no. 5, 1951, pp. 551–556, https://doi.org/10.1016/0002-9343(51)90036-8.

Sabel, Michael S., and Sonya Dal Cin. "Trends in Media Reports of Celebrities' Breast Cancer Treatment Decisions." *Annals of Surgical Oncology*, vol. 24, no. 3, 2016, pp. 1–7, https://doi.org/10.1245/s10434-016-5202-7.

Said, Edward W. *Culture and Imperialism*. Knopf, 1993.

Saint Augustine. *Confessions. 354–430*. Translated by. Henry Chadwick, Oxford UP, 2008.

Salam, Maya. "For Serena Williams, Childbirth was a Harrowing Ordeal. She is not Alone." *The New York Times*, 11 Jan 2018. nytimes.com/2018/01/11/sports/tennis/serena-williams-baby-vogue.html.

Salter, Mark B. "Surveillance." *The Routledge Handbook of New Security Studies*, edited by J. Peter Burgess. Routledge, 2010, pp. 187–196.

Sanbhava, Padma. *The Tibetan Book of Death: Liberation through Understanding in the Between*. Translated by Robert A.F. Thurman. Bantam Books, 1993.

Sarasin, Philipp. *Reizbare Maschinen: Eine Geschichte des Körpers 1765–1914*. Suhrkamp, 2001.

Saunders, Cicely. "The Evolution of Palliative Care." *Journal of the Royal Society of Medicine*, vol. 94, 2001, pp. 430–432, https://doi.org/10.1177/014107680109400904.

Saunders, George. *Tenth of December*. Random House, 2013.

Savage Brosman, Catherine. "Theories of Collectivities in Sartre and Rousseau." *South Central Review*, vol. 2, no. 1, 1985, pp. 25–41, https://doi.org/10.2307/3189408.

Sawyer, Robert. *Frameshift*. Tor Books, 1997.

Scarry, Elaine. *The Body in Pain. The Making and Unmaking of the World*. Oxford UP, 1985.

Schaupp, Simon. "Measuring the Entrepreneur of Himself: Gendered Quantification on the Self-Tracking Discourse." *Lifelogging: Digital Self-tracking and Lifelogging– Between*

Disruptive Technology and Cultural Transformation, edited by Stefan Selke, Springer, 2016, pp.249-266.

Schleifer, Ronald. *Intangible Materialism: The Body, Scientific Knowledge, and the Power of Language*. Minnesota UP, 2009.

Schlesinger, Arthur M. "The Lost Meaning of 'The Pursuit of Happiness'." *The William and Mary Quarterly*, vol. 21, no. 3 1964, pp. 325–327, https://doi.org/10.2307/1918449.

Schmeck, Harold M. "Nixon Signs Cancer Bill; Cites Commitment to Cure." *The New York Times*, 24 Dec. 1971, *New York Times Archives.com*, 1996, https://nytimes.com/1971/12/24 /archives/nixon-signs-cancer-bill-cites-commitment-to-cure.html.

Schneider, Patrick A., Christine M. Zainer, Christopher Kevin Kubat, Nancy K. Mullen, and Amberly K. Windisch. "The Breast Cancer Epidemic: 10 Facts." *The Linacre Quarterly*, vol. 81, no. 3, 2014, pp. 244–277, https://doi.org/10.1179/2050854914Y.0000000 027.

Schoch-Spana, Monica. "Bioterrorism: US Public Health and a Secular Apocalypse." *Anthropology Today*, vol. 20, no. 5, 2004, pp. 8–13, https://jstor.org/stable/i370667.

Schoch-Spana, Monica. "The People's Role in US. National Health Security: Past, Present, and Future." *Biosecurity and Bioterrorism*, vol. 10, no. 1, 2012, pp. 77–88, https://doi.or g/10.1089/bsp.2011.0108.

Schröder, Ariane. *Biological Inf(l)ections of the American Dream: Contagious Disease and Narrative Containments in U.S. American Literature and Culture*. LIT Verlag, 2020.

Schweik, Susan. *The Ugly Laws: Disability in Public*. New York UP, 2009.

Seagals, Steven T. *It's a Bird*. Vertigo, 2004.

Seale, Clive. *Constructing Death: The Sociology of Dying and Bereavement*. Cambridge UP, 1998.

Seale, Clive. "Media Constructions of Dying Alone: A Form of Bad Death." *Social Science and Medicine*, vol. 58, 2004, pp. 967 -974, https://doi.org/10.1016/j.socscimed.2003.10 .038.

Seale, Clive, and Sjaak van der Geest. "Good and Bad Death: Introduction." *Social Science and Medicine*. vol. 58, 2004, pp. 883–885, https://doi.org/0.1016/j.socscimed.2003.10 .034.

Sedgwick, Eve Kosofsky and Adam Frank, editors. *Shame and Its Sisters: A Silvan Tomkins Reader*. Duke UP, 1995.

Sedgwick, Eve Kososky. *Touching Feeling: Affect, Pedagogy, Performativity*. Duke UP, 2003.

Sedgwick, Eve Kososky. "White Glasses." *The Yale Journal of Criticism*, vol. 5, no. 3, 1992, pp. 193–208, https://doi.org/10.1080/0950236032000050744.

Seife, Charles. "23andMe Is Terrifying, But not for the Reasons the FDA Thinks." *Scientific American*, 27 Nov. 2013, https://scientificamerican.com/article/23andme-is-terrifyin g-but-not-forw-reasons-fda/.

Selke, Stefan. *Lifelogging: Wie die Digitale Selbstvermessung Unsere Gesellschaft Verändert*. Econ, 2004.

Selke, Stefan. "Introduction: Lifelogging – Disruptive Technology and Cultural Transformation – The Impact of a Societal Phenomenon." *Lifelogging: Digital Self-tracking and Lifelogging– Between Disruptive Technology and Cultural Transformation*, edited by Stefan Selke, Springer, 2016, pp. 1–21.

Senate of the United States. "Breast Cancer Education and Awareness Requires Learning Early Act", 111th Congress, 1st session, 7 May 2009, https://congress.gov/bill/111th-congress/senate-bill/994/text?r=31&s=1.

Shakespeare, Tom. "'Losing the Plot?' Medical and Activist Discourses of Contemporary Genetics and Disability." *Sociology of Health and Illness*, vol. 21, no. 5, 1999, pp. 669–688. https://doi.org/10.1111/1467-9566.00178.

Shakespeare, Tom. "Social Model of Disability." *Disabilities Studies Reader*, edited by Lennard Davis. Routledge, 2006, pp. 197–204.

Sharp, Lesley A. "The Invisible Woman: The Bioaesthetics of Engineered Bodies." *Body and Society*, vol. 17, 2011, pp. 1–30, https://doi.org/10.1177/1357034X10394667.

Shelley, Mary Wollstonecraft. *Frankenstein; or, The Modern Prometheus*. 1818. Mockingbird Classic Publishing, 2014.

Shostak, Sara. "Marking Population and Persons at Risk: Molecular Epidemiology and Environmental Health." *Biomedicalization: Technoscience, Health, and Illness in the U.S.*, edited by Adele E. Clarke, Laura Mamo, Jennifer Ruth Fosket, Jennifer R. Fishman, and Janet K. Shim, Duke UP, 2010, pp. 242–262.

Shouse, Eric. "Feeling, Emotion, Affect." *Journal Media and Culture*, vol. 8, no. 6, Dec. 2005, https://doi.org/10.5204/mcj.2443.

Shryock, Richard H. "Eighteenth Century Medicine in America." *American Antiquarian Society Proceedings*, vol. 59, no. 2, 1949, pp. 275–292.

Shryock, Richard H. "The Significance of Medicine in American History." *The American Historical Review*, vol. 62, no. 1, 1956, pp. 81-91, https://jstor.org/stable/1848513.

Shteyngart, Gary. *Russian Debutante's Handbook: A Novel*. Riverhead Books, 2002.

Shteyngart, Gary. *Absurdistan*. Random House, 2006.

Shteyngart, Gary. *Super Sad True Love Story*. Random House, 2010.

Shteyngart, Gary. "Only Disconnect." *The New York Times*. 16 July 2010, https://nytimes.com/2010/07/18/books/review/Shteyngart-t.html.

Siebers, Tobin. "Disability in Theory: From Social Constructionism to the New Realism of the Body." *The Disabilities Studies Reader*, edited by Lennard Davis, 2006. Routledge, 2006, Pp. 173–183.

Sinclair, Upton. *The Jungle*. 1906. Bantam reissue, 2003.

Singleton, Rivers Jr., and D. Heywar Brock. "Teaching Bioethics from an Interdisciplinary Perspective." *The American Biology Teacher*, vol. 44, no. 5, 1982, pp. 280–285 + 313, https://jstor.org/stable/4447504.

Skloot, Rebecca. *The Immortal Life of Henrietta Lacks*. Random House, 2010.

Slater, Jen, Embla Ágústsdóttir, and Freya Haraldsdóttir. "Becoming Intelligible Woman: Gender, Disability and Resistance at the Border Zone of Youth." *Feminism and Psychology*, vol. 28, no. 3, 2018, pp. 409-426, https://doi.org/10.1177/0959353518769947.

Smith, Rogers M. "The 'American Creed' and American Identity: The Limits of Liberal Citizenship in the United States." *The Western Political Quarterly*, vol. 41, no. 2, 1988, pp. 225–251, https://jstor.org/stable/448536.

Snow, Charles Percy. *The Two Cultures and the Scientific Revolution*. 1959. Cambridge UP, 1961.

Sontag, Susan. *Illness as Metaphor and AIDS and Its Metaphors.* New York: Picador, 1990. [*Illness as Metaphor* first published 1977, 1978. *AIDS and Its Metaphors* first published 1988,1989.].

Spivak, Gayatri Chakravorty. "Can the Subaltern Speak?" *Marxism and the Interpretation of Culture*, edited by Cary Nelson and Lawrence Grossberg. Illinois UP, 1988, pp. 271–313.

Staff, Fitbit, et al. "Earn up to $1,500 for Healthy Behavior with Fitbit's New Healthcare Integration." *Fitbit Blog*, 3 May 2017, https://blog.fitbit.com/fitbit-charge-2-healthca re-integration/.

Stannard, David E. "Death and Dying in Puritan New England." *The American Historical Review*, vol. 78, no. 5, 1973, pp. 1305–1330, https://jstor.org/stable/1854094.

Stanton, Elizabeth Cady. "Declaration of Sentiments and Resolutions." *Seneca Falls Convention*, 1848, https://sjsu.edu/people/cynthia.rostankowski/courses/HUM2BS14/so /Womens-Rights.pdf.

Starr, Paul. *The Social Transformation of American Medicine.* 1982. Basic Books, 2008.

Steedman, Carolyn. *Landscape for a Good Woman: A Story of Two Lives.* 1986. Virago, 2003.

Stern, Alexandra Minna. *Eugenic Nation: Faults and Frontiers of Better Breeding in Modern America.* U of California P, 2005.

Stevenson, Robert Louis. *The Strange Case of Dr. Jekyll and Mr. Hide.* 1886. Dover Publications, 1991.

Sturgeon, Theodore. *More than Human.* 1953. Gateway, 2000.

Sunder Rajan, Kaushik. *Biocapital: The Constitution of Postgenomic Life.* Duke UP, 2006.

Sunder Rajan, Kaushik. "Introduction: The Capitalization of Life and the Liveliness of Capital." *Lively Capital*, edited by Kaushik Sunder Rajan. Duke UP, 2012, pp. 1–41.

Susann, Jacqueline. *Valley of the Dolls.* Grove Press, 1966.

Svendsen, Lars. *A Philosophy of Fear.* Translated by John Irons, Reaktion Books, 2008.

Tatum, Edward Lawrie. "Nobel Lecture: A Case History in Biological Research." *The Nobel Prize.* 11 Dec. 1958, https://nobelprize.org/prizes/medicine/1958/tatum/lecture/.

Tatum, Edward Lawrie. "Molecular Biology, Nucleic Acids, and the Future of Medicine." Perspectives in Biology and Medicine, vol. 10, no. 1, 1966, pp. 19–32, https://doi.org/1 0.1353/pbm.1966.0027.

Taylor, Diana. *The Archive and the Repertoire: Performing Cultural Memory in the Americas.* Duke UP, 2003.

Thacker, Eugene. "The Thickness of Tissue Engineering: Biopolitics, Biotech, and the Regenerative Body." *Theory and Event*, vol. 3, no. 3, 1999, pp. 1–16, https://muse.jhu.edu/ article/32555.

Thacker, Eugene. "Redefining Bioinformatics: A Critical Analysis of Technoscientific Bodies." *Enculturation*, vol. 3, no. 1, 2000, https://enculturation.gmu.edu/3_1/thacker .html.

Thacker, Eugene. "The Science Fiction of Technoscience: The Politics of Simulation and a Challenge for New Media Art." *Leonardo*, vol. 34, no. 2, 2001, pp. 155–158, https://jsto r.com/stable/1577019.

The Fifth Element. Directed by Luc Besson, Columbia Pictures, 1997.

The Island. Directed by Michael Bay, Dream Works Pictures, 2005.

"The Scar Project: Breast Cancer is not a Pink Ribbon: Home." *The SCAR Project*, https://th escarproject.org/.

This American Life. "It Says So Right Here." *This American Life*, 25 Oct 2013, https://thisam ericanlife.org/509/it-says-so-right-here.

This American Life. "Dr. Gilmer and Mr. Hyde." *This American Life*, 12 April 2013, https://th isamericanlife.org/492/dr-gilmer-and-mr-hyde.

Thrift, Nigel. "Intensities of Feeling: Toward a Spatial Politics of Affect." *Geografiska Annaler*, vol. 85B, no. 1, 2004, 57–78.

Tobell. Dominique A. *Pills, Power, and Policy: The Struggle for Drug Reform in Cold War America and Its Consequences*. U of California P, 2012.

Tobell. Dominique A. "'Who's Winning the Human Race?': Cold War as Pharmaceutical Political Strategy." *Journal of the History of Medicine and Allied Sciences*, vol. 64, no. 4, 2009, pp. 429–473, https://doi.org/10.1093/jhmas/jrp012.

Tomes, Nancy. "Merchants of Health: Medicine and Consumer Culture in the United States, 1900–1940." *The Journal of American History*, vol. 88, no. 2, 2001, pp. 519–547, https://doi.org/10.2307/2675104.

Tomes, Nancy. *The Gospel of Germs: Men, Women, and the Microbe in American Life*. Harvard UP, 1998.

Tomes, Nancy. *Remaking the American Patient: How Madison Avenue and Modern Medicine Turned Patients into Consumers*. U of South Carolina P, 2016.

Tomkins, Silvan. "What are Affects." *Shame and its Sisters: A Sylvan Tomkins Reader*, edited by Eve Kosovsky Sedgwick, and Adam Frank, Duke UP, 1995.

Tomkins, Silvan. *Affect, Imagery, and Consciousness: The Positive Affects*. Springer, 1962.

Trapp, Brian. "Super Sad True Melting Pot: Reimagining the Melting Pot in a Transnational World in Gary Shteyngart's Super Sad True Love Story." *MELUS: Multi-Ethnic Literature of the U.S.*, vol.41, no. 4, 2016, pp. 55–75, https://jstor.org/stable/44155283.

Treichler, Paula A. *How to Have Theory in an Epidemic. Cultural Chronicles of AIDS*. Duke UP, 1999.

Tremain, Shelley. "On the Government of Disability: Foucault, Power, and the Subject of Impairment." *The Disabilities Studies Reader*, edited by Lennard Davis. Routledge, 2006, pp. 185- 196.

Tuttle, Todd M., Elizabeth B. Habermann, Erin H. Grund, Todd J. Morris, and Beth A. Virnig. "Increasing Use of Collateral Prophylactic Mastectomy for Breast Cancer Patients: A Trend Toward More Aggressive Surgical Treatment." *Journal of Clinical Oncology*, vol. 25, no.33, 2007, pp. 5203–5209, https://doi.org/10.1200/JCO.2007.12.3141 .

U.S. Children's Bureau. "Is Your Child's Birth Recorded?" 1945. Washington, DC: U.S. Government Printing Office, 4pp, https://mchlibrary.org/history/chbu/20937-1945.pdf.

U.S. Food and Drug Administration. "Mobile Medical Applications: Guidance For Industry and Food and Drug Administration Staff." *FDA*, 25 Sept. 2013, https://fda.gov/do wnloads/MedicalDevices/.../UCM263366.pdf.

U.S. Food and Drug Administration. "FDASIA Health IT Reports: Proposed Strategy and Recommendations for a Risk Based Framework." *FDA*, 1 April 2014, https://fda.gov/ media/87886/download.

U.S. Food and Drug Administration. "Ultrasound Imaging." *FDA*, https://fda.gov/radiat ion-emitting-products/medical-imaging/ultrasound-imaging.

UPMC Center for Health Security. "Atlantic Storm Interactive." *UPMC*, 14 Jan. 2006, https://centerforhealthsecurity.org/our-work/events-archive/2005_atlantic_storm/flash/index.htm.

UPMC Center for Health Security. "Dark Winter: About the Exercise." *UPMC*, 2001, https://centerforhealthsecurity.org/our-work/events-archive/2001_dark-winter/about.html.

UPMC Center for Health Security. "Dark Winter: Final Script." *UPMC*, 2001, https://centerforhealthsecurity.org/our-work/events-archive/2001_dark-winter/Dark%20Winter%20Script.pdf.

UPMC Center for Health Security. "Dark Winter: Overview." *UPMC*, 2001, https://centerforhealthsecurity.org/our-work/events-archive/2001_dark-winter/index.html.

Van Dijck, José. *The Transparent Body: A Cultural Analysis of Medical Imaging.* U of Washington P, 2005. [Series: *In Vivo*].

Van Dijck, José. *Imagenation: Popular Images of Genetics.* New York UP, 1998.

Vanouse, Paul. "Relative Velocity Device." UW Henry Art Gallery, Seattle, WA. April, 2002, https://paulvanouse.com/rvid.html.

Vaz, Paulo, and Fernanda Bruno. "Types of Self-Surveillance: from Abnormality to Individuals 'at Risk'." *Surveillance and Society*, vol. 1, no. 3, 2003, pp. 272–291, https://doi.org/10.24908/ss.v1i3.3341.

Verbrugge, Martha H. *Able-Bodied Womanhood: Personal Health and Social Change in Nineteenth-Century Boston.* Oxford UP, 1988.

Vine, Barbara. *The House of Stairs.* Viking Press, 1989.

Vogel, Vigil J. *American Indian Medicine.* U of Oklahoma P, 1970. [Series: *The Civilization of the American Indian Series*].

Völz, Johannes, and Russell A. Berman. "Introduction." *Telos*, vol. 170, 2015, pp.3-6, https://doi.org/10.3817/0315170003.

Völz, Johannes. "The Aspiration for Impossible Security." *Telos*, vol. 170, 2015, pp. 23–45, https://doi.org/10.3817/0315170023.

Völz, Johannes. "Aestheticizing Insecurity: A Response to Security Studies and American Literary History." *American Literary History*, vol. 29, no. 3, 2017, pp. 615–624, https://doi.org/10.1093/alh/ajx018.

Völz, Johannes. "A Nation of Fugitives: Harriet Jacobs's Incidents in the Life of a Slave Girl and the Narrativization of (In)security." *eTransfer*, vol. 2, 2012, pp. n.pag, https://hsozkult.de/journal/id/zeitschriftenausgaben-7242.

Von Feigenblatt, Otto F. "Exploring Human Insecurity through Phenomenological Research: A Brief Review." *RCAPS Working Paper*, no. 09–8, January 2010.

Vonnegut, Kurt. *Galapagos.* Dell Publishing, 1985.

Waddington, Simon N., et al. "A Broad Overview and Review of CRISPR-Cas Technology and Stem Cells." *Curr Stem Cell Rep*, vol. 2, 2016, pp.9-20, https://doi.org/10.1007/s40778-016-0037-5.

Wald, Priscilla. "Future Perfect: Grammar, Genes and Geography." *New Literary History*, vol. 31, no. 4, 2000, pp. 681–708, https://doi.org/10.1353/nlh.2000.0051.

Wald, Priscilla. "What's in a Cell?: John Moore's Spleen and the Language of Bioslavery." *New Literary History*, vol. 36, 2005, pp. 205–225, https://jstor.org/stable/20057889.

Wald, Priscilla. *Contagious: Cultures, Carriers, and the Outbreak Narrative*. Durham, London: Duke UP, 2008.

Wald, Priscilla. "American Studies and the Politics of Life." *American Quarterly*, vol. 64, no.2, 2012, pp. 185–204.

Waldby, Catherine. *The Visible Human Project: Informatic Bodies and Posthuman Medicine*. Routledge, 2000.

Waldschmidt, Anne. "Disability goes Cultural: The Cultural Model of Disability as an Analytic Tool." *Culture, Theory, Disability: Encounters between Disability Studies and Cultural Studies*, edited by Anne Waldschmidt, Hanjo Berressem, and Moritz Ingwersen. transcript, 2017, pp. 19–27.

Wallace, Maeve, et al. "Separate and Unequal: Structural Racism and Infant Mortality in the US." *Health and Place*, vol. 45, 2017, pp. 140–144, https://doi.org/10.1016/j.healthplace.2017.03.012.

Walker, Julia A. "Why Performance? Why Now? Textuality and the Rearticulation of Human Presence." *The Yale Journal of Criticism*, vol. 16, no. 1, 2003, pp. 149–175, https://doi.org/10.1353/yale.2003.0011.

Walter, Tony. *The Revival of Death*. Routledge, 1994.

Walzer Leavitt, Judith. "Birthing and Anesthesia: The Debate over Twilight Sleep." *Women: Sex and Sexuality Part 2*, special issue in *Sings*, vol. 6, no.1, 1980, pp. 147–164, https://jstor.org/stable/3173972.

Walzer Leavitt, Judith. *Typhoid Mary: Captive to the Public Health*. Beacon Press, 1997.

Waples, Emily. "Emplotted Bodies: Breast Cancer, Feminism, and the Future." *Theorizing Breast Cancer Narratives, Politics, Memory*, special issue in *Tulsa Studies in Women's Literature*, vol.32/33, no.2/1, 2013/2014, pp.47-70, https://jstor.org/stable/43653276.

Ward, Jamie A. "Monitoring the Mundane: Wearable Computing and our Growing e-Legacy." *Building Material*, vol. 17, 2007, pp. 48–49, https://jstor.org/stable/i29792319.

Warren, Charles. "Fourth of July Myths." *The William and Mary Quarterly*, vol. 2, no. 3, 1945, pp. 237–272, https://doi.org/10.2307/1921451.

Washington, Booker T. *Up From Slavery*. 1901. The Floating Press, 2009.

Watson, David. "Beautiful Walls: A Response to Johannes Völz." *American Literary History*, vol. 29, no.3, 2017, pp. 625–628, https://doi.org/10.1093/alh/ajx015.

Watson, David. "Introduction: Security Studies and American Literary History." *American Literary History*, vol. 28, no. 4, 2016, pp. 663–676, https://doi.org/10.1093/alh/ajw049.

Watson, James D. *The Double Helix: A Personal Account of the Discovery of the Structure of DNA*. 1968. Touchstone, 2001.

Weinbaum, Alys Eve. "Racial Aura: Walter Benjamin and the Work of Art in a Biotechnological Age." *Literature and Medicine*, vol. 26, no. 1, 2007, pp. 207–239.

Weinstein, Cindy. "The Invisible Hand Made Visible. 'The Birth-Mark'." *Nineteenth-Century Literature*, vol. 48, no.1, 1993, pp.44-73, https://jstor.org/stable/2933940.

Wells, H.G. *The Island of Dr. Moreau*. 1898, Penguin Classics, 2005.

Wentersdorf, Karl P. "The Genesis of Hawthorne's 'The Birthmark'." *Jahrbuch für Amerikastudien*, vol.8, 1963, pp.171-186, https://jstor.org/stable/41155034.

Westworld. Created by Lisa Joy, and Jonathan Nolan, season 1 and 2, HBO, 2016, 2018.

White, Hayden. *Metahistory: The Historical Imagination of Nineteenth Century Europe*. 1973. John Hopkins UP, 1975.

White House. "National Security Strategy 2006." *The White House: President George W. Bush*, Mar. 2006, https://georgewbush-whitehouse.archives.gov/nsc/nss/2006/.

White House. "National Security Strategy 2010." *The White House: President Barack Obama*, 27 May 2010, https://nssarchive.us/wp-content/uploads/2020/04/2010.pdf.

Wibben, Annick T.R. *Feminist Security Studies: A Narrative Approach*. Routledge, 2011. [Series: *PRIO New Security Studies*].

Williams, Raymond. *Marxism and Literature*. Oxford UP,1977.

Willmetts, Simon. "Digital Dystopia: Surveillance, Autonomy, and Social Justice in Gary Shteyngart's Super Sad True Love Story." *American Quarterly*, vol. 70, no.2. 2018, pp. 267–289, https://doi.org/10.1353/aq.2018.0017.

Wineapple, Brenda. *Hawthorne: A Life*. Alfred A. Knopf, 2003.

Werlin, Nancy. *Double Helix*. Dial Books, 2000.

Wexler, Alice. *Mapping Fate: A Memoir of Family, Risk, and Genetic Research*. U of California P, 1996.

Wexler, Alice. "Mapping Lives: 'Truth,' Life Writing, and DNA." *The Ethics of Life Writing*, edited by John Paul Eakin, Cornell UP, 2004, pp. 163–173.

Wexler, Alice. "Huntington's Disease in Popular Culture: A Brief Historical Perspective." *Journal of Huntington's Disease*, vol. 3, 2014, pp1-4, https://doi.org/10.3233/JHD-149002 .

Wexler, Alice. "Eugenics, Heredity, and Huntington's Disease: A Brief Historical Perspective." *Journal of Huntington's Disease*, vol. 1, 2012, pp.139-141, https://doi.org/10.3233/JHD-129007.

Wexler, Nancy S. "Huntington's Disease: Advocacy Driving Science." *Annual Review Medicine*, vol. 63, 2012, pp. 1–22, https://doi.org/10.1146/annurev-med-050710-134457.

WNYC. "What are you doing for the test of your life?" *Youtube*, uploaded by WNYC, 22 Oct. 2013, https://youtube.com/watch?v=I26oysXly2E.

WNYC. "DNA Secrets: The Antidote." *WNYC*, 25 Oct. 2013, https://wnyc.org/story/dna-secrets-what-you-want-know/.

Woodward, Kathleen. "Statistical Panic." *A Journal of Feminist Cultural Studies*, vol. 11, no. 2, 1999, pp. 177–203, https://muse.jhu.edu/journals/dif/summary/v011/11.2woodward.html.

Woodward, Kathleen. *Statistical Panic: Cultural Politics and Poetics of Emotion*. Duke UP, 2009.

Woodward, Kathleen. "Concepts of Identity and Difference." *Identity and Difference*, edited by Kathleen Woodward. Sage Publication, 1997, pp. 7–62.

Woodward, Kathleen. "Calculating Compassion." *Compassion: The Culture and Politics of an Emotion*, edited by Lauren Gail Berlant. Routledge, 2004.

Wolf, Gary. "Know Thyself: Tracking Every Facet of Life, from Sleep to Mood to Pain, 24/7/365." *Wired*, June 22, 2009, https://wired.com/2009/06/lbnp-knowthyself/.

Wolf, Gary. "The Data Driven Life." *The New York Times*, 28 April 2010, https://www.nytimes.com/2010/05/02/magazine/02self-measurement-t.html.

Wolf, Gary. "The Quantified Self." *TED Talks*, June 2010, https://ted.com/talks/gary_wolf _the_quantified_self.

Wolfe, Cary. *What is Posthumanism?* University of Minnesota Press, 2010.

World Health Organization. "Basic Documents." 1948. 48th Edition, *WHO*, 31 Dec. 2017, https://apps.who.int/gb/bd/PDF/bd48/basic-documents-48th-edition-en.pdf #page=1.

World Health Organization. "The World Health Report 2007 – A Safer Future: Global Public Health Security in the 21st Century." *WHO*, 2007, https://who.int/whr/2007/whr0 7_en.pdf?ua=1.

World Health Organization. "mHealth: New Horizons for Health through Mobile Technologies." *Global Observatory for Health Series*, vol. 3, 2011, https://who.int/goe/publica tions/goe_mhealth_web.pdf?ua=1%3E.

Wouters, Cas. "The Quest for New Rituals in Dying and Mourning: Changes in the We-I Balance." *Body and Society*, vol. 8, no. 1, 2002, pp. F 1–27, https://doi.org/10.1177/13570 34X02008001001.

Young, Iris Marion. "Gender Seriality: Thinking about Women as a Social Collective." *Signs*, vol. 19, no. 3, 1994, pp. 713–738, https://jstor.org/stable/3174775.

Young Survivor Coalition. "Survivor Stories." *Young Survival Coalition*, https://youngsurv ival.org/blog/survivor-stories.

Zamyatin, Yevgeny. *We*. 1924, Translated by Natasha Randall, Modern Library, reprint 2006.

Zanger, Jules. "Speaking of the Unspeakable: Hawthorne's 'The Birthmark'." *Modern Philology*, vol. 80, no.4, 1983, pp.364-371, https://jstor.org/stable/437071.

Zola, Irving Kenneth. "Medicalization as an Institution of Social Control." *Ekistic*, vol. 41, no. 245, 1976, pp. 210–214, https://doi.org/10.1111/j.1467-954X.1972.tb00220.x.

23andMe. "Welcome." *23andMe*, 2014, 23andme.com/.

23andMe. "Find out What Your DNA Says About Your Health, Traits, and Ancestry." *23andMe*, 2019, https://www.23andme.com/en-int/dna-ancestry/.

23andMe. "23and Me 'This is Me' TV Ad: Portraits of Health" *Youtube*, uploaded by 23andMe, Aug. 2013, https://youtu.be/ToloqU6fCjw.

23andMe Blog. "23andMe as seen on TV." 5 Aug. 2013, https://blog.23andme.com/news/ 23andme-as-seen-on-tv/.